Medicine Science and Dreams

David A. Schwartz, MD

Editor

Medicine Science and Dreams

The Making of Physician-Scientists

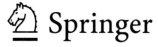 Springer

Editor
David A. Schwartz, MD
National Jewish Health
1400 Jackson St.
Denver, CO 80206
USA
schwartzd@NJHealth.org

ISBN 978-90-481-9537-4   e-ISBN 978-90-481-9538-1
DOI 10.1007/978-90-481-9538-1
Springer Dordrecht Heidelberg London New York

Library of Congress Control Number: 2010937017

Cover illustration:
Photo 1. The late Mark Feinberg (age 15) and brother Andy (age 11) with their mathematics projects for the central Pennsylvania Science Fair.
Photo 2. Laurie Glimcher in 1953.
Photo 3. The officers of the East Meadow High School (1970–1971) student Government Organization (left to right): The Late Larry Grabin, David Schwartz, and Jesse Reece.
Photo 4. Jeffrey Murray examining a child in the Philippines.
Photo 5. Bart Haynes with Dhaval Patel (left) a Duke MD-PhD graduate and rheumatology fellow who trained with Dr. Haynes.

Printed on acid-free paper

Springer is part of Springer Science+Business Media (www.springer.com)

To my entire family, especially my eternally supportive parents Jane and Sol Schwartz, my devoted wife and confidante Louise Sparks, and my unpredictable and amazing children Tziporah, Samuel, and Kiera, whose unwavering belief in me has encouraged me to dream.

Preface

I've always wondered what pushes or pulls people toward one career or another. Life choices make for life consequences, but what goes into these choices? The daily encounters, chance meetings, and derived opportunities, combined with the inherent individual values and attributes, allow one to weave through this complex maze of choices and settle on a life theme. While the fortune (or misfortune) of our families can, and oftentimes does, affect the breadth of our experiences, shape our values, and affect the scope of our options, I have been impressed that chance encounters with people outside the family have also shaped my values and have had a profound effect on my personal career opportunities and choices. In fact, these chance encounters do not represent random unrelated events but rather are influenced by a number of social, economic, geographic, cultural, and genetic factors that are integrally related to and derivative of each other. Despite this complexity, these daily, seemingly unrelated encounters serve to shape and reshape our lives, some events having far more impact than others.

It is these encounters and experiences that compose the stepping stones of our careers and that create traction and direction in our lives that I would like to explore as a way of understanding what moved me and others toward careers as physician-scientists. What were the high impact encounters? How did these encounters fundamentally affect our thinking? What are the inherent tradeoffs in the career of a physician-scientist? What are the events and responses that drew us to and keep us committed to these two somewhat disparate worlds of medicine and science? And are the worlds of medicine and science really that disparate?

Physician-scientists are unusual creatures. While we are drawn to medicine and the clinical challenges of our patients, we are also drawn to the opportunities that our patients' medical problems bring to science. For a physician-scientist, going back and forth between medicine and science is natural and almost necessary. Both medicine and science stimulate each other, and it is the integration of these two disciplines that makes our work so unique and exciting. So while a physician-scientist might both practice medicine and explore novel scientific concepts, all of us strive to integrate medicine and science to create new knowledge. For us, one without the other just doesn't work.

Although the future of physician-scientists remains a subject of debate and concern, the conceptual combination of medicine and science lies at the very heart of the practice of medicine. Science is a major component of medicine, and most people who go into medicine are fundamentally excited by science. However, the practice of medicine is often referred to as an art because it involves understanding people and placing that perception into a scientific context. The "art" of medicine involves integrating human behavior, social context, and science, and helping the patient make the best decision for his or her future. While we keep getting better at the science, we also need to continue to improve our skills in understanding the patient, his or her family, and his or her unique situation. Fundamentally, the life of a physician involves combining medicine and science to benefit the patient. My belief is that every medical student has the potential and ability to become a physician-scientist.

In editing this book, I could have chosen to put these choices and decisions in a historical context, conducted structured interviews with my colleagues, and analyzed the data. I could have structured the contributions of each author to address specific motivating experiences or conceptual issues. Given my own scientific background, this might seem like the most reasonable approach. However, I have specifically decided to focus on personal experience, to recognize the unique path that each of us has taken, and to allow our collective biographies to highlight the turning points, encounters, choices, and drivers that have led us to choose and commit our lives to this hybrid career. Although these stories may help us understand what brought us to this highly specialized occupation, I sincerely hope that our personal experiences also move younger generations to seriously consider this spectacular profession. I trust this goal is shared by my co-authors.

While my own personal tale might seem altruistic, altruism was not the driving force. My choices (and I suspect those of my colleagues) were somewhat self-serving. While I wanted to help others, my career has been guided by my curiosity, which has been stimulated by a limited understanding of the world of health and disease that I have routinely encountered as a person and as a physician. I was drawn to the interface between science and medicine to understand medical problems that simply could not be understood by relying only on the conventional wisdom of clinical medicine. However, as I dove more deeply into my career, I found that while science could be used to understand medicine, medicine could also be used to make sense of science.

Each essay in the book has been written by an accomplished physician-scientist. The stories we have told are those of people and circumstances that have had profound effects on our creative opportunities, our career decisions, and our lives. Some of these people were traditional mentors; others were family, friends, teachers, or patients. While all of these encounters and events were quite distinct, all were meaningful encounters and each contributed in a unique way to give shape and substance to our careers.

The stories in this book are as different as we are. However, despite our diverse social, economic, geographical, and cultural backgrounds, there are common threads that are shared by physician-scientists. We work hard, are persistent and competitive, and have enough confidence to display our ignorance. We are dedicated to understanding life and fixing others, and we believe strongly in the common good. While we strive to enrich the lives of others, each of us have ourselves been greatly enriched by others, and we think boldly and plan for where science and medicine will take us.

My primary reason for editing this book is to enhance the public understanding of our career decisions and how our unique paths were necessary to enable our accomplishments. Our work is supported by the public, our research impacts the public, and the public should be able to understand what drives us and how they have supported us to develop our careers. However, an equally important reason for this book is to move people from medicine to science and from science to medicine.

Denver, Colorado   David A. Schwartz, MD
January, 2010

Acknowledgements

This book was a group effort. I am indebted to my distinguished colleagues for their contributions and their belief in my vision. The collective biographies are extraordinary and represent genuine experiences that brought meaning to the careers and lives of the authors. Our shared belief in the past, present, and future of the physician-scientist is what led to our combined dedication to this text. Speaking for all of the authors, I would like to extend my heartfelt gratitude to our mentors, trainees, and families for providing the guiding lights and unwavering support that has allowed each of us to develop a unique and fulfilling career path.

In addition to the authors, I would like to acknowledge the outstanding support and unusual commitment and loyalty that Linda Neese, my executive assistant, has provided throughout this project. Jennifer Kemp, PhD has contributed to every page of this book by editing each sentence and considering the relevance of each word. Finally, I need to thank my publisher, Tamara Welschot, for her belief in me and my vision for this text and for her sustained support throughout all phases of this project.

Contents

Contributors

Edward J. Benz, Jr., MD Department of Medical Oncology, Dana-Farber Cancer Institute, Boston, MA, USA, edward_benz@dfci.harvard.edu

Moira Chan-Yeung, MD Department of Medicine, University of British Columbia, Vancouver, BC, Canada; Department of Medicine, The University of Hong Kong, Hong Kong, China, myeung@unixg.ubc.ca

Andrew P. Feinberg, MD Center for Epigenetics Johns Hopkins University, Baltimore, MD, USA, afeinberg@jhu.edu

Laurie H. Glimcher, MD Department of Immunology, Harvard School of Public Health, Boston, MA, USA; Department of Medicine, Harvard Medical School, Boston, MA, USA, lglimche@hsph.harvard.edu

Gilad S. Gordon, MD Department of Medicine, University of Colorado Health Sciences Center, Denver, CO, USA, ggordon@orragroup.com

Barton F. Haynes, MD Department of Medicine, Duke Human Vaccine Institute, Duke University, Durham, NC, USA, hayne002@mc.duke.edu

Ralph I. Horwitz, MD Department of Medicine, Stanford University School of Medicine, Stanford, CA, USA, ralph.horwitz@stanford.edu

Michael D. Iseman, MD Division of Mycobacterial Diseases and Lung Infections, National Jewish Health, Denver, CO, USA, isemanm@njhealth.org

Stephen I. Katz, MD, PhD National Institute of Arthritis and Musculoskeletal and Skin Diseases, National Institutes of Health, Bethesda, MD, USA, katzs@od.niams.nih.gov

Talmadge E. King, Jr., MD Department of Medicine, University of California, San Francisco, CA, USA, tking@medicine.ucsf.edu

Philip J. Landrigan, MD, MSc, DIH Departments of Preventive Medicine and Pediatrics, Children's Environmental Health Center, Mount Sinai School of Medicine, New York, NY, USA, phil.landrigan@mssm.edu

Fernando D. Martinez, MD Arizona Respiratory Center University of Arizona, Tucson, AZ, USA, fernando@arc.arizona.edu

Jeffrey C. Murray, MD Departments of Pediatrics, Epidemiology and Biological Sciences, University of Iowa Carver College of Medicine, Iowa, IA, USA, jeff-murray@uiowa.edu

Gilbert S. Omenn, MD, PhD Departments of Medicine, Human Genetics, and Public Health, Center for Computational Medicine and Bioinformatics, University of Michigan, Ann Arbor, MI, USA, gomenn@umich.edu

David S. Pisetsky, MD, PhD Departments of Medicine and Immunology Duke University Medical Center, Durham, NC, USA; Durham VA Medical Center, Durham, NC, USA, dpiset@duke.edu

Robert W. Schrier, MD University of Colorado Denver, Aurora, CO, USA, robert.schrier@ucdenver.edu

David A. Schwartz, MD Departments of Medicine, Pediatrics and Immunology, Center for Genes, Environment, and Health, National Jewish Health, Denver, CO, USA; Department of Medicine and Immunology, University of Colorado Denver, Denver, CO, USA, schwartzd@NJHealth.org

Moisés Selman, MD Instituto Nacional de Enfermedades Respiratorias, Universidad Nacional Autónoma de, México, México, mselman@yahoo.com.mx

Erika von Mutius, MD Department of Asthma and Allergy, Munich University Children's Hospital, Munich, Germany, erika.von.mutius@med.uni-muenchen.de

R. Sanders Williams, MD The J. David Gladstone Institutes, University of California, San Francisco, CA, USA, rswilliams@mc.duke.edu

About the Authors

Edward J. Benz, Jr., MD is a pioneering academic hematologist whose early work showed that messenger RNA defects caused a common congenital anemia, thalassemia. This was the first demonstration that molecular biology could be applied to the study of human diseases. He has subsequently achieved international renown for his research in the areas of human red cell disorders, gene regulation, and membrane biology. He remains an active NIH-funded investigator and clinician.

As an educator, Dr. Benz has been an active teacher and mentor throughout his career. He has trained over 50 mentees in his laboratory, many of whom now hold senior faculty or leadership positions in academia, industry, or private practice. In recognition of his contributions as a mentor, he was named winner of the 2007 American Society of Hematology Mentoring Award in Basic Science.

Dr. Benz has also had an impact as a national leader, having served as President of the prestigious American Society of Clinical Investigation and President of the American Society of Hematology. Currently, he is the President of the Association of American Cancer Institutes. He has co-edited the top-rated textbook in the field of hematology and educated an entire generation about the application of molecular biology to clinical medicine through his lectures, review articles, and essays. In November of 2000, Dr. Benz was appointed President of the Dana-Farber Cancer Institute. He holds the Richard and Susan Smith Professorship in Medicine and is a Professor of Pediatrics and a Professor of Pathology at Harvard Medical School.

Moira Chan-Yeung, MD is currently a Professor Emeritus in the Department of Medicine at the University of British Columbia and an Honorary Professor in the Department of Medicine at the University of Hong Kong. She graduated from the University of Hong Kong, where she received her postgraduate training in internal medicine. She also received training in the Clinical Allergy Unit of the Cardiothoracic Institute at Brompton Hospital in London, England. She was appointed as an Assistant Professor in 1973 and became Professor of Medicine at the University of British Columbia in 1982. She has headed the Occupational and Environmental Lung Diseases Unit at the University since 1980.

Dr. Chan-Yeung is a leading authority on occupational asthma. Her research has led to occupational asthma being recognized as a compensable disease in Canada. She was instrumental in obtaining permanent disability pension for those patients who did not recover from this disease and for obtaining a more equitable assessment of respiratory impairment/disability in patients with asthma. The permissible concentrations of Western red cedar dust and grain dust were reduced to the current low levels based on the results of her studies. Her research interests have included occupational lung disease, environmental and genetic risk factors in asthma, and the primary prevention of asthma in childhood.

In 1998, Dr. Chan-Yeung returned to her alma mater as a Chair Professor in Respiratory Disease. In addition to heading several epidemiological studies of different lung diseases, including Severe Acute Respiratory Syndrome, she worked with local chest societies to promote respiratory health through education and public health policy.

A member on several research grant review committees, Dr. Chan-Yeung has also served as the Chairperson of the Assembly of Environmental and Occupational Health, American Thoracic Society and as a member of the Pulmonary Disease Advisory Committee for the National Heart, Lung, Blood Institute, National Institutes of Health, USA. In addition, she has served as the Chairperson of the Respiratory Diseases Section of the International Union Against Tuberculosis and Lung Disease and is the Editor-in-Chief (lung disease) of the official Journal of the Union. She is a consultant to the World Health Organization and is at present a member of the working group on Prevention of Chronic Respiratory Diseases and of the Global Alliance Against Respiratory Diseases.

She has published 350 peer-reviewed articles, numerous essays, and is an Editor of the books *Asthma in the Workplace* and *Respiratory Disease—An Asian Perspective*.

She received the Alice Hamilton Award for "Major and Lasting Contribution in Occupational Health" from the American Industrial Hygiene Association in 2000 and the Distinguished Achievement Award from the American Thoracic Society in 2008 in recognition of her contributions.

Andrew P. Feinberg, MD studied mathematics and humanities at Yale in the Directed Studies Honors Program, and he received his BA degree in 1973 and MD in 1976 from the accelerated medical program at Johns Hopkins University, as well as an MPH from Johns Hopkins in 1981. He performed a postdoctoral fellowship in developmental biology at the University of California in San Diego, clinical training in medicine and medical genetics at University of Pennsylvania, and genetics research and clinical training at Johns Hopkins.

Dr. Feinberg discovered epigenetic alterations in human cancer and is the leading pioneer of the epigenetic basis of human disease, including the discovery of human-imprinted genes, loss of imprinting (LOI) in cancer, and the molecular basis of Beckwith–Wiedemann syndrome (BWS), the paradigm of epigenetic cancer syndromes. His discovery of epigenetically-altered progenitor cells has led to a paradigm shift in our understanding of carcinogenesis, and his contributions reach into all areas of genetics, from technology to development to disease. He has pioneered studies of the epigenetic basis of disease generally, establishing the first epigenome center in the USA and discovering that one's epigenome changes over one's lifetime. He is also the inventor of random priming and methods for genome-scale epigenetic analysis.

Dr. Feinberg is King Fahd Professor of Medicine, Molecular Biology & Genetics and Oncology, and he holds an Adjunct Professorship at the Karolinska Institute in Sweden. Dr. Feinberg is also Director of the Center for Epigenetics, an NHGRI-designated Center of Excellence in Genome Sciences. His honors include election to the American Society for Clinical Investigation, the Association of American Physicians, the Institute of Medicine of the National Academy of Sciences, and the American Academy of Arts and Sciences, as well as membership on the ISI most cited authors list, a MERIT Award of the National Cancer Institute, a Doctor of Philosophy (Hon. Caus.) from Uppsala University, and the President's Diversity Recognition Award of Johns Hopkins University.

Laurie H. Glimcher, MD is the Irene Heinz Given Professor of Immunology at the Harvard School of Public Health and Professor of Medicine at Harvard Medical School. She received her BA degree from Radcliffe College and her MD from Harvard Medical School. Dr. Glimcher did her residency in internal medicine at the Massachusetts General Hospital (MGH). She received her postdoctoral training at Harvard and in the Laboratory of Immunology at the Institute of Allergy and Infectious Diseases in Bethesda. She is board certified in Internal Medicine and Rheumatology and is a Senior Rheumatologist at the Brigham and Women's Hospital. She heads the Immunology Program at Harvard Medical School and the Division of Biological Sciences program at the Harvard School of Public Health. She is a Fellow of the American Academy of Arts and Sciences, a Member of the Institute of Medicine of the National Academy of Sciences, and a Member of the National Academy of Sciences. She is the former President of the American Association of Immunologists. Dr. Glimcher is also a member of the American Asthma Foundation, Immune Diseases Institute, Health Care Ventures, Burroughs-Wellcome Fund, and Memorial Sloan Kettering Cancer Center Scientific Advisory Boards, and she serves on the Cancer Research Institute Fellowship Committee. She is on the Corporate Board of Directors of the Bristol-Myers Squibb Pharmaceutical Corporation and the Waters Corporation.

Dr. Glimcher's laboratory uses biochemical and genetic approaches to elucidate the molecular pathways that regulate CD4 T helper cell development and activation. The complex regulatory pathways governing T helper cell responses are critical both for the development of protective immunity and for the pathophysiologic immune responses underlying autoimmune diseases. Dr. Glimcher's laboratory has studied the transcriptional pathways that control this important immune checkpoint. The laboratory defined the genetic bases of both IL-4 and IFNγ expression in T cells. Her group identified the proto-oncogene c-maf as the transcription factor responsible for Th2-specific IL-4 expression. Subsequently, her group discovered the first Th1-specific transcription factor, T-bet, and demonstrated that this single factor is a master-regulator of IFNγ gene expression and the Th1 phenotype. Recent studies have demonstrated that T-bet controls Type 1 immunity in cells of both the adaptive and innate immune systems. Her laboratory has focused on the function of

T-bet in dendritic cells in mucosal immunity and tumorigenesis, with an emphasis on inflammatory bowel disease. She has expanded her interest in lineage commitment in lymphocytes to the B cell with the discovery of a transcription factor, XBP-1, that controls plasma cell differentiation and the Endoplasmic Reticulum Stress Response. Her laboratory has provided evidence for a link between ER stress and proinflammatory/autoimmune diseases. Skeletal biology is a separate interest of the Glimcher laboratory, having arisen from her discovery of a novel protein, Schnurri-3, that controls adult bone formation. Large scale screens have identified new proteins that control osteoblast and osteoclast commitment and activation in skeletal biology.

Gilad S. Gordon, MD received an AB in Biochemistry from Harvard College in 1979, an MD from the Division of Health Sciences and Technology at Harvard Medical School and the Massachusetts Institute of Technology in 1983, and an MBA from the University of Washington in 1988. He completed an internship and residency in Internal Medicine at the University of Colorado Health Sciences Center in 1986 and was a Senior Fellow in the Robert Wood Johnson Clinical Scholars Program at the University of Washington from 1986 to 1988. He has held academic medicine appointments in the Department of Medicine at the University of Indiana Medical School from 1988 to 1992 and is currently a Clinical Assistant Professor of Medicine at the University of Colorado Health Sciences Center and an attending physician at the Denver Veteran's Administration Hospital.

Dr. Gordon's career began at the Eli Lilly Company in Indianapolis, Indiana. At Lilly, his primary focus was undertaking cost-effectiveness studies, both from the perspective of the costs and effectiveness of individual drugs as well as the costs and effectiveness of drugs in the overall health care budget. In this capacity, he developed new methodologies for undertaking cost-effectiveness and quality-of-life studies as part of traditional Phase I through III clinical trials in both the USA and Europe. In 1991, Dr. Gordon moved to Colorado to work at Synergen, a biotechnology company developing drugs for sepsis and inflammation. In this role, he worked on incorporating health economic studies and quality-of-life studies into early phase trials of biotechnology products. From 1995 to 1998, Dr. Gordon worked in organizations which were developing clinical information systems and medical software designed to better understand and improve the provision of health care. Much of the work involved developing and then analyzing large databases to better understand how guidelines for care of certain diseases improved outcomes.

Since 1999, the main focus of Dr. Gordon's work has been on the clinical development of new chemical entities. He has worked with both large and small organizations to help them design innovative and appropriate multicenter Phase I through IV clinical trials for new novel molecules. The aim of these trials is to demonstrate the safety, efficacy, and economic and quality-of-life impacts of the new products in the treatment of hard-to-treat diseases.

Dr. Gordon has published over 65 articles and abstracts in peer-reviewed journals. His work on evaluating the role of guidelines in improving outcomes in the treatment of pneumonia was awarded the *Cecile Lehman Mayer Research Award* (best research paper) by the American College of Chest Physicians in 1996. In addition, Dr. Gordon has served on several editorial boards and a number of advisory panels. He is currently a member of the Board of Directors of the not-for-profit Caring for Colorado Foundation.

Barton F. Haynes, MD received his undergraduate education at the University of Tennessee-Knoxville and his medical education from Baylor School *cum laude*. After internal medicine residency training at Duke University Hospital, he trained at the NIH NIAID Laboratory of Clinical Investigation from 1975 to 1980, receiving training in infectious diseases, allergy, and clinical immunology. He joined the medicine faculty at Duke in 1980, served as the chief of the rheumatology and immunology division from 1987 to 1995, and was chair of medicine from 1995 to 2002. He is currently the Frederic M. Hanes Professor of Medicine and Immunology and Director of the Duke Human Vaccine Institute.

Dr. Haynes has been recognized for his discoveries of human cell surface molecules important in the human immune response, deciphering the developmental ontogeny of the human thymus, and developing technology for successful human thymus transplantation. He has worked on the problem of HIV vaccine development for over 25 years and is recognized as a research team leader who can bring disparate groups together to work on complex scientific problems. He currently serves as Director of the Center for HIV/AIDS Vaccine Immunology, a large international virtual consortium funded by the NIH to overcome roadblocks that hinder development of a successful HIV vaccine.

At Duke, Dr. Haynes has been awarded the Distinguished Faculty Award and the Diversity Award for Lifelong Commitment to Improving Ethnic and Gender Diversity of faculty and staff at Duke. He has been awarded Distinguished Investigator Awards from both the American Federation of Clinical Research and the American College of Rheumatology, in addition to the Lee Howley, Sr. Prize in Basic Research from the Arthritis Foundation. He is a member of the Institute of Medicine of the National Academy of Sciences and a fellow of the American Academy of Arts and Sciences.

Ralph I. Horwitz, MD arrived as scheduled on June 25, 1947. He grew up in Philadelphia, PA. at 2865 N. 8th Street where his parents owned a candy and convenience store. He was expected to pursue a career in law or medicine and to have a useful life. His choice of medicine took him first to medical school at Pennsylvania State University at Hershey, and subsequently to training in Internal Medicine at McGill (Royal Victoria Hospital), Massachusetts General Hospital, and Yale University for a fellowship in the Robert Wood Johnson Clinical Scholars Program.

Horwitz is internationally known for his pioneering research that helped to establish the field of clinical epidemiology and outcomes research. He has made numerous contributions to the fundamental methods of clinical investigation and in the application of those methods to the studies of the risk of disease and recovery from illness.

Horwitz joined the Yale faculty in 1978 as Co-Director of the Robert Woods Johnson Foundation Clinical Scholars Program, a position he held until leaving Yale in 2003. In this role, he helped to train a generation of leaders in patient-oriented research and health policy in medicine, pediatrics, surgery, and psychiatry. He was appointed Chief of the General Medicine Section in 1982, Harold H. Hines, Jr. Professor in 1991, and Chair of Internal Medicine in 1994. As a chair, he created a world-class program of clinical research and established the nation's first PhD program in a clinical department for physicians devoted to careers in biomedical science (Investigative Medicine Program).

In 2003, Horwitz was appointed Dean of the Case Western University School of Medicine (including the Cleveland Clinic Lerner College of Medicine) and was the founding Director of the Case Research Institute. Horwitz moved to Stanford University in 2007 as Arthur L. Bloomfield Professor and Chair of the Department of Medicine. Horwitz is an elected member of the American Society for Clinical Investigation, the Institute of Medicine of the National Academy of Sciences and the Association of American Physicians (AAP). He was Chair of the American Board of Internal Medicine (2003), President of the AAP, and is a Master of the American College of Physicians.

Michael D. Iseman, MD graduated with honors in history from Princeton in 1961. He then received his doctorate in 1965 from Columbia University, where he also received his residency training in internal medicine, as well as his fellowship training in pulmonary medicine.

Dr. Iseman joined the faculty at the University of Colorado in 1972 and National Jewish Medical and Research Center in 1982. He is currently Professor of Medicine with appointments in both pulmonary medicine and infectious diseases.

Dr. Iseman holds the Girard & Madeline Beno Chair in Mycobacterial Diseases and is well known for his work in the management of drug-resistant tuberculosis and other mycobacterial diseases. In addition to providing patient care on the ward and clinic, he has been the Director of a thrice-yearly, week-long course held at National Jewish on the management of tuberculosis—over the past 21 years, nearly 6,000 physicians and nurses from across the USA and around the world have attended. Dr. Iseman has been a consultant for the Colorado State Health Department, the US Centers for Disease Control, and the World Health Organization. A member of the Advisory Board of Partners in Health, Dr. Iseman has taught Partners in Health courses in Peru and Russia. He also has lectured in 47 states and 34 foreign countries. From 1997 to 2002, he was Editor-in-Chief of the *International Journal of Tuberculosis and Lung Disease*, which is published in Paris, France. In addition to contributing chapters to eight different textbooks, he has recently completed a single-authored book, *A Clinician's Guide to Tuberculosis.*

Dr. Iseman's program offers free consultation services for clinicians, public health officers, families, and patients affected by complicated or multi-drug-resistant tuberculosis, or disease due to nontuberculous mycobacteria. The consultation service started in 1988 and receives more than 1,000 requests per year.

Dr. Iseman received the Edward Livingston Trudeau award from the American Thoracic Society and the American Lung Association in 2005. The Trudeau medal recognizes lifelong major contributions to the prevention, diagnosis, and treatment of lung disease through leadership in research, education, or clinical care. Other awards include the Gold Medal for Clinical Excellence of the Columbia Alumni Association (1995), election to the Colorado Pulmonary Hall of Fame (1997), the Governors' Community Service Award from the CHEST Foundation (2004), and the Robert W. Schrier Award for Excellence from the Department of Medicine of the University of Colorado (2007).

Stephen I. Katz, MD, PhD has been Director of the National Institute of Arthritis and Musculoskeletal and Skin Diseases since August 1995 and is also a Senior Investigator in the Dermatology Branch of the National Cancer Institute. After attending the University of Maryland, where he graduated with honors, he graduated from Tulane University Medical School with honors in 1966. He completed a medical internship at Los Angeles County Hospital and did his dermatology residency at the University of Miami Medical Center. He served in the US Army at Walter Reed Army Medical Center from 1970 to 1972. From 1972 to 1974, Dr. Katz did a postdoctoral fellowship at the Royal College of Surgeons of England and obtained a PhD degree in immunology from the University of London in 1974. He then became Senior Investigator in the Dermatology Branch of the National Cancer Institute and in 1980, he became Chief of the Branch, a position he held until 2002. In 1989, Dr. Katz also assumed the position of Marion B. Sulzberger Professor of Dermatology at the Uniformed Services University of the Health Sciences in Bethesda, Maryland, a position that he held until 1995.

Dr. Katz has focused his studies on immunology and the skin. His research has demonstrated that skin is an important component of the immune system, both in its normal function and as a target in immunologically mediated disease. In addition to studying Langerhans cells and epidermally derived cytokines, Dr. Katz and his colleagues have added considerable new knowledge about inherited and acquired blistering skin diseases.

Dr. Katz has trained a large number of outstanding immunodermatologists in the USA, Japan, Korea, and Europe. Many of these individuals are now leading their own high-quality, independent research programs. He has served many professional societies in leadership positions, including as a member of the Board of Directors and President of the Society for Investigative Dermatology, on the Board of the Association of Professors of Dermatology, as Secretary-General of the 18th World Congress of Dermatology in New York in 1992, and as Secretary-Treasurer of the Clinical Immunology Society. Dr. Katz has received many honors and awards, including the Master Dermatologist Award and the Sulzberger Lecture Award of the American Academy of Dermatology, the National Cancer Institute's Outstanding Mentor Award, the Harvey J. Bullock, Jr. EEO Award in recognition of his extraordinary leadership in scientific, programmatic, and administrative arenas, the Excellence in Leadership Award from the International Pemphigus Foundation, the "Change It" Champion Award from Parent Project Muscular Dystrophy, and election into the Institute of Medicine of the National Academy of Sciences (USA). He has also received the Alfred Marchionini Gold Medal, the Lifetime Achievement Award of the American Skin Association, Doctor Honoris Causa Degrees from Semmelweis University in Budapest, Hungary, Ludwig Maximilian University in

Munich, Germany, and the University of Athens in Greece. He also received the Rothman Award for distinguished service to investigative cutaneous medicine and the Kligman/Frost Award. Dr. Katz has twice received the Meritorious Rank Award and has also received the Distinguished Executive Presidential Rank Award, the highest honor that can be bestowed upon a civil servant.

Talmadge E. King, Jr., MD held a professorship in medicine at the University of Colorado and was a senior faculty member at the National Jewish Medical and Research Center. In 1997, Dr. King became the Constance B. Wofsy Distinguished Professor and Vice Chair of the Department of Medicine at the University of California, San Francisco (UCSF), and Chief of Medical Services at San Francisco General Hospital (SFGH).

Dr. King is recognized as a superb researcher, teacher, clinician, and administrator. As a scientist, he has contributed to the fundamental understanding of interstitial lung diseases and has more than 240 publications. He has co-authored 12 books, including the acclaimed reference book *Interstitial Lung Disease*, now in its fifth edition.

Dr. King is an active member of a number of professional societies and is a past President of the American Thoracic Society. He has served on the Lung Biology and Pathology Study Section of the NIH, the Board of the American Board of Internal Medicine, the Pulmonary and Allergy Drugs Advisory Committee of the FDA, the Board of Governors of the NIH Warren Grant Magnuson Clinical Center, and the Board of Extramural Advisors of the National Heart, Lung and Blood Institute (NHLBI). He has been a member of the editorial boards of *American Journal of Respiratory and Critical Care Medicine*, *Annals of Internal Medicine*, *THORAX*, and *UpToDate*^{TM} *In Pulmonary and Critical Care*.

In all of these roles, Dr. King has not only excelled as a clinician and academic, but has taken a leading role in calling attention to the inequality of health care and lack of diversity in its own ranks. He led a group of faculty at SFGH in writing a textbook, *Medical Management of Vulnerable & Underserved Patients: Principles, Practice, Population*, the only reference available that focuses on the treatment of patients living with chronic diseases in poor and minority populations.

Dr. King has received numerous awards, including the Trudeau Medal, the highest honor of the American Thoracic Society. He has been elected to the Institute of Medicine of the National Academy of Sciences and the Association of American Physicians. He is a Master of the American College of Physicians and has been included on multiple lists of the finest doctors in the USA.

Currently, Dr. King holds the Julius R. Krevans Distinguished Professorship in Internal Medicine and is Chair of the Department of Medicine at UCSF. The Department is the largest of the 26 academic departments of the School of Medicine, ranks top among the top departments of medicine in research dollars granted by the NIH, and is ranked third in the 2009 *U.S. News & World Report* specialty rankings survey.

Dr. King lives with his wife, Mozelle, in Oakland, California. Their elder daughter, Consuelo, is a writer and editor living in Denver. Their younger daughter,

Malaika, is an executive at an insurance company and lives with her husband, Chad Kattke, and their daughter, Madison, in South Elgin, Illinois.

Philip J. Landrigan, MD, MSc, DIH graduated from Boston Latin School in 1959, from Boston College in 1963, and from Harvard Medical School in 1967. He completed an internship in medicine/pediatrics at Cleveland Metropolitan General Hospital and a residency in pediatrics at Children's Hospital Boston. He received a Masters degree in Science of Occupational Medicine and a Diploma of Industrial Health from the London School of Hygiene and Tropical Medicine at the University of London. He served for 15 years as an Epidemic Intelligence Service Officer and Medical Epidemiologist at the Centers for Disease Control and Prevention (CDC) and the National Institute for Occupational Safety and Health (NIOSH). While at CDC, Dr. Landrigan participated in the Global Campaign for the Eradication of Smallpox. Dr. Landrigan directed the national program in occupational epidemiology for NIOSH. At CDC, he was responsible for creating the unit that has evolved into CDC's National Center for Environmental Health. He was awarded the Meritorious Service Medal of the US Public Health Service.

In 1987, Dr. Landrigan was elected as a member of the Institute of Medicine of the National Academy of Sciences. He served as Editor-in-Chief of the *American Journal of Industrial Medicine* and Editor of *Environmental Research*. He has published more than 500 scientific papers and five books. He has chaired committees at the National Academy of Sciences on *Environmental Neurotoxicology* and on *Pesticides in the Diets of Infants and Children*. The NAS report that he directed on pesticides and children's health was instrumental in securing passage of the Food Quality Protection Act, the only environmental law in the USA that contains explicit provisions for the protection of children. From 1995 to 1997, Dr. Landrigan served on the Presidential Advisory Committee on Gulf War Veteran's Illnesses. In 1997 and 1998, he served as Senior Advisor on Children's Health to the Administrator of the US Environmental Protection Agency and was instrumental in helping to establish a new Office of Children's Health Protection at EPA.

Dr. Landrigan served from 1996 to 2005 in the Medical Corps of the US Naval Reserve. He retired in 2005 at the rank of Captain. He served in Korea and Ghana and was Officer-in-Charge of the West Africa Training Cruise, a medical humanitarian mission to Senegal in July 2004 that saw over 11,000 patients. He was awarded the Navy Commendation Medal (three awards), the National Defense Service Medal, and the Secretary of Defense Medal for Outstanding Public Service for his work on the Armed Forces Epidemiological Board. He continues to serve as Surgeon General of the New York Naval Militia, New York's Naval National Guard.

Dr. Landrigan is known for his many decades of work in protecting children against environmental health threats, most notably involving lead and pesticides. His pioneering research on lead toxicity at low levels persuaded the US government to mandate removal of lead from gasoline and paint, actions that have produced a 90% decline in incidence of childhood lead poisoning over the past 25 years. Dr. Landrigan has been a leader in developing the National Children's Study, the largest study of children's health and the environment ever launched in the USA. He has been centrally involved in the medical and epidemiologic studies that followed the destruction of the World Trade Center on September 11, 2001, and he has consulted extensively for the World Health Organization.

Fernando D. Martinez, MD obtained his "Licensure in Medicine" in 1971 at the University of Chile in Santiago. He subsequently obtained his medical degree at the University of Rome, Italy in 1975. He trained in pediatrics and pediatric pulmonary medicine at the University of Rome and was a general pediatric practitioner in Viterbo, Italy between 1981 and 1987. In 1987, Dr. Martinez became a Research Associate at the Arizona Respiratory Center, and in 1991, he became an Assistant Professor in the Department of Pediatrics, University of Arizona. In 1997, he was named Director of the Arizona Respiratory Center and the Swift-McNear Professor of Pediatrics at the University of Arizona.

Dr. Martinez has published more than 200 papers and reviews about the epidemiology, treatment, natural history, genetics, and gene-environment interaction of asthma and related traits. In 2008, he delivered the J. Burns Amberson Lecture at the Annual Meeting of the American Thoracic Society. He is currently a Regents' Professor at the University of Arizona and the Director of the BIO5 Institute, which fosters interdisciplinary research among investigators in the basic sciences, pharmacology, biomedicine, agriculture, and bioengineering.

Jeffrey C. Murray, MD is a pediatrician and medical geneticist who divides his time between patient care, teaching, and research into the genetic and environmental causes of pediatric disorders. He did his undergraduate studies at MIT, medical school and residency at Tufts, and a postdoctoral fellowship under Arno Motulsky at the University of Washington. He has been at the University of Iowa since 1984 and is currently Professor of Pediatrics, Biology, Epidemiology, Dentistry, and Nursing. His research has included directing a human genome center that built detailed human genetic maps and a craniofacial anomalies research center. He currently directs a program in Perinatal Health. He was elected as a Director of the American Society of Human Genetics and to the Institute of Medicine.

Dr. Murray's research is globally oriented with ongoing projects in Argentina, Brazil, Denmark, India, and the Philippines, with a focus on using large population datasets and genomics to identify genetic and environmental causes of cleft lip and preterm birth. He has trained over 20 graduate students and 35 postdoctoral fellows. His work fits into the niche of international health, common complex disorders, genetics, social justice, and the environment. He currently serves on the Advisory Committee to the Director of the NIH and on the Executive Steering Committee of the National Children's Study.

Gilbert S. Omenn, MD, PhD served as an Executive Vice President for Medical Affairs and as Chief Executive Officer of the University of Michigan Health System from 1997 to 2002. He was Dean of the School of Public Health and Professor of Medicine and Environmental Health at the University of Washington, Seattle, from 1982 to 1997. His research interests include cancer proteomics, biomedical informatics, public health genetics, science-based risk analysis, and health policy. He was principal investigator of the beta-Carotene and Retinol Efficacy Trial (CARET) of preventive agents against lung cancer and heart disease, Director of the Center for Health Promotion in Older Adults, and creator of a university-wide initiative on Public Health Genetics in Ethical, Legal, and Policy Context while at the University of Washington and Fred Hutchinson Cancer Research Center. He served as Associate Director, Office of Science and Technology Policy, and Associate Director, Office of Management and Budget, in the Executive Office of the President during the Carter Administration. He is a longtime Director of Amgen Inc. In 2006, he was the President of the American Association for the Advancement of Science (AAAS).

Dr. Omenn is the author of 463 research papers and scientific reviews and author/editor of 18 books. He is a member of the Institute of Medicine of the National Academy of Sciences, the American Academy of Arts and Sciences, the Association of American Physicians, and the American College of Physicians. He chaired the presidential/congressional Commission on Risk Assessment and Risk Management, served on the National Commission on the Environment, and chaired the NAS/NRC/IOM Committee on Science, Engineering and Public Policy.

He earned his BA degree at Princeton, MD at Harvard, and PhD in Genetics at the University of Washington. His internal medicine residency was at the Massachusetts General Hospital. He is active in cultural and educational organizations, and is a musician and tennis player.

Dr. Omenn is the recipient of the following honors and awards: US Public Health Service Special Fellow; National Genetics Foundation Fellow; Research Career Development Award, National Institute of General Medical Sciences; White House Fellow, US Atomic Energy Commission; Fellow, American College of Physicians; Member, Institute of Medicine, National Academy of Sciences; Fellow, Hastings Center Institute of Society, Ethics and Life Sciences; Fellow, Collegium Ramazzini; Fellow, American Association for the Advancement of Science; Member, National Academy of Social Insurance; Member, Western Association of Physicians; Member, American Academy of Arts and Sciences; Member, Association of American Physicians; President's Award, American Occupational and Environmental Medicine Association; White House Fellows Association John Gardner Legacy of Leadership Award; National Associate, National Academies/National Research Council; Member, Society of Fellows, NIH National Center for Minority Health & Health Disparities; Ambassador, Paul G. Rogers Society for Global Health Research; Distinguished Service Award, Human Proteome Organization (HUPO); Institute of Medicine Walsh McDermott Medal for Distinguished Service; Honorary Member, Society of Toxicology; and elected Fellow, American Medical Informatics Association.

David S. Pisetsky, MD, PhD received his BA degree in Biochemical Sciences from Harvard College *magna cum laude* in 1967 and his PhD and MD degrees from the Albert Einstein College of Medicine in 1972 and 1973. He was then an intern and resident in Internal Medicine at the Yale-New Haven Hospital from 1973 to 1975. From 1975 to 1978, he was a Clinical Associate at the National Cancer Institute.

He joined the faculty of the Duke University Medical Center in 1978 as Chief of Rheumatology at the Durham VA Hospital, where he has remained since. He became a Professor of Medicine in 1990.

For over 30 years, Dr. Pisetsky has been an active investigator in the field of autoimmunity, focusing on the pathogenesis of systemic lupus erythematosus (SLE) and the immunological properties of nuclear macromolecules. His laboratory was the first to demonstrate that the sera of normal humans contain antibodies to bacterial DNA, contrary to the dogma in the field at that time, which posited that only patients with SLE can respond to DNA. His laboratory subsequently demonstrated the mitogenic activity of bacterial DNA and the ability of synthetic oligonucleotides to both stimulate and inhibit immune responses. This work was important in reconceptualizing the role of DNA in both normal and aberrant immunity and led to new models for the pathogenesis of SLE. More recently, he has investigated the immune activities of HMGB1, a nuclear protein with alarmin activity. He has published almost 300 papers or essays and has had funding from the NIH, VA, and private foundations. In 2001, he was awarded the Howley Prize from the Arthritis Foundation for his work.

Dr. Pisetsky served as Chief of Rheumatology at the Duke University Medical Center from 1996 to 2007 and remains as the principal investigator of the NIH-sponsored training program in inflammatory diseases. Dr. Pisetsky has taught extensively at the preclinical and clinical levels. He conducts two major clinics each week in rheumatology and serves as an attending on General Medicine each year. In his laboratory, Dr. Pisetsky has had more than 30 students as well as MD and PhD fellows. Of these, many have gone on to major academic positions as well as careers as independent scientists in industry. Dr. Pisetsky lectures extensively throughout the country and world.

Dr. Pisetsky has served on numerous committees for the NIH, VA, American College of Rheumatology (ACR), Arthritis Foundation, and the Lupus Research Institute. His service to the ACR has been very extensive. He was a Section Editor of the *Journal of Immunology* from 1995 to 2000, and from 2000 to 2005, he served as Editor of *Arthritis and Rheumatism*, the leading journal in the field of rheumatology, and he currently serves as the Physician Editor of *The Rheumatologist*. In addition to his scientific writing, Dr. Pisetsky has published over 60 narratives and short stories on medicine, including articles in *Annals of Internal Medicine* and *JAMA*.

Robert W. Schrier, MD Professor of Medicine, was formerly Chairman of the Department of Medicine at the University of Colorado School of Medicine for 26 years and Head of the Division of Renal Diseases and Hypertension for 20 years. In 1989, he was elected a member of the Institute of Medicine of the National Academy of Sciences. He has been President of the Association of American Physicians, the American Society of Nephrology, the National Kidney Foundation, and the International Society of Nephrology. Dr. Schrier is a Master of the American College of Physicians and an Honorary Fellow of the Royal College of Physicians. He has authored over 900 scientific papers and edited numerous books, including editions in internal medicine, geriatrics, drug usage, and kidney disease. His research contributions center on autosomal dominant polycystic kidney disease, pathogenesis of acute renal cell injury, hypertension and diabetic nephropathy, and renal and hormonal control of body fluid volume in cirrhosis, cardiac failure, nephrotic syndrome, and pregnancy. He brings to his research interests a unique combination of expertise in body fluid control mechanisms, renal function, and cardiovascular function. He has advanced a unifying hypothesis of sodium and water regulation in health and disease, stimulating worldwide interest in the biomedical science community. Dr. Schrier's research has been funded by the National Institutes of Health for over 35 years.

During Dr. Schrier's 26 years as Chairman of Medicine at the University of Colorado, the full-time faculty increased from approximately 75 to 500. The total annual research funding obtained by the Department's full-time faculty rose from approximately $3 to 100 million, including the faculty's contributions to the General Clinical Research and Cancer Centers. The housestaff and fellow training programs also became nationally prominent. Thirty endowed research chairs between $1.5 and $2.0 million each were established. For these contributions, Governor Owens announced an Honorary Proclamation designating May 4, 2002 as Robert W. Schrier Day in Colorado, and Mayor Wellington Webb proclaimed May 4, 2002 as Robert W. Schrier Day in the City and County of Denver. In 2002, Dr. Schrier also received the prestigious Belle Bonfils-Stanton Award for Contributions in Science and Medicine.

Dr. Schrier has received honorary degrees from DePauw University, the University of Colorado, the University of Silesia, and the University of Toledo. He has received the highest awards of the American College of Physicians (John Phillips Award), the National Kidney Foundation (David Hume Award), the American Society of Nephrology (John Peters Award), the International Society of Nephrology (Jean Hamburger Award), the German Society of Nephrology (Franz Vollhard Award), the Western Society of Clinical Investigation (Mayo Soley Award), the Association of Professors of Medicine (Robert H. Williams Award), the American Kidney Fund (National Torchbearer Award), the Association of American Physicians (Francis Blake Award), Acute Renal Failure Commission (Bywaters Award), the New York Academy of Medicine (The Edward N. Gibbs Memorial Award), the University of Strasburg (Louis Pasteur Medal), the Grand Hamdan International Award for Medical Sciences, and the Alexander von Humboldt Research Award for his contributions in biomedical research, education, and clinical medicine.

David A. Schwartz, MD has made numerous contributions toward understanding the role that biological and genetic determinants play in the onset of diseases that are influenced by environmental exposures. His research has identified endotoxins or lipopolysaccharide (LPS) as an important cause of airway disease among those exposed to agricultural dusts. He is recognized for identifying a specific genetic variation in the Toll-4 gene that is associated with a diminished response to LPS, placing individuals at higher risk of sepsis and lower risk of atherosclerosis. Dr. Schwartz has also recently identified variations in a mucin gene that place individuals at increased risk of developing interstitial lung disease. His research in epigenetics has demonstrated that the epigenome is exquisitely responsive to environmental stress and that this has a profound effect on immunobiology and the development of allergic airway disease. Dr. Schwartz's interest in environmental lung disease has provided new insights into many other areas, including the pathophysiology and biology of asbestos-induced lung disease, pulmonary fibrosis, environmental airway diseases, and innate immunity.

Prior to joining National Jewish Health in 2008, Dr. Schwartz served as Director of the National Institute of Environmental Health Sciences (NIEHS) and the National Toxicology Program (NTP) at the National Institutes of Health (NIH) between 2005 and 2008. During his tenure at the NIH, he guided the development of the Genes, Environment and Health Initiative, the Epigenomics and Human Health Initiative, and a program in translational research in environmental sciences. Between 2000 and 2005, Dr. Schwartz served at Duke University, where he held concurrent positions at the Medical Center including Vice Chair of Research and Director of Pulmonary and Critical Care Medicine. While at Duke, Dr. Schwartz played a pivotal role in establishing three interdisciplinary centers in Environmental Health Sciences, Environmental Genomics, and Environmental Asthma, illustrating his commitment to bringing together an array of scientific expertise with state-of-the-art technology to tackle critical health concerns and public health issues.

Dr. Schwartz has authored more than 250 peer-reviewed research papers and numerous essays. He has served on several editorial boards, scientific study sections, and advisory panels. He is a member of the American Society for Clinical Investigation and the Association of American Physicians and the recipient of the 2003 American Thoracic Society Scientific Accomplishment Award.

A native of New York, Dr. Schwartz earned his BA degree in Biology from the University of Rochester in 1975. He received his medical degree from the University of California, San Diego, in 1979. After completing a residency and chief residency in Internal Medicine at Boston City Hospital, he completed a fellowship in Occupational Medicine at the Harvard School of Public Health. While at the University of Washington, Dr. Schwartz completed a research fellowship in the Robert Wood Johnson Clinical Scholars Program and a Pulmonary and Critical Care fellowship. Dr. Schwartz currently serves as Provost and Director of the Center for Genes, Environment, and Health at National Jewish Health.

Moisés Selman, MD Throughout his career, Dr. Selman has made important scientific contributions in the complex field of interstitial lung diseases, primarily in idiopathic pulmonary fibrosis and hypersensitivity pneumonitis. In the latter, he was one of the first investigators to demonstrate that this disorder could evolve to fibrosis with the subsequent destruction of lung architecture. Also, he described a new clinical/pathological entity called airways-centered interstitial fibrosis, which was previously confused with hypersensitivity pneumonitis. Dr. Selman's research has revealed different molecular and cellular mechanisms involved in the pathogenesis of hypersensitivity pneumonitis and has contributed to the identification of its transcriptional signature.

His seminal contribution in the area of idiopathic pulmonary fibrosis was a *position paper* published in 2001 in which he proposed a new hypothesis for the understanding of the pathogenesis of this devastating disorder. Although it was previously considered a classical inflammatory-driven fibrosis, Dr. Selman and his colleagues, supported by clinical observations and experimental studies, proposed a new model for the pathogenesis of this disease based on epithelial-fibroblast profibrotic inter-communication. This has lead to a major shift in the paradigm of our understanding and thus treatment of idiopathic pulmonary fibrosis. More recently, with evidence obtained from gene expression studies, he suggested that the pathogenesis of idiopathic pulmonary fibrosis may be at least partially explained by aberrant activation of developmental pathways.

Dr. Selman has served his entire professional career at the National Institute of Respiratory Diseases in Mexico City. In addition to his own interest and work in fibrotic lung disorders, he established and headed the Research Unit of this Institute during the early 1980s. Here he mentored numerous young pulmonary fellows and biologists in the field of lung science and encouraged the development of translational research. His talent and outstanding efforts resulted in the formation of several productive research groups that are currently working on a wide variety of topics in respiratory medicine.

Dr. Selman has authored more than 180 peer-reviewed research papers, numerous reviews, editorials, and essays, and two books. He has served on several editorial boards and advisory panels and is a member of the Protocol Review Committee of Idiopathic Pulmonary Fibrosis at the National Institutes of Health. He is a member of numerous Clinical Societies and recipient of the 2008 National Prize of Science and Arts, México, and the 2008 American Thoracic Society Scientific Accomplishment Award.

A native of Chile, Dr. Selman received his medical degree from the University of Chile in 1970. After completing a residency and chief residency in Thorax Hospital at the National Medical Center of the IMSS in México, he concluded a mastership in Molecular Biology at the National Autonomous University of Mexico. In 1978, he joined the National Institute of Respiratory Diseases, where he became Director of Research. In 1979, he was also appointed as Adjunct Professor at the Faculty of Medicine and the Faculty of Sciences in the National Autonomous University of Mexico.

Dr. Erika von Mutius, MD has focused her research on the epidemiology of childhood asthma and allergies, reflecting her education in pediatrics (LMU Munich) and epidemiology (Harvard School of Public Health, USA). Her primary interest was in the role of air pollution in the development these diseases. Her group was the first to show that, contrary to all expectations, asthma and allergies were less prevalent in the polluted areas of East Germany than in the much less polluted western part of the country. Subsequently, her group was the first to replicate David Strachan's observation, which inversely related the number of siblings to the occurrence of hay fever and atopy, three years after his publication, thereby instigating the "hygiene hypothesis." In collaboration with Swiss and Austrian colleagues, her group was also the first to propose a protective effect of a farm childhood, substantially corroborating the notions of the "hygiene hypothesis." This observation has since been widely replicated in Europe and around the world. Through interdisciplinary collaboration with epidemiologists, clinicians, immunologists, geneticists, statisticians, microbiologists, veterinarians, and milk hygienists, she has elaborated specific protective farm exposures in large, mostly EU-funded cross-sectional and longitudinal prospective surveys.

In 2004, Dr. von Mutius accepted a professorship in pediatrics at the Munich University Children's Hospital, where she has been the Head of the Asthma and Allergy Department since 1993. Her research interests have focused on the epidemiology of pediatric respiratory and allergic diseases. She has worked in several multicenter and interdisciplinary projects addressing the potential role of genetic and environmental risk factors for atopic illnesses. She has longstanding experience with design, implementation, and data analysis of large, multicenter, epidemiological studies on pediatric respiratory diseases and allergies, including birth cohort studies.

Dr. von Mutius has been the recipient of several prestigious awards. She serves on a number of international committees and is an active editorial board member of national and international journals such as the *New England Journal of Medicine* and the *Journal of Allergy and Clinical Immunology*. Among others, she is a member of the European Respiratory Society (ERS) and the European Academy of Allergology and Clinical Immunology (EAACI). She has authored more than 200 peer-reviewed journal articles and review papers and over 20 essays on a variety of topics in the field of asthma and allergy.

After receiving her medical degree from the University of Munich in 1984, Dr. von Mutius completed her internship and residency training in the Department of General Pediatrics, Neonatal and Pediatric Intensive Care. During 1992 and 1993, she was a research fellow at the Respiratory Sciences Center at the University of Arizona, Tucson, USA, with Professor Fernando Martinez. She also received training in Clinical Effectiveness at the Harvard School of Public Health in Boston, USA during 1997 and 1999, and she received a Master of Science in Epidemiology from the School in 2000.

R. Sanders Williams, MD is Professor of Medicine at the University of California, San Francisco and President of the J. David Gladstone Institutes. He was educated and received postdoctoral training in public and international affairs, internal medicine, cardiology, biochemistry, and molecular biology at Princeton University, Duke University, Harvard University (Massachusetts General Hospital), Oxford University, and the Cold Spring Harbor Laboratory. He served on the faculty of Duke University and of the University of Texas before assuming the role of Dean of the School of Medicine at Duke in 2001. He was promoted to Senior Vice Chancellor in 2007 and took on the leadership of the University's global strategy in 2008. In 2010, Dr. Williams began serving as the President of the J. David Gladstone Institutes.

As a scholar and scientist, Dr. Williams discovered genes, proteins, and pathways that control development, proliferation, cell size, and differentiation of cardiac and skeletal muscle cells (myocytes). His laboratory defined basic principles of how these cells adapt to changing physiological demands associated with exercise or disease states. As an educator, he has been continuously active in classroom teaching up to the present, and he has served as primary mentor to over 40 graduate students and postdoctoral fellows, many of whom have become distinguished faculty at major colleges and universities.

Dr. Williams led the Duke School of Medicine as Dean during a period that was highlighted by its ascendance in the national rankings of NIH grant support, a near doubling of its annual budget to over $800 million, enhancement of its physical plant by the addition of six new academic buildings, an increased rate of election of faculty to the National Academy of Sciences, the first appointments of department chairs who were female or African-American, and the founding of successful multidisciplinary, University-wide institutes in genome sciences, brain sciences, global health, and translational medicine. He has been a University leader in globalization of academic programs, serving as founding Dean of the Duke-NUS Graduate Medical School of Singapore.

On the national stage, Dr. Williams has served as the President of professional societies, on editorial boards of leading academic journals such as *Science*, and in government service on the Director's Advisory Committee of the National Institutes of Health and the Board of External Advisors to the National Heart, Lung and Blood Institute. Dr. Williams has been honored by election to the Institute of Medicine of the National Academy of Sciences, Alpha Omega Alpha, the American Society for Clinical Investigation, and the Association of American Physicians. He is a Fellow of the American Association for the Advancement of Science. In 2005, he received the Pioneer Award from the Samuel Dubois Cook Society for his work on behalf of social justice.

List of Acronyms

AAAS	American Association for the Advancement of Science
AAP	Association of American Physicians
ABCD	appropriate blood pressure control in diabetes
ACR	American College of Rheumatology
AEC	Atomic Energy Commission
AFB	acid-fast bacilli
ALL	acute lymphoblastic leukemia
AMA	American Medical Association
ATS	American Thoracic Society
BAL	bronchoalveolar lavage
BC	British Columbia
BHAT	beta-blocker heart attack trial
BP	bullous pemphigoid
BSL-4	biosafety level 4
BUN	blood urea nitrogen
BWS	Beckwith–Wiedemann syndrome
cAMP	cyclic adenosine monophosphate
CARET	beta-carotene and retinol efficacy trial
CCHS	Central Catholic High School
CCIF	Cancer Center Isolation Facility
CCU	coronary care unit

CDC	Centers for Disease Control and Prevention
CEPH	Center for the Study of Human Polymorphisms
COMGAN	Commission for the Global Advancement of Nephrology
COPD	chronic obstructive pulmonary disease
CPK	creatine phosphokinase
CTSA	Clinical and Translational Science Award
DGH	Denver General Hospital
EAAC	European Academy of Allergology and Clinical Immunology
EIS	Epidemic Intelligence Service
EPA	Environmental Protection Agency
ERS	European Respiratory Society
EVPMA	Executive Vice-President for Medical Affairs
FFBS	flexible-fiberoptic bronchoscope
FQNs	fluoroquinolone
GDR	German Democratic Republic
GI	Government Issue
GSF	Gesellschaft für Strahlenforschung
GTRs	government travel requisitions
HHMI	Howard Hughes Medical Institute
HIV	human immunodeficiency virus
HKU	University of Hong Kong
HMS	Harvard Medical School
HP	hypersensitivity pneumonitis
HST	health science and technology
HTLV-I	human T cell lymphotrophic virus type I
HTLV-1	human T-cell leukemia virus-1
HUPO	Human Proteome Organization
ICU	intensive care unit
ILD	interstitial lung disease
IPF	idiopathic pulmonary fibrosis

ISN	International Society of Nephrology
LAV	lymphadenopathy-associated virus
LC	Langerhans cells
LCI	laboratory of clinical investigation
LOI	loss of imprinting
LPS	lipopolysaccharide
MBA	masters of business administration
MCHR	Medical Committee for Human Rights
MD	medical degree
MGH	Massachusetts General Hospital
MHC	major histocompatibility complex
MIT	Massachusetts Institute of Technology
MMP	matrix metalloproteinase
MPH	Master's of Public Health
MRCP	Membership of the Royal Colleges of Physicians
mRNA	messenger RNA
MSTP	Medical Scientist Training Program
NCI	National Cancer Institute
NHLBI	National Heart, Lung and Blood Institute
NIAID	National Institute of Allergy and Infectious Diseases
NIAMS	National Institute of Arthritis and Musculoskeletal and Skin Diseases
NICU	neonatal intensive care unit
NIEHS	National Institute of Environmental Health Sciences
NIH	National Institutes of Health
NIOSH	National Institute for Occupational Safety and Health
NJH	National Jewish Health
NSBH	nonspecific bronchial hyperresponsiveness
NTP	National Toxicology Program
NYU	New York University

OMB	Office of Management and Budget
OSHA	Occupational Safety and Health Administration
OSTP	Office of Science and Technology Policy
OVA	Ovalbumin
PAS	para-aminosalicylate sodium
PHS	public health service
PKA	protein kinase
PMU-6	preventive medicine unit 6
QS	Quacquarelli Symonds
RAG	recombination activating gene
RNA	ribonucleic acid
ROTC	reserve officer training corp
RWJ	Robert Wood Johnson
SAT	scholastic aptitude test
SCID	severe combined immunodeficiency disease
SFGH	San Francisco General Hospital
SHAD	shipboard hazard and decontamination
SLE	systemic lupus erythematosus
SSSP	Summer Studies-Skills Program
TRP	transient receptor potential
UBC	University of British Columbia
UCHSC	University of Colorado Health Sciences Center
UCSF	University of California, San Francisco
UIP	usual interstitial pneumonia
UM	University of Michigan
UNC	University of North Carolina at Chapel Hill
USPHS	US Public Health Service
UT	University of Texas
UT	University of Tennessee
UTEP	University of Texas, El Paso

V	variable
VA	Veterans Administration
WCB	Workers' Compensation Board
WRAMC	Walter Reed Army Medical Center
WRGH	Walter Reed General Hospital
WWII	World War II
WWS	Woodrow Wilson School
XBP1	X-box binding protein 1

One
The Loneliness of the Physician-Scientist

Fernando D. Martinez

1.

I awake startled.
Frightened.
There is noise again coming from my mom and dad's bedroom.
I am sweating. I'm cold.
Dad shouts.
BREATHE CALMLY.
She has asthma again.
I can hear her.
The door is closed.
I will put my ear on the door.
I can hear her now.
I told Mrs. Toovey about my mom. She said you can practice writing asthma on your notebook.
Write my mom has asthma she said.
It's cold and I am shivering.
Suddenly Dad opens the door.
WHAT ARE YOU DOING HERE?
I see Mom. Her eyes are popping out, she looks like a lizard. Or a frog without a neck. Her mouth is open and makes noises.
She is squeezing a red rubber balloon with her hand a lot.
GO BACK TO BED.
I asked Mrs. Toovey if Mom will die. "I don't know," she said "but pray for her."
"I will cure asthma Mrs. Toovey," I said. She smiled and caressed my cheek.

F.D. Martinez (✉)
Arizona Respiratory Center, University of Arizona, Tucson, AZ 85719-1109, USA
e-mail: fernando@arc.arizona.edu

D.A. Schwartz (ed.), *Medicine Science and Dreams*,
DOI 10.1007/978-90-481-9538-1_1, © Springer Science+Business Media B.V. 2011

2.

I was born and raised in Chile and, from the time I was a young child, I became aware of the shame of poverty. In the neighborhood where we lived, destitute women carrying hungry children wearing no shoes or even clothes often knocked on our door asking for a dime. "They will use it for booze," Mom said to my sister and me. We lived in what were then the middle-class outskirts of Santiago, where slums mixed with the first suburbia, and the streets were quiet but edgy. From behind our house's fence I could see men stumbling out of the cheerless bar on the street corner. On Fridays, just before my father came back from his evening shift at the Children's Hospital, six or seven canutos, the derisive name we used for evangelicals, stood just outside the bar, first shouting how Jesus had saved them from alcoholism and then singing His praises with their guitars and drums. I never saw them leave for their shanty homes nearby; perhaps they sang all night I thought. Nobody listened.

Starting in elementary school, my parents enrolled me in an American boys' school, called Saint George's College, established in Chile in the 1930s by the Catholic Congregation of the Holy Cross. My classmates were mostly sons of rich merchants and landowners. "You are the future leaders of this country," Father Huard, the Rector, often told us. "Compassion and faith," he repeated. For a while, my life was immune to the misery that smothered our city.

Soon, however, the shielded peace collapsed. Around our home, the vacant lots were illegally occupied by poor families escaping crime and disease just a few hundred yards away. There were not enough police to evict them all, and soon our new neighbors lived in shacks made of used cardboard boxes and construction discards, among ravenous dogs and children of filth and lice. "Time to leave," Dad said after I was bitten by one of those dogs and had to be treated with painful abdominal injections for rabies. We moved to an apartment close to city center, hoping to get away from the foreboding surroundings.

3.

By the time I reached high school, what had surrounded us became part of our lives. The Cuban revolution inspired and instigated massive strikes and uprisings among the working poor and the disenfranchised. Peasant families migrating from the forsaken rural areas occupied large swats of land demanding public services and were brutally repressed. Many young Catholics embraced the Theology of Liberation, a left-wing movement that first emerged in Brazil and extended throughout Latin America. They demanded better wages for the working poor and supported an agrarian reform that would give land ownership to the peasants. Contrary to the Cuban regime, however, they aspired to preserve freedom and human rights. By the time I was 14, I was deeply attracted to the ideas of the Liberation Theologians (we did not call ourselves that way, but I like how it sounds, as if from a book by the great Chilean author Roberto Bolaño).

At school, there didn't seem to be anybody else who dared open his mouth then. They will do like in Cuba, many of my wealthy classmates said, they will steal our land and our factories and exile us to Miami. A center-left party supported by the Catholic Church, and which included the Liberation Theologians, won the presidential elections in 1964. I did not hide my quixotic enthusiasm for the timid agrarian reform started by the new government, but it cost me dearly; I was bullied and ostracized for years. One of those bullies my classmate since first grade with whom I had a gruesome fistfight in the school's aseptic restroom, would soon become a fatal protagonist of our country's history.

4.

Periodically, my mother still had her terrible asthma attacks. One evening in the early 1960s, when I was finishing elementary school, my father announced jubilantly that he had met a German physician who was giving a conference in his hospital. Dr. Weidenslaufer had a new treatment for mom's asthma, he said. As always, my mother said nothing, looking back at him with resignation and muted submission. "What would that be?" I asked, and my father went on and on about how great German medicine had been. They also discovered allergies, he said, and almost all the allergic reactions and tests have the names of German scientists. Dr. Weidenslaufer studied with them, he said, and brought all the German techniques with him. A few days later, Weidenslaufer came home with my father late in the afternoon. He was in his sixties then, and he was still robust and tall. He used the thickest eyeglasses I had ever seen. I always thought he really didn't need them; he was, for all real purposes, blind. He wore clothes that looked old to me and his shoes were inadequately shiny for their age. He sat in our dining room in front of my mother and started asking her questions in a mingled language: "When do you have asthma attacks?" "Only in spring," mother said. "How do you feel between your attacks?" "I am well," she said. "What do you think causes your asthma?" "I fear warm days in spring," she said. Weidenslaufer listened impassibly while staring at the windows, as if paying attention to the roaring traffic below. He remained silent for a few minutes. He then opened his thick and withered bag, and very tentatively extracted from it ten or more little bottles with murky liquids of different colors in them. "What are those?" I asked. My father fulminated me with his stare; he had allowed me to stay and watch; now he probably regretted it. Weidenslaufer did not answer; he slowly and mysteriously palpated my mother's forearm, as if searching for something lost, and suddenly, right above her elbow he stopped: hier, he muttered. He then palpated carefully each of the bottles with the cloudy liquids, diese, he said triumphantly, and meticulously placed one with a greenish fluid in front of him. He again searched for something in his bag and finally took out what looked to me like an old syringe. "I sterilized it at home," he told my father. He cleaned the rubber at the top of the little bottle with alcohol my father brought for him and inserted the needle into the bottle, missing his finger by a few millimeters. He found again the same point on the back of my mother's arm, sterilized it, and finally injected the ugly liquid in.

He smiled, staring now vacuously into the self-portrait of my Aunt Matilde that hung there, ever unwatched and unwatchable. Years later, my mom finally and surreptitiously removed the portrait from the wall, hoping nobody would notice, but the next time Matilde visited us she surely did, because she died without ever again speaking to my father.

I could not stop looking anxiously at my mother's arm, and finally, after 15 or 20 anxious and silent minutes during which nobody moved and Weidenslaufer never stopped staring at Matilde's face, I noticed a reddish color flare up at the spot of the injection. "It itches," mother said, and "I feel light-headed." Weidenslaufer awoke suddenly; his hands stumbled on the parade of little bottles and reached the spot on my mother's arm. Yah, he mumbled in throaty German, and smiled. I will have to give her some epinephrine, just as a precaution, he told my father, pronouncing epinephrine directly in German. He proceeded as before, blindly searching in his bag, extracting another bottle, this time one made of dark glass, and injected some of its liquid into my mother's other arm. After some minutes, he declared the operation concluded. "You are lucky," he told my bewildered mother, "I can treat your asthma. You are allergic to *Platanus orientalis*," he said, "and I have developed an extract in my laboratory that will cure you. I will inject you once a week for the next months in my office." I watched him in awe. "You can cure all asthmatics?" I asked. He looked through his eyeglasses and through me for a moment, "No, Sohn," he said, while he gathered his bottles and syringes. "Your mother is allergic only to *Platanus*, the tree that you see in almost all streets in Santiago. Most are not that fortunate." "How do you know?" I insisted. "I know," he said, irritated. I was going to ask what he did for persons with asthma who were not like my mother but my father interrupted us. "Can I take you home?" he offered. "No," Weidenslaufer said, "I have my car parked downstairs." He stumbled toward our front door, searched clumsily for the knob, and left with his arm extended, gingerly descending the stairs one by one.

I never saw Weidenslaufer again, but for two years my mother regularly attended his clinic on Wednesday mornings. After two years of injections, my mother stopped having asthma attacks. For the first time, she could leave the apartment in springtime and even come with us to fly kites in Manquehue hill in late September. Weidenslaufer had recommended three years of therapy, but he died before he could complete it.

His therapy became mythical in my imagination, but when I learned a few years later about the Nazis and the holocaust, a doubt started to loom: who was Dr. Weidenslaufer? Pictures of concentration camps and brutal experiments conducted on prisoners there crossed my mind. Had he been part of them? Finally, I could not resist and asked my father. "I never asked, and he never said anything," father said. "Many persons came from Germany to Chile," he explained, "some before the war, usually Jews persecuted by the Nazis, some after the war, many of them Nazis escaping the allies or soldiers freed from prisoner camps. I don't know to which group he belonged," he said. "He used to live in the south of the country and had just moved to Santiago when I met him." I kept asking my father for further explanations to no avail. "What would we gain by knowing?" he demurred.

And that is where I left Weidenslaufer. Our only encounter still haunts me, shrouded in his astonishing cure for my mother's asthma, the same disease I treat and study today, but also in the evil that I hanged in my fantasy to his unknown past. If he was perpetrator or victim, I will probably never find out.

5.

My last years of high school were marked by loneliness and rejection, dubbed "the revolutionary" and scorned with other silly nicknames. My greatest distraction and relief was long-distance running, and I practiced it obsessively. Our biology lessons were antiquated and boring, and never was Darwin or DNA ever mentioned in our classrooms. Still, I was convinced that I had to complete the work Weidenslaufer and his German teachers had started; I would cure all asthmas. Shortly after the end of my senior year, I applied directly to medical school, as was and still is the system in Chile, and was accepted. I had just turned 17.

From the very beginning, medical school was a house of wonders for me. The faculty at the University of Chile was the best trained in Latin America. Our Associate Professor of Biochemistry, Hermann Niemeyer, published regularly in *Nature* and *Journal of Biological Chemistry*. Humberto Maturana, a faculty member in the Department of Biology, had made major contributions to the understanding of movement detection by the retina and had several papers in *Science*. I soon realized that I was living one more contradiction, difficult to fathom and explain: the helplessly poor country with the beleaguered and aloof elite that I had encountered at school had a first-class medical school, which was practically free of charge. The University was the highest source of reputation back then. All the best clinicians in the country were proud to teach at the medical school and thought of that as their true profession. Many (including my father) considered private medical practice a necessary evil to supplement their meager academic salaries.

During my first years of medical school, the environment was one of constant challenge and discussion, and the fact that I spoke fairly good English helped me participate in the journal clubs to which the faculty invited interested students. I was often charged with reading a scientific paper and commenting on it. One of those articles brilliantly showed intracellular formation of lamellar bodies containing surfactant in lung epithelial cells. The paper was in *Science* and speculated that mitochondria were the source of surfactant. At the time, I had no way to know or care about the paper's authors, but I was fascinated by the beautiful electron microscopy technology, revolutionary for the time, and by the idea that mitochondria were involved. The idea somehow got stuck in my brain. A quarter of a century later, while I was being recruited for a position at the University of California in San Francisco, I was interviewed by John Clements, one of the pioneers in surfactant research, in his tiny office full of papers and books at the Cardiovascular Research Institute. While he was animatedly telling me about how he came to understand surfactants from studies of the effects of chemical weapons for the Army, I suddenly remembered the article I had reviewed as a student. "We've come a long way," I said to break the silence while he was guiding me to my next appointment. "There was a time when people thought surfactant was made by mitochondria." I could not see Clements, who was following me in a narrow corridor. I could only hear him say wryly, "Yes, I've often been wrong." At first I did not understand what he meant but then, suddenly, I had a harrowing illumination. I distractedly went through the rest of the morning interviews and asked to skip lunch and be taken to the library. I hurried through the large Index Medicus tomes in use before PubMed could even be imagined and found the *Science* paper from 1962. John Clements, the same John Clements, was the last author. I thought to go back to his room and apologize for the involuntary snafu, but I was so profoundly embarrassed that I did not dare. The next day, at the wrap-up interview, my host said, you really impressed Clements, and showed me a handwritten note he had received from him that morning: "Hire him now!" it said.

6.

Still a teenager, I was euphorically enthralled by the larger than life characters I encountered almost daily in medical school. During the first year, I was a student volunteer in Dr. Elias Motles' lab. There and then, I fell in love with science. Motles was a respiratory physiologist who had trained in New York with Andre Cournand. After Motles had left, Cournand was awarded the Nobel Prize for having transferred heart catheterization into clinical practice. That's how strange science is, Motles used to say, Cournand was never interested in the heart; he wanted to know about pulmonary perfusion and that is why he developed cardiac catheterization. "It was when I was at Columbia that he realized the clinical importance of what he was doing," Motles added, and hooked up with the cardiologist. I used to joke with Motles that perhaps he gave Cournand the idea, and Motles, always wise and humble, chuckled.

We performed experiments in which we measured surface tension after pouring lung lavage from prematurely delivered rats on a small tub in which a piston slowly moved a bar, which in turn decreased or increased the liquid surface over which the surfactant was distributed. The main reason I had volunteered with Motles was an idea that came to me when he lectured us on lung mechanics: Perhaps surfactant deficiency could have a role in asthma. Soon, however, I was overtaken by the mysterious nature of what we were observing on that tub: hysteresis. When the bar moved in the direction of expanding the surface in which the lavage was distributed, surface tension (measured with a balance system invented by John Clements, something I did not know then!) was very low and remained low for a while until it quite suddenly increased and achieved a new plateau, similar to that of saline. When we contracted the surface, however, something for me totally unexpected occurred. The inked pen that traced the surface tension on lab paper did not follow the same track. Surface tension remained high for a longer period of time and then suddenly dropped when the surface was much smaller than when it had increased, as the bar moved in the opposite direction. For Motles, obviously, this was perfectly natural, but for me this was unexplainable. How could the same number of molecules distributed on the same tub surface, all things equal, show a completely different behavior depending on the direction of the piston's movement? Not only did Motles not deride my astonishment, he explained very simply with a metaphor: When you start from the narrowest surface, all surfactant molecules are vertical and they have to snap to the horizontal position in order for surface tension to increase. This snapping occurs suddenly to a large number of molecules at the same time and late during expansion. In the opposite direction, the horizontal molecules snap to the vertical position late, thus keeping surface tension high. As you can imagine, he added teleologically, this makes not only inspiration possible but also expiration much easier. There were many more discussions about these mysterious surface tension phenomena between Motles and me. My objection that his was a simple description and did not explain what the mechanism was that allowed the snapping was answered with an encouragement to "go talk to the biophysicists at the College of Science." I never did. I reasoned that this dynamic dependency had to be a general property of biology if not of matter, and therefore, a great challenge to our capacity to know and understand biological processes, any temporal cross-section of a biological phenomenon could be enormously deceiving. I did not know or even suspect then that many more contexts other than time could affect biological outcomes, but I intuited that a lot was hidden behind the beautiful hysteresis curves drawn by the china pen in Motles' lab.

Concomitant to my experience in Motles' lab, I attended what was then a required Introduction to Biology course by Professor Maturana, the retina researcher. Maturana was (and still is) a short man with a thick beard, thick eyeglasses, and thick mind, who spoke slowly and almost secretively in a low-pitched voice. Maturana challenged us to look at biological phenomena from 10,000 feet; what is it that is common to all forms of life? After cogently arguing against all of our naïve answers (and prions had not even been described then!), he concluded that a new concept he had invented needed to be created to describe the essential nature of biological phenomena: autopoiesis. And he drew this big circle on the blackboard from which an arrow emerged and returned back to the circle. I do not have enough space (a subterfuge perhaps to hide the inadequacy of my remembrance and acumen!) to attempt to further describe Maturana's disquisitions. Suffice to say that his ideas were espoused and expanded by his brilliant student Francisco Varela, and are explained in their book *Tree of Knowledge*. For years, recalling Maturana's lessons evoked wonder and boundless awe in me. I heard him speak recently after a 30-year hiatus and I read *Tree of Knowledge*. Although I greatly admired his logical "post-rational" proposals and I had goose bumps when I heard him talk again about autopoiesis, he was unable to meet the mythical standards that the mind of a 17-year-old medical student had unfairly imposed on him.

Maturana's lessons obviously added to the intrigue with which I followed Motles' experiments, but they did not address the basic problem I still saw: How could autopoiesis be studied experimentally? Could we learn biology by studying each component, one at a time, without a method to understand the whole?

During those months I had become very friendly with my medical school class-mate and fellow Liberation Theologian Juan Pablo Jimenez. Although he had been in the Catholic Seminary for 2 years before changing his mind about priesthood, he has never stopped being an intensely spiritual, almost metaphysical person. He had had intense instruction in philosophy at the Seminary and thus he immediately grasped my conundrums. We spent hours discussing hysteresis and autopoiesis and their implications. We read together each of the thousand pages of the Guyton *Textbook of Medical Physiology*, competing feverishly to best interpret the true "meaning" of each phenomenon described, well beyond the requirements of our class. I soon understood that both Maturana and Motles were right. It was essential to understand the primordial physical phenomena that make up biology: ion move-ments, membrane properties, energy accumulating reactions. But the closer we got to them, the less we understood how they organized by themselves into something with a biological "meaning." "You have a philosophical mind," Jimenez said, "you need to study epistemology." I had not heard the word before and had no idea what he was talking about. I decided to heed his advice and was accepted in the Masters in Philosophy program at the Catholic University in Santiago. During my second year of medical school, I studied about propranolol and *Hymenolepis nana* during the day and about Kant, Wittgenstein, and symbolic logic four evenings a week.

7.

Those first two years at the university, I am certain, left an indelible seal on me. From 30 years away, they emerge flooded with reckless joy, quests unending, and energizing epiphanies. I do not know what trajectory my life would have taken if the tragic events I lived later had not occurred. I do know, however, that the insight I had then—that all occurrences in biology are context-dependent—has permeated all my work and even my thought processes since. Devoid as I am of any mystical imagina-tion, fascinated by, but completely unable to understand Prajapati and Protogonos, the Hindu and Greek deities who presided over nothingness before anything was, I am left with the only source of spirituality my senses can detect: the endless diver-sity and creativity of the human individual. I have always thought of humans as eager accumulators of past contexts, endowed at birth with a capacity that certainly not only limits us but also allows us to overcome the cages of predetermination and bestows on us the potential to be free.

Very recently, the genetic revolution engendered the expectation (and the promise) that all complex phenotypes with a strong genetic component could be one day predicted to a significant degree with relatively simple tests of inherited variation. This dogma appeared to challenge the primordial concept of human cre-ativity and freedom that I had so simply learned watching a lab container. Could it be that the most elemental human characters are bestowed mechanically by genes? Not wanting to be fixated in my self-imposed orthodoxy, my conviction flickered. Could I have been wrong all along? Could there truly be a *primum movens* of life, Dawkins' selfish gene, Borges' Aleph of perfect understanding? I like to ask my most enlightened friends the simplest of questions: Could a computer one day compose de novo Mendelssohn's octet (one of my favorite pieces of music), note by note? Invariably, all of them have the same answer: of course! It's just a combinatorial riddle, is it not? "Yes, there are octillions of possible combinations in 30 minutes of music," one friend said, "but a strong computer, starting from Mendelssohn's genes, will 1 day recompose the octet by limiting the likelihood landscape." No way, is still invariably my answer, unless you can reproduce not only Mendelssohn's genes, quite an easy task these days, but also all his life history up to age 16, when he composed the octet: his music-loving Jewish family, their conversion to Christianity when he was a young boy, his encounters with Goethe, who convinced him he was the new Mozart, and so forth. How can you model this individual and unique road?

I confess that I was paradoxically relieved when I saw the results last year of a meta-analysis of scores of genome-wide studies of height, a human phenotype that has one of the strongest hereditary components. Even when hundreds of thousands of persons are studied, only a small fraction, not more than 5%, of the variability of height in the population is directly explained by known genetic variations. There is still a possible "genetic" explanation for this failure: There are many low-frequency variants still undiscovered. I cannot rule out this possibility, but much more plausible seems to me the contention that genetic determination is context-dependent. Yes, perhaps only Mendelssohn's genes could have composed the octet, but without his life history, no octet would have been possible either.

Who knows, perhaps my grandchildren or their grandchildren will solve the enigma of Mendelssohn's octet.

8.

Politics had a minor role in these first years of my medical school. Among my basic science teachers, who almost invariably had trained in the USA, eyes were turned north. The war in Vietnam was raging and was followed in the lab with wrath and anxiety; we all wanted the war to end, the students lingering in the labs for still vague ideological reasons, our teachers mostly because many of the friends they had made during training had children, teenagers like me, fighting in Southeast Asia. An image is engrained in my brain: November 1968—all my teachers and some of my fellow students and postdocs listening to the Voice of America on shortwave radio and following the results of the presidential elections in an auditorium adjacent to the new labs we had recently moved into. It was warm already in the southern spring but we had no air conditioning. The traffic noise coming from the open windows facing Independencia Street in Santiago made the fickle radio signal even more difficult to understand. Finally, Nixon was declared the winner, and we all were left terribly disappointed. We could not even suspect, however, how the effects of that election result would resonate fatefully in those same corridors just a few years later.

Returning recently to visit my family and friends in Chile for Christmas, as I do every year, I nostalgically went back to see those same labs again. I entered the area that was brand new then, old-looking and antiquated now. The room where we gathered that early November morning was still there, but it was now called Julio Cabello Hall. He was one of the teachers who gathered that day around the shortwave radio, and he had died unexpectedly two years later. I could see him still, a large man with booming voice, sitting close to Niemeyer, his most admired assistant, lamenting the lack of wisdom of the American voters.

9.

If I try to recall what happens next, the sense I get is that of a mesmerizing cataclysm, similar to what I felt more recently, after 9/11. Bafflingly, that cataclysm is strongly linked in my memory to another 9/11 ... 9/11 of 1973.

10.

When I was in the third year of medical school in 1969, the echoes of the student uprisings in the USA and Europe bounced in our classrooms and labs and gripped us all with a commotion that nobody could have predicted just a few months earlier. Student assemblies gathered almost daily and fierce orators proclaimed the need to reform the University. The barons who despotically controlled all departments had to be dethroned, they shouted. Faculty and students had to have a say in the University affairs. Soon we were on an indefinite strike.

It was impossible not to get caught in the vortex of incendiary speeches and supposedly unattainable dreams. I still belonged to the Liberation Theologians, and we started participating in the gatherings and adhered to the strike. One of the main objectives was to tie the medical school to the needs of the poor. The Theologians wanted the students to go practice from very early in the slums. The full professors, who governed the autonomous university and were the only members of the faculty senate, fiercely opposed any changes and accused students of wanting to destroy the intellectual jewel that our school was. Motles called me one day and told me how disappointed he was. "You will be a great scientist one day. Choose," he told me, "you either learn science and epistemology or work in the slums, there is no time for all three." "No," I insisted, "we want to use the school and its prestige to change the world." My admired mentors privately supported us, but fearful of reprisals from the full professors, seldom participated in the assemblies. Finally, the center-left administration mediated and imposed a referendum among faculty, students, and staff, and the results were overwhelmingly favorable to the reformers. We had won!

11.

A new progressive dean and a faculty senate were elected, and the new curriculum fostered the integration of medical students into the network of pediatric clinics that the administration had established in the slums. Soon I was attending one of those clinics, in the southernmost periphery of Santiago. Although my mother often lent me her car to go to school, the only physician that staffed the clinic told me not to drive at first. It is too dangerous if they don't know who you are, take the bus instead. So once a week I traveled for an hour and then walked two miles each way to reach the clinic in a slum called Villa O'Higgins.

What I saw there once a week for two years changed all my life's premises. The clinic was located in one of the fields occupied mostly by poor peasants in years past, as I described earlier, and with time the meager sheds had become permanent residencies of large, extended families. Some dwellers had built clumsy brick homes with government loans, but most still lived in crowded and filthy conditions. Most dwellings had no running water or sewage, and electricity, when available, was often surreptitiously stolen from nearby, high-tension electric towers, at great risk for the countless children that roamed the streets. Unemployment, malnutrition, alcoholism, and crime were rampant. Dozens of young mothers stood in line every day at 4 AM hoping to get one of the few tickets that were distributed for the day's visits. Those who were not lucky often stood there, with their sick babies in their arms waiting to see if we could squeeze them between two visits. Dr. Francisco Mardones, the clinic's doctor, an idealistic young man, was a Liberation Theologian himself. "There is no time for a lot of teaching," he said on my first day. "You'll do immunizations. Just stick as many children as you can. Only if the nurse cannot help you, ask me."

I started in early summer, and soon I had to leave immunizations to the only nurse available, and there I was, a 19-year-old boy treating extremely malnourished children, often intensely dehydrated due to acute diarrhea. Calling the district hospital was all but useless: "We are full up to the corridors," they said, "do as best as you can." Even if there were free beds, there was no fast way to transport the patients to the hospital, no ambulance, no parents or neighbors who owned cars. Fortunately, Mardones had trained a group of teenage girls and they administered the oral rehydrating fluids to the patients, whom we lined in their mothers' arms outside the clinic until we had to close in the evening. I am sure we saved many lives then. But the winter was the true nightmare. Dozens of half-starved children died in front of our eyes of severe airway obstruction due to bronchiolitis, and we were completely helpless: there was no oxygen, no radiology to ascertain pneumonia, and antibiotics were scarce. "Spare the antibiotics for meningitis," Mardones used to tell me. At least we will decrease contagion.

That experience made me conclude that Motles could not be right; what good could it make to become a scientist if more than half of the population lived in misery, if 12% of all children died in the first year of life of malnourishment and treatable diseases? From this new fulcrum, Kant's a priori categories of knowledge seemed thickheaded, and the hours I often needed to try to figure out but one Proposition of the *Tractatus Logico-Philosophicus* a waste of my time. I abandoned the Philosophy program and the labs and became more and more involved in the student movement.

12.

By 1970, we Liberation Theologians had become profoundly disappointed with the center-left administration. Not enough had been done and children were still dying of hunger. Things had to change. We decided that we would support the candidate of the left, Salvador Allende, in the presidential elections that year. Allende was a socialist physician who admired Castro but promised to respect democracy and the constitution. He won a plurality of votes and by law, the Chilean Congress had to choose between the two largest vote-gainers. The extreme right opted for a strategy of terror to constrain the military to intervene against Allende. A week before the day in which Congress in full session would vote, the Army Chief of Staff, who respected the constitution, was ambushed and shot while being driven on a central street in Santiago. He died a few days later. Investigators soon identified the individuals who had participated in the ambush. One of the alleged assassins was my classmate, the bully I had had to fight against in high school.

Allende was finally voted for by Congress. I not only continued medical school but also became very active politically. I was elected president of the medical student council. We supported the changes the new government was fostering and looked at the future with great hope. Perhaps I could return to becoming the scientist I always dreamed to be, the one who would complete Weidenslaufer's job to cure asthma.

But chaos ensued. In part due to the pressures and machinations of the Nixon administration, who wanted to overthrow Allende from the very beginning, in part due to the plotting of the extreme left, who wanted a socialist revolution à la Castro at all costs, the government lost control of the economy and of the country. All transportation was paralyzed by the truckers' strike, funded by the CIA, and basic products were impossible to find; many factories and farms were forcefully taken from their rightful owners by workers instigated by the extreme left. We all wished for a peaceful outcome, but soon it became clear that a military "solution" was inevitable.

13.

September 11, 1973.
I awake startled.
Frightened.
There is noise coming from the large deep hole they are digging for the freeway right in front of our apartment.
Sounds like shots.
They are shots.
I look out the window.
Fifty or more soldiers walk tentatively along the wide construction crevice. They look toward the apartment buildings and every now and then shoot randomly toward them.
One of them looks toward our window. He sees me. He shoots. I drop to the floor.
Frightened.
They are shooting, I shout. I am sure they are on their way to take the presidential palace, three blocks away.

I listen to the radio. Almost all stations have military music. The Marxist government has been deposed, they say.

Every now and then lists of persons who are summoned to surrender to the military are read.

Two of my fellow student leaders are among them. I will probably be named soon.

We have to get out of here. But we are surrounded by troops.

I am sweating.

The presidential palace will be bombed by the Air Force, the radio announces. All those living around the palace should evacuate immediately.

Curfew in two hours.

We run out of the building with tens of others. There are soldiers all around. That way, they shout pointing their guns.

A group of prisoners surrounded by troops is advancing slowly from the palace. Some seem severely wounded and bleed. Walk, goddamn sons of bitches.

We run.

14.

I left the country a few weeks later for Italy, exiled. Many of my fellow student leaders were not as lucky. They disappeared without a trace, even some of those who had voluntarily surrendered to the military.

In subsequent years, I became a physician-scientist.

Most of the training needed to become one I had already obtained by then.

Two
Gamow, Guppies, and the Search for GOD

David S. Pisetsky

The term physician-scientist is one of those compound words that has been created to unite disparate elements. Our language has others: student-athlete, warrior-statesman, and player-coach. The hyphen is a convenient way to keep the words together, but the hyphen cannot obscure the inherent contradictions that fight within. At that core, physicians and scientists (just like scholars and athletes) are worlds apart. Becoming a physician-scientist demands a union that can take years to forge and is often tenuous and unnerving.

In my experience, the careers of physician-scientists are more varied, unpredictable, and quixotic than those of either a scientist or a physician. Like me, most physician-scientists spend their lives jumping between identities and life styles. While a very rewarding and exciting venture, the life of a physician-scientist requires a special personality, an unusual gestation period, and a multitude of academic parents who can have wildly different aspirations and expectations for their offspring.

The compound words I noted have two interesting features. The first is that each describes a person of action—physician, warrior, athlete, or player—in conjunction with a person of thought—scientist, statesman, student, or coach. The second feature is that the order of the two words seems to matter, and, in all but one case, the action person precedes the thought person. Only for the student-athlete does the work of the mind take precedent. I think that this positioning is intentional and allows the National Collegiate Athletic Association to create the illusion that the athlete's focus is on education rather than scoring points or winning games.

To this day, my own identity can seem uncertain. When asked what I do by someone at a reunion, a cocktail party, or in a bygone era, a meeting of the Parent-Teacher Association, I have never said that I am a physician-scientist. Instead, with ordinary people, I say that I am a doctor while, with other physicians, I say that I am a rheumatologist. If more explanation is needed, I will say that I do research or I am

D.S. Pisetsky (✉)
Departments of Medicine and Immunology Duke University Medical Center, Durham, NC 27705, USA; Durham VA Medical Center, Durham, NC 27705, USA
e-mail: dpiset@duke.edu

D.A. Schwartz (ed.), *Medicine Science and Dreams,*
DOI 10.1007/978-90-481-9538-1_2, © Springer Science+Business Media B.V. 2011

in academics. While physician-scientist describes perfectly my career, I do not use this designation.

Why not say, "I am a physician-scientist" if that is what I am? In part, I think that my reluctance reflects the inherent ambiguity that comes from a fragmented life. Also, in looking at my own career, I have to wonder whether I am physician-scientist or a scientist-physician, although I have absolutely never heard the latter term.

In my years on the faculty at the Duke University Medical Center, I have read hundreds of essays from applicants to our various programs: medical school, graduate school, MSTP (Medical Scientist Training Program), house staff, and fellowship. Perusing more than my share of, "Why I want to be a doctor (or rheumatologist or immunologist)" treatises, I have noticed that essays from the MD and PhD applicants differ in describing how they reached their career choice. The MD applicants usually describe a dramatic occurrence, an event in which a physician intervenes decisively in the life of the applicant or his or her family. Whatever the outcome of the intervention is, the applicant reports a transformative and inspirational moment when he or she decides to become a doctor.

In contrast, the PhD applicants start out their essays with statements like, "I always wanted to know how things work," or, "I have always been a very curious person." Few of these essays describe a discovery or revelation of knowledge gained. At best, the applicant reports that he was spared discipline when Dad found the television set completely disassembled. Few of these essays describe a role model or exposure to the work of a scientist, since scientists are not commonly encountered by young people. Nor do most scientists produce strong impressions like physicians, who literally can rescue someone from the dead or staunch the bleeding.

Rather, the impressions left by scientists are often bland or indistinct, since their work is cerebral and the topics of their inquiry are often obscure. What drives the PhD applicant is something internal, a fundamental curiosity about the world that can be satisfied by the applicant's own thinking or reading. In the life of a scientist, a book or a lecture may be as influential as a person. Even though scientists work with their hands and sometimes utilize machines as big as a bulldozer, they are people of the mind, and what leaves an impression for them are ideas as much as people or action.

Becoming a physician-scientist really involves the acquisition of three identities: physician, scientist, and physician-scientist. The timing for these stages is very variable, although I think that, for many physician-scientists, the science part comes first. You can play with a chemistry set when you are 10 years old, but you cannot do a cardiac cath in the basement. For me, the science part was clearly first. I always enjoyed school and always liked to think and ponder. On the other hand, I have always had a taste for engagement, public service, and a life involved with other people, wanting the opportunity to have an impact and do good in the world in a way that science alone could not provide.

How were these elements put together so that I became a genuine physician-scientist, both an MD and PhD, who attends on general medicine, sees patients, and does basic science with as much energy now as ever before? My honest answer is that I do not know how I got to where I am today, but I am happy that I did.

Autobiography is often subject to revisionism if not fiction, since memory can put lipstick on the proverbial pig of the past. In this brief journey into the past, I will try to be honest and describe the moments in my life when my identity as a scientist took hold and why dual citizenship in the world of science and medicine still gives me a thrill. Alas, much will be missing in this account: a long and happy marriage, two wonderful children, and collaborations and adventures with scores of trainees, colleagues, and friends. This article is Genesis. Since I am not on Facebook, for the rest, Pubmed and Google may provide what details may be there.

Born in 1945, I grew up during a time in history when both science and medicine probably gave the world more hope than ever before and where medical research was one of the most esteemed and prestigious callings imaginable. Furthermore, in my family, which had emerged from successive traumas of the Depression and World War II, the profession of medicine was the aspiration for the children. Indeed, there seemed to be little reason to think of another calling, since medicine had it all. When I asked my mother's Aunt Jenny if she thought I should become something other than a doctor, she looked with disbelief and laughed uproariously, "What? A plumber?"

I spent my early life in and around New York City, a part of the world which has more Jews than just about any other, certainly so after World War II when European Jewry was almost completely destroyed. The intellectual tradition and devotion to scholarship of Jews are thousands of years old, but in Europe it was confined to Talmudic study led by the rabbis. As Jews came to America, opportunity grew, and science and medicine became new paths through which the drive for scholarship could be expressed.

The path of Jews to medicine was often constrained by anti-Semitism and financial limitation. Nevertheless, many American Jews became physicians, although, like my father, they went to Europe for their medical education. My father Joseph attended the University of Berlin medical school from 1930 to 1936 and had a whale of a good time. He learned from the giants of German medicine, wrote a thesis on the neuropathology of systemic lupus erythematosus, and savored the vibrant culture of Berlin. Fortunately, he got out well in advance of the terrible events of the Holocaust.

With help from friends, he obtained a house staff position in New York. There, he met my mother Lillian, who had worked her way through Hunter College, earning $3 per day as a salesperson at Macy's on 34th Street. The Depression had a big impact on her thinking and she became committed to helping the underdogs in life, serving first as a home-bound teacher for sick children. My parents were married just as the War started.

During the War, my father was a Captain in the Army, serving stateside in Wyoming and Oregon, and then my family returned to New York where my father became a staff physician at the Bronx VA Hospital. The Bronx VA was then a great research institution where Roslyn Yalow worked with Sol Berson on the immunoassay of insulin, a discovery that led to a Nobel Prize. In another wing of the hospital,

Ludwig Gross defined the inheritance of cancer in mice. The world was filled with optimism and, while the war produced the bomb, it also led to important medical advances. Peace created the momentum for further research. The future looked very bright. Medicine was in the vanguard, and my parents wanted their children to be in that vanguard.

My parents devoted themselves to the education of my sister Estelle and me. We went to the Museum of Natural History, the Metropolitan Museum of Art, Broadway, and everything else that was culturally worthwhile and affordable. My father, who probably would have been a physician-scientist had circumstances allowed, always engaged Estelle and me in projects. When I was in the first grade and my sister in the third grade, he conjured the idea of using television to help blind people see and worked with us on a project for the New York City Science Fair.

Our television was a cigar box, with the lens cut from the cardboard interior of a toilet paper roll. As part of our entry for "The Blind Shall See," my sister held the camera from which emerged wires attached to my head by a harness of plastic tubing. The idea was that the TV sent a signal from the box to my head where electric zaps on my scalp would be perceived as a visual image. During the competition, Estelle explained the concept to a judge. She must have done a very good job since we won a first prize. Either that or we were very cute. More science fair projects followed and, a few years later, my father helped me to build a guidance system for a rocket ship, with a gyroscope positioned inside a scaffolding of plexiglass. We were all thrilled when a picture of me assembling this contraption made the front page of the local newspaper (Fig. 2.1).

In looking back on this time, the lives of two Jewish New Yorkers became major stories and, in different ways, were each an impetus for success and good deeds. This was especially true for the drive, not always clearly enunciated, to have Jews gain a position of pride and accomplishment. On the negative side, there was Julius Rosenberg, who along with his wife Ethel was accused of selling atomic secrets to the Russians. The Rosenbergs lived within a few miles of our apartment building on the Grand Concourse in the Bronx. The execution of the Rosenbergs in 1953 is one of the most vivid memories of my childhood. The whole story is a terrible tragedy of treason, fear, and vengeance. It fueled anti-Semitism and was a further motivation for Jews to be even better than other Americans.

As a polar opposite to the Rosenbergs, there was Jonas Salk, a man of science and medicine whose vaccine changed the world. People today do not usually know polio beyond the story of Franklin D. Roosevelt or contact with an increasingly rare person who was a victim of that dread disease. Before the polio vaccines, every summer was a time of oppressive fear and, when a child in the area came down with polio, swimming pools emptied and parents became terrified that their child too would be grievously struck. Salk changed all that and, within a few years and the addition of the Sabin vaccine, polio essentially disappeared. Whether Salk's work was worthy of a Nobel Prize has been much debated, but he became a great hero, especially so for Jews who had to contend with the shadow of the Rosenbergs.

Salk's vaccine showed powerfully the importance of medical research to change the world and, if polio could be conquered, optimism soared that cancer and other

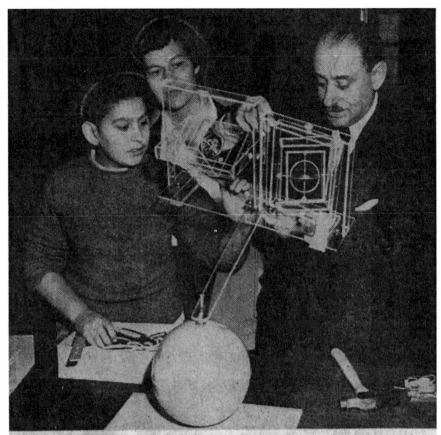

STABLE PLATFORM for outer of his parents Mr. and Mrs. Jo- of the local students exhibiting space is set up by David Piset- seph Pisetsky. The platform con- at the fair which will be ope sky, twelve, student at Albert sists of a globe with two gyro- to the public Thursday and Fri Leonard Junior High School, at scopic gadgets suspended above day—Staff Photo by Dante Ra the Westchester Science Fair in it on lucite arms. Davis is one faell. the County Center, with the help

Fig. 2.1 Big day at the Westchester Science Fair. My whole family was very excited when we saw this picture on the front page of The Standard-Star, the local paper of New Rochelle, on April 16, 1958, the day the fair opened. The newspaper cost 7 cents. The other big story concerned a possible tax cut by a President everyone called Ike

dread diseases would soon be contained. One of the lessons of Salk's work, often highlighted, is the value of basic research. Without basic research in tissue culture and viral propagation, polio as a disease would have been approached technologically, as engineers tinkered with iron lungs to make them smaller and more efficient. In contrast, basic research, by providing the scientific underpinning for vaccine development, shifted the paradigm and completely eliminated the need for the iron lungs.

While the 1950s had very dark moments, the post-war period was a heady time and science was at the top. With a role model like Salk and the support of parents and family, even in elementary school, a career plan was forming in which I would become a medical researcher. In 1954, when I was in the fourth grade, my family moved to New Rochelle, a suburb of New York City renowned for its public school system. New Rochelle had a strong commitment to education, and the Roosevelt School on North Avenue was a much more enjoyable place for me than PS 46 of the Bronx, where Irish-Catholic teachers had wanted to clobber me for what they thought were my rebellious ways. My interest in science was congruent with everything around me and, throughout the last two years of elementary school, junior high, and high school, I enjoyed myself immensely, doing well academically.

I have always been a reader, and, during junior high school, I read my way through the books of George Gamow, starting with "One, Two, Three...Infinity," buying them in paperback editions for 50 cents in a book shop in the slowly deteriorating New Rochelle downtown. Gamow was a physicist and, while I liked cosmology and cosmogony, I wanted to read more biology. I went to the public library and found what looked like a very interesting book on evolution. Alas, when I went to the check-out desk, I was refused. It turns out that one of the book's illustrations showed naked Neanderthal women with breasts exposed, albeit obscured by dense body hair. Nevertheless, the exposed breasts made the book *verboten*, and a duller substitute was provided. This was a time when *Lady Chatterley's Lover* was banned and *Peyton Place* was notorious. Who knew that the *Evolution of Man* ranked with such scandalous works?

After my mother died in 2007, I went to New Rochelle to pack up mementos of my childhood, including a list of books I read at that time (Fig. 2.2). I am not sure why I kept a list, but the focus on science it illustrated is startling. Whereas boys of my age were supposed to be reading science fiction, I was reading the real item, working my way through texts on electronics, chemistry, and space science. I loved rocketry and could name the thrust of every rocket then known. When I showed this list to my daughter, she laughed, saying, "You certainly were a nerd." "Still am," I said, knowing that physician-scientists have more than a touch of nerds about them.

Among the events of this time, the one I consider the most significant was a science fair project when I was a junior in high school. Over the years, I had done projects with my father but I was ready to strike out on my own. At that time, I kept tropical fish and, as I like to say, I had a green thumb when it came to my aquarium. In my aquarium, algae flourished, the water was a dark green, and the glass walls of the aquarium were coated with a thick paste of vegetal growth. I kept the tank filled with guppies, but the guppies died at an appalling rate. Fearing their inevitable extinction, I consulted a book about tropical fish and learned that guppies ate their young. Intrigued by this seeming biological anomaly, I pored through books at the main library of New Rochelle, which was fortuitously located near a favorite pizza restaurant named Giovanni's. After a hard Saturday afternoon in the library, I would meet a friend and we would share one of Giovanni's finest pies, which cost about one dollar.

Reading about motherhood, I came across research on prolactin, which is the mammalian hormone that regulates milk production. I put two and two together and

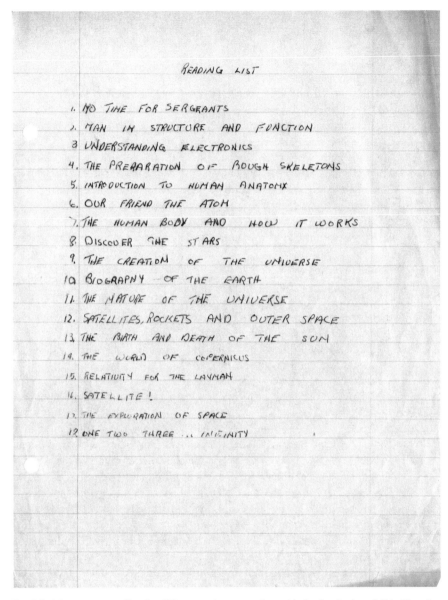

READING LIST

1. NO TIME FOR SERGEANTS
2. MAN IN STRUCTURE AND FUNCTION
3. UNDERSTANDING ELECTRONICS
4. THE PREPARATION OF ROUGH SKELETONS
5. INTRODUCTION TO HUMAN ANATOMY
6. OUR FRIEND THE ATOM
7. THE HUMAN BODY AND HOW IT WORKS
8. DISCOVER THE STARS
9. THE CREATION OF THE UNIVERSE
10. BIOGRAPHY OF THE EARTH
11. THE NATURE OF THE UNIVERSE
12. SATELLITES, ROCKETS AND OUTER SPACE
13. THE BIRTH AND DEATH OF THE SUN
14. THE WORLD OF COPERNICUS
15. RELATIVITY FOR THE LAYMAN
16. SATELLITE !
17. THE EXPLORATION OF SPACE
18. ONE TWO THREE ... INFINITY

Fig. 2.2 My summer reading list. What surprises most about this list is why I read "No Time for Sergeants"

decided that, if the guppies were given prolactin, their feelings of motherhood would surge and that they would cherish and not devour their little offspring. Knowing that the Westchester Science Fair was coming up, I decided on a project. I would set up two tanks of fish. I would treat one with prolactin and keep the other as the control.

The outcome measure would be the number of surviving baby guppies. I then went to a pet store for supplies and set up another fish tank, carefully positioning the bubbler that kept oxygen in the water to keep the guppies alive, although in my case, it seemed to make the algae thrive.

With everything ready to go and baby fish on the way, I went to the local pharmacy to buy the needed prolactin for the experiment. Suffice it to say, my request was greeted incredulously since not only did I not have a prescription for prolactin, but prolactin for human use did not exist. I explained the situation to the pharmacist, who had nothing else to offer. I was disappointed if not despondent, both because I would not have an entry for the science fair and also because I was genuinely interested in the results of this experiment. Having read about the miracle powers of prolactin, I wanted to see whether it could make mama guppy more nurturing.

With the deadline for the science fair looming, I asked my father for help. As a hospital psychiatrist, he had access to psychotropic medications and he suggested that we use Thorazine instead of the prolactin. The substitution seemed more than reasonable since, at least in humans, Thorazine can dramatically alter behavior. If this agent could make psychotic people tranquil, perhaps it could make guppies less likely to make the next generation a happy meal. I was overjoyed that my project would go on and that I would have a bona fide hypothesis for testing.

My father brought home a vial of Thorazine from the hospital along with some syringes as I waited for the arrival of the baby guppies. How do you dose a fish with an antipsychotic, especially when it will be put into tank water thick with algae? Empiricism would rule and I decided that, with only one experimental tank to play with, I would dose escalate once the baby guppies arrived. With the Thorazine in the refrigerator and a syringe ready to squirt, I waited in anticipation of the birth of the babies.

One day I came home from high school and was excited to see the tanks filled with little babies. The moment of the experiment had arrived and, with great excitement, I got the Thorazine from the refrigerator and filled up the syringe with the liquid to start the dose escalation. I put in a few drops into the tank and was shocked by what happened next. Both the mother and babies started to gyrate madly—the fish equivalent of a grand mal-seizure—and within seconds, the carnage was over as mother and babies all succumbed. My experiment was over, a dismal failure that would shock an Institutional Animal Care and Use Committee today. Having run out of time and without any more fish to test, all I could do for the science fair project was to prepare a very circumscribed and morose account of an experiment gone awry. On 5 × 7 white cards, I drew pictures of fish shaking and floating dead, but this project did not fare well. Unlike "The Blind Shall See," there were no prizes. I did get a certificate of participation, however (Fig. 2.3).

Like many incidents from my childhood and adolescence, there is an amusing and bittersweet quality to this account of my first independent project, but I am very proud of the whole event. Importantly, the idea was mine. It came from the literature. It had a testable hypothesis and I knew I needed controls. Modulating behavior by drugs is now the vogue and, with a limited repertoire of reagents, I made a good choice. This was by no means the first idea of mine that did not

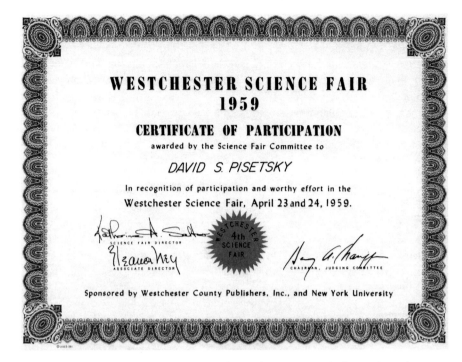

Fig. 2.3 Certificate from Westchester Science Fair. After my success in first grades, prizes were elusive and all I got were certificates of participation

pan out, but I was very excited to read many years later that fish have their own version of prolactin that regulates salt and water metabolism. If I had only measured urinary output instead of maternal behavior, I would have hit the jackpot in high school, although I must say measuring the urinary output of a guppy in a 10 gallon fish tank would have been a challenge.

The early 1960s had an extraordinary emphasis on science. The Russians launched Sputnik in 1957, and America, afraid of losing its technology edge, made huge investments in science education. Science became probably the most important subject in my junior high and high school, and I couldn't have been happier. I excelled in science classes (albeit not math) and did well because I enjoyed the material. In junior high, I had a terrific science teacher named Mr. Bonagur who had charisma and could motivate even the most recalcitrant student. One of the challenges of Mr. Bonagur's classes was the unscheduled exams called blitzes. Rather than announcing quizzes or exams, he would spring them unannounced, often with great fanfare such as having them pop out of the window blinds as he rolled them down.

"Pencils out. Books away," he would say gleefully as he read out the questions.

No one had ever gotten 100 on a Bonagur blitz and I wanted to be the first. I studied hard, but these quizzes were hard. While I was often at the top of the class, my grades hovered around 95. I intensified my efforts for an exam on biochemistry and, when the blitz came, I rolled through the questions, sensing that I could achieve the previously unachievable. I got to the last question, which was the formula for the fatty acid oleic acid. I debated whether the formula should end with "COOH" or "COO" and, perhaps nervous or tired or maybe reluctant to enter a realm no student had gone before, put down "COO."

I got a 98, and I remember Mr. Bonagur's sad expression when he told the class how close I had come. Even though 100 was supposed to be beyond reach, knowing how much I liked his class and how hard I worked, he really wanted me to get that 100. As it turned out, I worked with fatty acids during my graduate work and realize now how silly my error was. I still wonder what would have happened if I had gone with my instinct and added that extra H for the hydrogen and, as they say, tread where no one had ever tread before.

After tenth grade, I attended a National Science Foundation camp at the Choate School to study biology and scientific Russian (my counselor was Keith Brodie who later became President of Duke) and, after eleventh grade, I went to Cornell University on another science program to take a course in bacteriology. Part of that course was an independent research project, and I developed the idea to test whether the cell wall of bacteria was essential for DNA synthesis. For this experiment, I wanted to treat bacteria with lysozyme to strip off the cell wall and then see if they could still divide. The professor of the course was dismissive of this idea and discouraged me from this project. We actually got into a serious argument, me the upstart eleventh grader tangling with a full professor at one of the nation's top universities. I told him that the purpose of the course was to help students to think independently and that I was annoyed that he wasn't going to let me test my idea. Even if the experiment was hopelessly naive, I thought that it was better to let me fail than to prevent me from trying.

The professor relented and I did my experiment. Once shorn of their cell wall, the bacteria, like my Thorazine-infused guppies, died promptly and there was no cell division to measure. Despite the failure, I was happy to have both developed my own idea and persevered despite opposition. I continued to read about the subject and eventually submitted a version of the project to the Westinghouse Science Talent Search and was very pleased to be a semi-finalist. I also wrote about this encounter for my essay for Harvard College and was incredibly happy when I was accepted.

When I graduated from New Rochelle high school, I was awarded a prize for the person most likely to become a physician. I was disappointed, since I had done very well in the science courses and Westinghouse competition and would have liked recognition. I had done nothing in high school that concerned medicine, although I had aced biology. What was it about me then that struck my teachers as a future doctor rather than a future scientist? I still do not know.

Starting in 1963 at Harvard College and continuing through 1973 when I graduated from the Albert Einstein College of Medicine with both my MD and PhD degrees, I was fortunate to have great teachers, mentors, and role models in science. At Harvard, although I was a pre-med, I took a highly selective course called Chem 11 and 12 for science majors with interest in physical and organic chemistry. High level P-chem was not my forte, and I suffered trying to learn orbital theory. The classes were tough and, among my classmates, there was a future Nobelist and at least two members of the National Academy of Science. Fortunately, the courses were curved, and my 30 or 40 out of 100 on an exam usually sufficed to get a B. After a particularly dismal performance, I went to see one of the course professors, Frank Westheimer, a legendary chemist, about what I could do to improve my performance. He asked me about my interests and plans. When I said I was pre-med, he shook his head and said that they made a mistake when they accepted me in this course (my 800 on the chemistry college board not withstanding).

I did better in biochemistry than chemistry, but on some exams, was only a shade above a Gentleman C (Fig. 2.4). Actually, my best grades at college were in philosophy, political science, and literature. Nevertheless, after a brief flirtation with a major in History and Literature, I elected Biochemical Sciences as a major and worked closely with some of the most influential people in my life. Dr. Maurice Pechet was what was called a tutor at Harvard. A physician at the Massachusetts General Hospital in endocrinology, Dr. Pechet ran a laboratory on hormone action. With Dr. Pechet, a group of students worked our way through a textbook on steroid biochemistry. While a physician, Dr. Pechet was a scientist at heart, and he encouraged me to get the best training in basic science that I could and graciously arranged for me to work with Dr. Klaus Biemann at MIT. Dr. Biemann was one of the pioneers of mass spectrometry and, as a junior, every week I took the Red Line to the Kendall station and then walked over to MIT where Dr. Biemann taught me how the structure of molecules could be identified from their fragmentation products. Considering the eminence of Biemann as a scientist (he is a member of the National Academy and won the Benjamin Franklin Medal of Chemistry in 2007), I remain amazed that he had time and patience to teach me one-on-one, especially since another great chemist said I was a mistake for this field.

The work with Biemann meshed perfectly with my summer work which I pursued with Dr. Sam Seifter at the Albert Einstein College of Medicine. Dr. Seifter, who died recently, was the father of one of my high school classmates, Madeleine, and he welcomed students into the laboratory. Dr. Seifter was one of the kindest, gentlest, and most dedicated scientists I have every known and he had a remarkable commitment to social justice and improving the lives of the less fortunate. In New York City, that meant African-Americans and Puerto Ricans, although, earlier in life, Dr. Seifter was active with labor groups. After the summers of my freshman, sophomore and junior years in college, I worked with Dr. Seifter on the structure of collagen and other biological macromolecules that are natural polymers. Mostly, I blundered, such as when I tried to remove the salt from a collagenase digest by dialyzing it. Of course, I also removed the digested peptides but Dr. Seifter was always understanding and patiently explained the right way to do the purification. He was a wonderful biochemist, and, for my college thesis, we decided to sequence peptides from earthworm cuticle collagen using techniques I learned in Biemann's lab. While the intent of the project was fine, I never got the peptides clean enough to sequence them on Biemann's machine using a nifty chemical known as Gagosian's reagent.

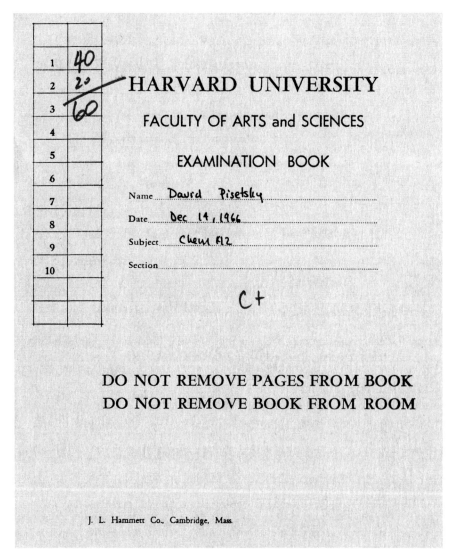

1	40
2	20
3	60
4	
5	
6	
7	
8	
9	
10	

HARVARD UNIVERSITY

FACULTY OF ARTS and SCIENCES

EXAMINATION BOOK

Name David Pisetsky

Date Dec 14, 1966

Subject Chem 42

Section

C+

DO NOT REMOVE PAGES FROM BOOK
DO NOT REMOVE BOOK FROM ROOM

J. L. Hammett Co., Cambridge, Mass.

Fig. 2.4 Exam book from senior year biochemistry. There were two questions on this exam. The one that gave me the real trouble was the second one: Describe experiments you would design to ascertain whether the heptadecenoic acid was metabolized by β-oxidation or by ω-oxidation plus β-oxidation. As my score of 20 indicates, I could not describe many experiments of this kind

Unlike today's medical school applicants, during college, I did not volunteer in hospitals, tutor underprivileged students, or nor do anything else that would be considered related to people. I was a full-fledged science major, a real wonk in the jargon of that era. Despite my enjoyment of science and my desire to do research, I still wanted to be a doctor, although I was absolutely clueless how I would accomplish this. Fortunately, the Medical Scientist Training Programs (MSTPs) were coming along and this seemed liked a perfect solution, since I could get training as a scientist and still be a doctor. At the time, Einstein had an outstanding faculty in cell and molecular biology and was one of the first MSTPs in the country. I dithered between New York University and Einstein, eventually deciding on Einstein since I knew the faculty and I liked the ethos. The decision turned out to be far more important since I met my wife Ingrid, also a medical student, during our first year.

The simultaneous training of an MD and PhD is a tricky business, since the professions are so different. MD training, certainly in its first phase, is about rote, memory, algorithms, and learning to do everything just as it has always been done before. "See one, do one, teach one." is a rubric that often characterizes clinical training on the wards. In contrast, PhD training is about thinking, innovation, and trying to do something that was never done before. More simply, such training could be reduced to "See one. Do something different."

Fortunately, the MSTP director at Einstein was the great pharmacologist Al Gilman, who was willing to listen to students to make the program a success. Our group of students, (called Mud-Fuds since we were going to get both degrees) met with Dr. Gilman (although Einstein was an informal place and some of us called him Al). Dr. Gilman also wanted to expose us to some exciting scientists and developed a seminar with a very bright young neurophysiologist named Alan Finkelstein, who taught us about the chemistry of membranes and his work on artificial lipid bilayers which could generate an electric potential. While I could not grasp the math, I was fascinated by the structure of membranes. Interestingly, I still work on membranes today.

At that time, the USA was in great turmoil because of Vietnam and civil rights. New York City was a wild, dangerous, and chaotic place, and 1968 witnessed the assassinations of Martin Luther King and Robert F. Kennedy. Einstein always had a strong social conscience and tradition of service, and, because its teaching hospitals were in the worst areas of the Bronx, the school worked hard to meet the medical needs of a very poor and disenfranchised population. Times were bad, however, and Einstein's good intentions were not appreciated. Community organizers literally threw the staff out of Lincoln Hospital and, one evening, Black Panthers took over a meeting of Einstein students and faculty, with very menacingly looking Panthers frightening the hell out of us before leaving.

In the face of a cry for immediate action to help the care of the poor, working in a basic science lab may have seemed a bit irrelevant. The faculty of Einstein, like Sam Seifter, nevertheless believed that improvement in life came from science and that learning to do research was an admirable response to social need. I have never been a political activist, but I was reassured that, as America's society was being reconstructed in the 1960s, that medical research was integral to a greater good.

First year medical school was predictably boring save for Dr. Finkelstein's lectures and, during the summer, Dr. Seifter arranged for me to work in a laboratory in Caracas, Venezuela, to study the structure of red blood cell membranes with one of his former post-docs. With no TV, I was completely cut off from the coverage of the Chicago riots, only learning about them upon my return to the USA. I had great fun making red blood cell ghosts in a mountaintop lab that opened directly into a tropical garden with large pink flowers and flitting humming birds.

When I returned to the USA, I had to begin to think about my thesis work and with whom I would work. This decision turned out to be very difficult, since I knew I wanted to do both clinical and bench work, and I felt I had to obtain training that would be relevant to my ultimate specialty. The trouble was that I did not know what type of specialty I wanted to pursue. In the Einstein program, students started their PhD training immediately after the first two years of medical school and did not have the benefit of at least the first set of clerkships to know where they would fit in clinically. While I assumed that I would be an internist (certainly not a surgeon!), it was possible that neurology or psychiatry would catch my fancy, and I was wide open when it came to medicine.

I spoke to Al Gilman and he told me to work with the best scientist I could and train in biochemistry, since biochemistry is applicable to every aspect of medicine. From Finkelstein's class, I had developed an interest in membranes, and the Department of Microbiology had recently hired a very well-trained molecular biologist named Tom Terry who had worked with the biophysicist Harold Morowitz at Yale. Tom was using *Mycoplasma laidlawii* to study the interactions of proteins and lipids in the membrane and had developed a very nice system to grow the organisms in different fatty acid-containing media. We decided to determine how the protein composition changed depending on lipid content, using a recently developed gel electrophoresis system. The project progressed very well and I got my first paper in *Biochimica et Biophysica Acta*. Unexpectedly, Tom decided to leave Einstein, leaving me in need of another lab, so I went back to Gilman for advice.

Of the scientists at Einstein at the time, Jerry Hurwitz had probably the greatest renown. Because of his discovery of RNA polymerase and other nucleic acid enzymes, he was on track for the National Academy of Science and possibly even a Nobel Prize. Jerry is a smart, tough and dynamic scientist who combines a fierce competitive spirit with unparalleled commitment to excellence. His laboratory had the reputation as a fearsome place, where people worked seven days a week and those who did not succeed were banished. Also, Jerry wanted the Mud-Fuds to train like regular PhD candidates, and I was not keen on spending four or five years in the lab, knowing that I was going to do house staff training.

With considerable anxiety, I met with Jerry to discuss potential projects if I joined his lab, and we agreed upon studying the role of the cell membrane in DNA synthesis in *E. coli*. Studies on a series of *E. coli* temperature sensitive mutants defective in DNA synthesis had shown that, with a block in replication, the organism became stuffed with sheets of lipid bilayers. I liked that project, since it meshed with my work with Tom Terry. My other project would involve the mechanisms by which the initial products of DNA synthesis, called Okazaki fragments, were joined. To study these processes, I was going to use an in vitro system in which *E. coli* were treated with toluene to permeabilize their membranes and allow a more precise dissection of the biochemical requirements for synthesis and joining.

Jerry always did his own laboratory work and was a phenomenal experimentalist, since he was both exceptionally smart and had great hands. His experiments, even those of a very complicated design, worked perfectly each and every time. This was an era of lots of tritium and P32 and, as we completed experiments on DNA synthesis, we precipitated the newly formed DNA with trichloracetic acid and collected it on a filter. We would then put the filters into vials of fluid that glowed luminously and then went to count them in a room with four Packard scintillation counters, waiting for our turn to get on the machines. The stuff was hot, and one-minute counts would be enough to indicate whether an enzyme was doing its thing. We would gaze at the counts the way investors look at stock prices. Whereas the experiments of others in the laboratory were going boom, my work was going bust. I could not get the toluene to open the cells, and there was no incorporation of radioactivity.

I worked right next to Jerry in the lab and he became annoyed and frustrated as my experiments languished. I had followed the protocol exactly but never observed any incorporation of the tritiated thymidine. Treating *E. coli* with toluene is not difficult. All that is necessary is to add a few drops and vortex. Nevertheless, my vortexing was not working, and day after day the printouts from the scintillation counter were depressingly flat. From where he worked, Jerry would look at me suspiciously, wondering whether the investment in this Mud-Fuds would ever pay off.

As a mentor, Jerry came from the Bear Bryant or Bobby Knight school, and, one morning, he rushed into the lab and literally threw a copy of *Nature* on my desk. In it was an article on exactly my project. Jerry was furious, and said that we had been scooped because I had failed to get the toluene system to work. Of course, that idea was preposterous since the work had been completed and the article was accepted well months before I started in the laboratory. I was not going to bring that up, however. Sitting right where Jerry worked as he simmered, I read the article carefully. I found flaws with the controls and realized that we hadn't been scooped after all. With trepidation, I pointed these issues out to Jerry who seemed mollified. I actually think that he was impressed that I had detected the problems, but he would never say that.

He volunteered to help me with the toluene treatment and, of course, he got it to work the first time, his suspicions about my capabilities as a scientist once again rising. I was given a reprieve and was able to churn out data for a while and join the crew in the counting room whose experiments were productive. Just at this time, another group published, an allegedly improved in vitro system for DNA synthesis in *E. coli*. This system involved lysozyme treatment of *E. coli* sitting on little pieces of cellophane under which a reaction mix was placed. The virtue of this system was that it eliminated the treatment with an organic solvent and allowed the *E. coli* to remain intact. To get material for the project, I went off into to a bombed-out area of the South Bronx where a company in a decrepit warehouse made large sheets of cellophane for industrial use.

Maybe the cellophane was dirty or not porous enough, but this system did not work the way it was touted and, when I got any counts at all for thymidine incorporation, they turned out to be bogus. I reported my results to Jerry, and this time, he was not forgiving and we had one of those famous meetings in his office which led to expulsion or at least a period of exile in another less demanding lab. In so many words, Jerry told me that I didn't know what I was doing, that I was throwing things around, and that I did not have the drive or talent of perseverance to do good research. He said that I might as well return to medical school to be a doctor and hang out a shingle in the Bronx. Near tears, as I saw my research career reaching an untimely end, I told Jerry that he was wrong and that I was a good scientist and that I would show him. I said that the problem was the cellophane and not me and, if he would let me return to the toluene system, I would produce something novel. Satisfied by the response, Jerry opened the door and let me go back to the lab.

Having gotten another second chance, I knew I had to do something important, and, like many scientists, I started thinking of new ideas only to realize that they wouldn't work. While Jerry did not set a time frame for success, I felt the clock ticking. Fearing ever increasing pressure, I searched for new ideas when one day, while eating a danish as I walked to work down Morris Park Avenue, the idea came to me. I would use the toluene system to study in vitro the closing of Okazaki fragments formed in vivo, using sucrose gradient centrifugation to separate out the replication products under various conditions.

The idea was neat and the system worked like a charm. Every week we discovered something new about DNA synthesis in E. coli, categorizing the effects of ATP on the joining of Okazaki fragments, the effects of nalidixic acid on replication, and the diverse fates of recently replicated DNA in the DNA-sensitive mutants (Fig. 2.5). The system was a gold mine, and soon I was the leader of the pack in the counting room. I was the one who had exciting new findings to discuss, and the others in laboratory wanted to know what I was doing. Jerry was pleased; I was pleased and work on my PhD moved swiftly along. The first paper on this system was published in the *Journal of Molecular Biology*, and I was as proud and excited as you can imagine. My only regret about this paper is that I did not separate out the study on nalidixic acid, since it really indicated the role of DNA gyrase.

During the course of my PhD research, both with Tom Terry and Jerry Hurwitz, I took courses in immunology with a trio of young assistant professors, all of whom have gone on to be stars in the field. Barry Bloom, Matt Scharff, and Stan Nathanson, like the entire Einstein faculty, were devoted to teaching and were very generous with their time. They convinced me that immunology, a field until then focused on crude immunization experiments in mice, was emerging as a scientific discipline which would soon be amenable to molecular techniques. Certainly, immunology represented one of those overarching endeavors which would be useful no matter what I did in medicine. Intrigued by the complexity of the immune system, including the role of GOD (more prosaically, the generation of antibody diversity) and the nascent field of tumor immunology, I decided that this would be the future direction of my work.

After finishing my PhD, I returned to the wards of Jacobi Hospital, which is one of those venerable city hospitals that in the movies is called Fort Apache. The place was a catastrophe but the medicine was exciting. I discovered quickly that, just as I liked research, I liked clinical medicine. From then on, I knew that I wanted patient care as part of my life, but it could never be a full-time activity. It simply did not

Fig. 2.5 Working in Jerry's lab. Once I had the toluenized cell system mastered, I had a great time setting up DNA synthesis reactions, using long 100-μl glass pipettes to deliver 5 μl aliquots into little glass tubes. Forty years later, I am still working on DNA

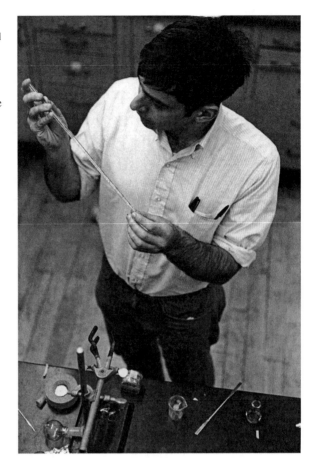

give me the same buzz as doing experiments. Ultimately, research is about thinking and creativity, my strengths, but clinical medicine is about compulsivity and ritual, which are less of my strengths.

After leaving Einstein, I joined the house staff training at the Yale-New Haven Hospital, worked every other night most of the time, learned to be a doctor but never had a mentor like my science mentors. Most of the teaching in house staff occurs on the wards with residents and fellows, and rounds involved an attending of the month club.

After Yale, I went to the NIH to study immunology with David Sachs in the National Cancer Institute. David is a wonderful scientist who can do both basic research as well as the most applied but innovative work in organ transplantation. With David, I worked on the genetics of the immune response in mice and the expression of genetic markers of unique antibody variable (V) regions called idiotypes. Idiotypes were a popular paradigm for elucidating the intriguing question of V gene diversity and allowed me to pursue my own search for GOD. My clinical work involved the treatment of patients afflicted with malignant melanoma with BCG to stimulate immune responses. While I had gone to NIH with the idea of doing tumor immunology, I decided that oncology was not for me. It was too sad and consuming.

Anyone studying immunology reads about the role of tolerance in autoimmunity, of which the disease systemic lupus erythematosus is the prime example. The signature autoantibodies of lupus are directed to DNA and, in one of those "Eureka" moments in life, I decided that I could combine my understanding of DNA with my understanding of immunochemistry to elucidate anti-DNA production in lupus. Although I had taken care of one patient with rheumatoid arthritis and one patient with lupus as a house officer, I decided to become a rheumatologist because I liked the science and wanted the challenge of understanding a mysterious disease. With great training from David and a vision emerging from the midst of post-doctoral fellowship, I went off to Duke to join what was then called the Division of Rheumatic and Genetic Diseases. Happily, my division chief was Ralph Snyderman, a preeminent physician-scientist and a giant of American medicine, who guided me through my beginning years at Duke. I started as Chief of Rheumatology at the Durham VA Hospital, a position that I still hold.

As trainees, physician-scientists are like the characters in the "Wizard of Oz," who are in search of a part: a heart for the Tin Man, a mind for the Scarecrow, and courage for the Lion. Actually, trainees need all three, but I think that for most of them, courage was the most crucial: the courage to be an outstanding scientist and an outstanding clinician at the same time and the courage to take risks in the laboratory to do something truly significant.

Throughout my career, I have been fortunate to work with genuine wizards, who gave me heart, mind, and courage. These mentors challenged me to ask fundamental questions, to think big thoughts, and to ask big questions. Importantly, they took my ideas seriously and engaged me as equals in any discussion of science as we pored over data or diagrammed models on a blackboard. We certainly had ups and downs, which is to be expected when strong minds and strong egos interact, but our differences ultimately related to the best way to find the truth and get the clearest answer.

My success in life relates strongly to my identity. As I have come to realize, I do not consider myself a physician-scientist. Rather, I consider myself both a physician and a scientist and that, even as I do clinical work, I approach problems with the curiosity, rigor, and intensity instilled in me by my teachers in the lab. Like many of the best scientists, I would rather fail asking a big question than succeed asking a small question. Still, I am doctor and would rather take care of people today while waiting for the fruits of basic research to come tomorrow.

Thirty years later, I am pursuing topics that had their beginning long, long ago. I study the fate of DNA during cell death, the structure of membranes released from cells as they die, the genetics of the immune response to DNA, the effects of cell death pathways on the immune response to tumors, and the development of tolerance-inducing treatment for rheumatoid arthritis. Only the use of prolactin to stop guppies from eating their babies has fallen by the wayside. Who knows, maybe with better preliminary data to write another grant, I may get back to that one too.

Three
The Epigenesis of an Epigeneticist

Andrew P. Feinberg

The Admission Director's Question

I'm going to begin this essay in the middle of the story, with a question the Johns Hopkins Medical School Admissions Director asked me in the spring of 1971, and also the question David Schwartz asked all of us in creating this book, namely, "Why did you want to become a physician-scientist?" I was a sophomore at Yale, and I had applied to medical school on a lark, really. The winter before the interview, a college friend and I drove to Baltimore to visit his cousin's family. We decided to visit the main campus of Hopkins, but got lost and wound up at the medical campus, so we figured we would walk around. I picked up a catalogue, and later read about the "2–5" program, in which you go to medical school for five years after two years of college. I had not really considered medicine seriously but thought—what the heck, why not apply? So when summoned for an interview, still not having thought about it much, I was probably the least worried of the 100 applicants because I wasn't sure I wanted this anyway. When I was ushered into the Admission Director's office he was sitting behind a large wooden desk, and a second interviewer, a psychiatrist—no kidding—was sitting at 90 degrees to me to watch my reactions. The Director actually picked up my thick folder and said, "Feinberg, you have science coming out of your ears. You can go to any graduate school you want. Medical school is boring, boring, boring, so why do you want to do that?" And then he tossed the folder onto his desk, and it slid (I think unintentionally) across the table with papers flying all over the room. I think it was my finest hour, as I looked him in the eye and said, "Dr. X, obviously you don't have a Jewish mother." Years later, he told me that I was likely going to get in anyway, but that the psychiatrist told him that they had to take me if for no other reason than to lighten Hopkins up a little.

The complete answer, though, has its roots several years before, when I was in high school, even though I did not realize at the time that my decisions were leading me down this path. I'll return to that period later, but first I want to complete this middle part of the story.

A.P. Feinberg (✉)
Center for Epigenetics, Johns Hopkins University, Baltimore, MD 21205, USA
e-mail: afeinberg@jhu.edu

D.A. Schwartz (ed.), *Medicine Science and Dreams*,
DOI 10.1007/978-90-481-9538-1_3, © Springer Science+Business Media B.V. 2011

The Decision Itself

What put medical school on the table for me was Mark Twain. I had been reading everything he ever wrote including *Letters from the Earth*, work that was so politically incorrect then, and now too, that Twain asked for it to be published posthumously, hence the title. There is something wonderfully alive, American, but at the same time universal about Twain—you feel in between books that you are not fully awake. The element of Twain that really got to me in that period— I was 18 during the events above—was that you could be very observant, very rational, very *scientific*, and yet be able to *do something*—literally do something practical with your hands, directly, that people understand. And if you didn't *do something*, well then maybe you would never be fully alive. The defining book of his, for me, was *Life on the Mississippi*, in which he relates the practical life of an accomplished steamboat pilot. He never could have observed human nature as well as he did, I believe, if he did not know how to do a particular practical thing very well. Piloting combined rational thinking, genuine scientific understanding of hydrodynamics, shipbuilding, and even biology, and I think he wrote of the virtue of mastering something practical. He said that knowing the skill of piloting informed every other aspect of his life. It gave a frame of reference for his abstract thoughts. This idea really resonated with me then, as I had been a young mathematician but could not see myself spending my life in a room with a pencil and paper. I thought I should have a "thing" I could do, such as examine anyone anywhere on the planet and figure out what is wrong and maybe fix it. So a major appeal to me of medicine was that you could be a scientist, but you could also do something—anywhere, to anyone, even if you did not share a language, probably—that really mattered to them. It seemed worth the extra trouble to get an MD, for my own sake, so I could fix something perhaps—albeit a living human being—or else I would be somehow just too theoretical. Anyway, that's the actual reason I had at age 18. And I did tell Dr. X this too after he got a good laugh from my wisecrack first answer. This was during Christmas break of sophomore year, and suddenly I might be going to medical school in six months. I was considering, for half a year really—two alternative lives—medical science, or some other scientific life. *And I never actually made the choice.* The final decision was made for me. I was spending the summer working for IBM in Paris. Although I had worked for IBM previously, I never would have gotten that summer job except for a strange accident of fate. Arthur Watson—of the family that created IBM and heavily endowed Yale (where I was going to school)—was then Ambassador to France. I did not know him, but at a dinner with IBM France executives he said, completely out of the blue (there's a doubly cryptic pun there), "You should have a Yale man working here this summer." I learned this later from someone who was at the dinner. He related that after the dinner the IBM people went into sheer panic until someone found my letter, asking for a job, buried in a file, and they called me in New Haven to offer me the job on the spot.

So I found myself living quite well, at IBM's expense, near the Arc de Triomphe in an IBM apartment in the 16th Arrondissement (very nice) in the summer of 1971. As is still common today, in fact happening again at this writing, the French postal service, which includes the telephone system, went on strike for weeks during the peak calling season of the summer. Apparently Hopkins had accepted me to the program while I was away, and required an answer within a week. My father opened the Hopkins letter sent to my home, and was unable to call me. Email wasn't even someone's dream yet. So my dad sent me a telegram addressed to IBM France. At the time, Western Union charged $20 for ten words, the equivalent of about $50 now, but they only charged $3 for nine words, so here is the complete text of his message—note that the word "STOP" was required by the telegraph company after each sentence. I have a vivid memory of the VP for research finding me in the big cubicle area in my Paris office, and handing me this tiny piece of yellow paper which read:

"ACCEPTED HOPKINS STOP SENT DEPOSIT STOP LOVE POP STOP"

And it was in this way it was determined I would be a physician.

Childhood: From Math to Computers to Neuroscience

The promised first part of this story begins in childhood. For me, and I think for many scientists, the decision to do science is made very early, and I already knew this was my future by 13 years of age. I had been doing recreational mathematics since I was 11, competing in local and regional science fairs (Fig. 3.1). It started with imitation of my older brother Mark, who died in a motorcycle accident when I was 15. He was quite talented, inventing "Tribonacci numbers," based on a

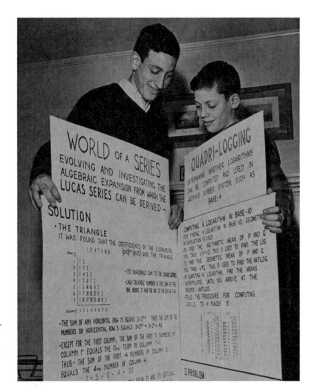

Fig. 3.1 The late Mark Feinberg (aged 15) and brother Andy (aged 11) with their mathematics projects for the central Pennsylvania Science Fair. Figure reprinted with permission from the Patriot News, Harrisburg, PA

generalization of a number sequence of Leonardo Fibonacci of Pisa, and he found some beautiful relationships which were published in the *Fibonacci Quarterly* while he was in high school. My first publication of any kind, at 19, was in the same journal. Like Mark, I was attracted to number theory, and I had the chance to present my work on Bernoulli numbers at a National Science Olympiad at Iowa State University when I was 15. I started a well trod path of not doing what everyone else was doing by leaving the group and looking up James A. Van Allen's laboratory while I was there. He made a huge impression on me. He took out his lab notebook from the Mercury rocket launch, in which he had recorded, in pencil, each analog reading of the earth's magnetic field, from which he reconstructed the Van Allen belts. I held the data in my hand! He then more or less fixed me up with one of the female undergraduates in the lab. So my first experience at seeing real data was coupled with girls! I don't know if there is a direct relationship, but on that day, I was hooked as a scientist.

After my junior year of high school, I took a year of college calculus in a special summer program at Cornell University. My professor was Elisha Netanyahu, the uncle of the brothers Yoni (a hero) and Benjamin (Prime Minister) Netanyahu, and he spent the summers with that family in Ithaca teaching people like me. I remember at the time thinking he was incredibly old but equally energetic, but I think he was then exactly my age now—57. We lived and breathed math for four hours of class and six hours of homework daily—it was fantastic. I remember some of the great moments of that class, and I realize this will seem strange to non-nerds but eminently reasonable to nerds. One of these moments was the application of parametric differential equations to solve cycloids (like the valve on a wheel that is rolling). It's insanely complicated if solved non-parametrically but very simple parametrically. Another memory is the proof that natural logs fall out of integration of $1/x$. Mr. Netanyahu was so excited by what he was showing us that he would shout and dance and even spit at the board. The third memory is of a sycophantic student, Y, from Bronx science who acted superior to me but knew less, but was still quite intimidating. After a really bad answer from Y one day, Mr. Netanyahu looked at him with contempt and said, "Y does not impress. Y does not impress." ...Yes! Math and science are fair, I thought then, and that is basically correct.

Also during that summer, I had my first exposure to mainframe computers, programming in Fortran using punch cards (!). I was running FORTRAN to plot functions from class. So during the next academic year, my senior year of high school, missing access to the powerful mainframes of the time (64K, clock time a little under a microsecond), I wrote to IBM headquarters in Armonk, NY, asking the following questions: "Why do computers just have to be at big companies or universities? Why can't everyone have one in his house? Would you please send me a used one that you don't need so I can see how that would work out?" Amazingly, they did not simply toss this letter. They passed it around a bit, and then I was asked to come to the local IBM sales office for a meeting. My dad came along as I could not drive yet. A nice fellow in a black suit, white shirt, black tie—that was the IBM look then—asked me a number of questions that were more mental health related than computer related. So I asked him if he was trying to determine if I were crazy. He admitted he was but wouldn't tell me why. I never knew whether the report to IBM was "crazy" or "not crazy," but whichever answer it was, it was the answer IBM wanted, as they invited me to work as an intern at their research facility at Yorktown Heights, NY for the summer.

The unit I was in worked on early artificial intelligence in two ways: trying to teach computers to "see" in three dimensions, by solving the "hidden line" problem, which my immediate boss actually did, and to "feel," which was my area—I worked on sensory devices, which eventually became part of touch pads for computers; but most interestingly to distribute information, and processing, over large distances. They were working out packet transmission, and they had conversations about how that would be like synapses in the brain sending neurotransmitters. I know that in the histories of the internet, IBM does not figure prominently, but I was there in 1969 when they were working on how to transmit information over distances between computers. Yorktown Heights was the first of many places I have worked, that did seem special to me at the time, but I did not realize how special. I met people at IBM who even then were trying to model computers to recreate the human brain. By the end of the summer, I had decided I wanted to know what the brain really is, what makes us think, and maybe recreate brains using computer circuits.

College, Briefly, or How I Became a Teenage Medical Student

Even before I chose neuroscience—bear in mind I'm not a neuroscientist, but more on that later—I knew I needed to study more than science alone, or even science mainly, for a while at least. In my junior year of high school I decided I wanted to go to Harvard as an undergraduate, but they sent me a very interesting letter on April 15, 1969. It said that normally they have too many qualified students for the available slots, but not that year. In fact, they felt that this time they could fill the class with the people who actually belonged there, and I wasn't one of them. So my choice was between MIT and Yale. MIT felt that they could recruit me by giving my high school library a check for $70 for a book allowance. Yale, on the other hand, offered me an extraordinary scholarly experience, but not in science. It was called "Directed Studies," or DS, primarily a humanities program. Seventy freshmen were admitted to special small tutorial classes for two years, with no more than a 10:1 student:teacher ratio. The emphasis was on original thinking, and you wrote a paper in every class every week—plus I was carrying math and physics classes outside the program. I worked about 14 hours a day, a habit I never lost. There was a wonderful biology class in DS, taught by Philip Applewhite. I remember trying to design a carnivorous plant, and also trying to figure out the thermodynamic balance of a cell (that was impossible actually). If I had taken a regular biology class with 300 students I never would have gone into biology or medicine.

In those two years at Yale, I was deeply influenced by Philosophy (taught by Roscoe Hill, the single teacher who influenced me the most), not only by the thoughts and the thought processes, but also by the whole concept of humanism. I became committed to the idea of combining humanism and science in what I did with my life. The "logical" philosophers Descartes and Kant, and later Russell, led me to believe that rationalism was correct, that almost anything could be reasoned out. Plato, too, excited me. I thought even then that he was wrong about many things, but the process of abstract thought and argument which he used was new to me. There was a moment, in fact, in my sophomore year, when I attended a graduate level Plato class, that I think I became an academic for life. The class was taught by the late Robert Brumbaugh, who used the Socratic method himself and was a great philosopher of education. It was the most amazing classroom experience I ever had, and I use the Socratic method to this day to teach genetics.

When my father telegraphed me that I was going to medical school, I thought it would allow me to be a philosopher scientist in ways that mathematics and computer science would not. So I didn't telegraph him back to say no. Of course, the deposit was already spent, too.

How I Unchose Neuroscience and Chose Genetics

In medical school, I quickly found myself within the orbit of the great Solomon Snyder, in whose lab I basically spent half of medical school. I had two high impact papers in *Proceedings of the National Academy of Sciences* and one unimportant paper in a second tier pharmacology journal. The problem was that the work in *Proceedings of the National Academy of Sciences* was not what Sol's lab really did (except for Sol himself obviously)—it was exciting, though. One of these studies was a model of opiate agonists and antagonists, and the other was a derivation, that proved correct, of the structure–activity relationship of antischizophrenic phenothiazines. It involved computer models of chemical structure that I had written the previous summer at a computational chemistry lab at Washington University. The unimportant paper was the bread and butter of the lab, which we called "grind and bind," or measuring affinities and receptor occupancies of neurotransmitter agonists and antagonists. There were future famous people in the lab doing terrific experiments like that, published in high profile journals, but to me it wasn't really neuroscience, at least my IBM version of it. Rather, it was good cell biology, and I did not see how that was going to explain how the brain really thinks, or if not that, allow me to design a biologically based computer, another of my dreams at the time.

In my last year of med school, I had matched to do an internship and had a choice of Neurology residency at Penn or Hopkins, but by then I knew I didn't want to practice the type of neuroscience that I had been exposed to. Worse, during my medicine internship at Penn, I disliked my neurology rotation, which was the fault of a very bad resident, not neurology or the attendings—but that is the damage junior mentors can do to their subordinate trainees. I even considered switching to Psychiatry, so I interviewed at Penn for their residency since I was already working there. The problem there was that they had me watch behind a mirror, with the house staff, a psychoanalytic session by a famous practitioner of that now largely discredited art. The patient was a Wharton Business school student, a woman, whose stated reason for getting advice was that men would lose interest in her when they saw how engaged she was in her profession. The analyst asked her about her job interviews in Chicago, particularly the size of the buildings, the gender of the interviewers, and the nature of the suits the interviewers wore. The answers obviously were: large, male, and pin-striped. After the psychoanalysis session, with great excitement, the psychiatrist and the residents fulminated over the phallic imagery of the interview. Even though I wasn't supposed to talk, I protested to the group that this was ridiculous, that the best firms are in tall buildings, the business world is dominated by men, and that all the suits are pin-striped. And furthermore, I said, the patient's dates were just jerks who didn't appreciate smart ambitious women, and the shrink should have told her she's normal and the world—at least the part she was seeing—was crazy. At this point, the psychiatrist asked me, "And have YOU read Freud's *Interpretation of Dreams?*" I told him I had, that I thought Freud fabricated some of the data (it turns out he did), and I asked the residents if they had read the book—none had. I quit the interview process on the spot. This was again I think very bad luck, as there were some terrific psychiatry residency programs then.

But still I had the dream of either decoding the brain or building one of my own, so I took a middle path. I interrupted my clinical training to go back to the lab, and I did a postdoctoral fellowship in Neuroscience at University of California, San Diego. It was an unusual program that allowed fellows to rotate through labs prior to settling down for sustained research. I found myself in an invertebrate neurophysiology lab. The experiments were just torture. We were supposed to understand "behavior" by measuring one neuron while stimulating another. To me, this had nothing to do with computers or thought, and it was so, so slow. Worse, the animals themselves, leeches, were confined in aquaria with duct tape, and they could dig through the tape, crawl across the floor, up your leg, and have a fine meal until you found them later that night. After 3 months, I shared my frustration with the Director of the postdoctoral program, Sam Barondes, and he replied that neurophysiology was like the "Charge of the Light Brigade," citing Tennyson's poem to me. But I was more taken with Bosquet's quip, "C'est magnifique, mais ce n'est pas la guerre," in other words, it's beautiful work but has nothing to do with the thinking brain and will almost certainly kill you before you're finished. So I moved to Sam's developmental biology lab and spent two years working on cell fate commitment and migration in the slime mold *Dictyostelium discoideum*, showing that it involves cell adhesion, not just chemotaxis. It was a great experience. Sam describes science as a high art form, and he's a master painter. He was also a great role model as he has a far reaching mind across many areas of science, but also in medicine (he's a psychiatrist) and humanities (hence the Tennyson quote). He's also like a little kid in a playground—playful is a good word—which is a lot of what science is.

I learned during those months in Sam's lab that I could invent new methods. In this case it was a method for purifying cells committed to differentiation into the two mature cell types—spore and stalk—while they were still undifferentiated slug cells but committed to their destiny. It was a great feeling and a key part of scientific innovation, almost like being a wizard, I think. It involves reading everything—everything—on a subject, and then being unafraid to try something completely different, and not getting upset when it doesn't work, which is absolutely positively what will happen.

Of course, at the end of this, I was an orphan from neuroscience, because the work wasn't really brain related, and I had no idea what I was going to do. I decided to spend a year in the National Health Service Corps working at a clinic in the slums of East Baltimore. It was an appealing program because the physicians were also appointed as junior faculty at Johns Hopkins, and admitted patients there as well as took part in the didactic program for house staff. *It was my year on the Mississippi River* (see Mark Twain above), in which I really felt that at least part of my studies were put to some good use. And it was fun. I learned and did all sorts of practical things that one normally does not do in a typical clinical medical residency, like how to reduce dislocations and set fractures, how not to kill someone in the acute management of an automobile accident, and how to tell without instruments which sick people are in danger of dying right away and which are not. I can think of three people—a patient in the care of another doctor in that clinic, a motorcyclist who had crashed near my apartment that year, and a little girl who was injured recently by an airbag two cars in front of me on the way home—who I know that I was able to save because of that year in East Baltimore. That's a pretty neat feeling.

But the work toward the end of this clinical year was boring, and I knew I needed to return to research, but really had no idea what to do other than medical science in some way. A friend told me about the MPH (Master's of Public Health) program at Johns Hopkins, and I enrolled and took courses in epidemiology, biostatistics, and biomedical engineering. At the same time, I continued my clinical training and my academic relationship as an Instructor in the Department of Medicine at Johns Hopkins. At the time, the public health year was something interesting to do, with no clear relationship to my career. However, without it I would never have been able to do the work I've been recently engaged in developing a new epigenetic epidemiology of common human disease. I'm also not sure whether without that training I would have thought so clearly about the cause–effect relationships in cancer epigenetics early in my ultimate choice of genetics. The most memorable part of the year for me was biostatistics, my first formal return to mathematics. In particular, I was taken with Tukey's idea that one must actually look at the data visually before even beginning to make sense of it statistically, that otherwise one is carefully measuring nonsense. It's more important to do the statistical test on the real differences that your eye can see, even if it's not so clear how to do that, than it is to do the easy statistical test on something relatively unimportant. The recent success of our epigenetics center is in large measure related to the involvement of Rafael Irizarry of the same Biostatistics Department, who is an intellectual descendant (mentee's mentee) of Tukey and looks at data exactly this way. I wouldn't have been able to appreciate what Rafa can do if I had not experienced that year.

That year I also became very interested in cancer genetics. I already had extensive research training, including a postdoc, and was eager to return to the lab. During the MPH year, I became interested in cancer. I had read a paper that bothered me, arguing that chromosome rearrangement syndromes specifically cause common cancers, while mutation syndromes cause skin cancer, and thus chromosome rearrangements are the proximate cause of solid tumors. By reexamining published case reports using age- and sex-adjusted cancer incidence rates, i.e., with good epidemiology, I found that those syndromes did not cause common cancer, that is, that author was wrong, but it was still true and unexplained that hereditary cancers were quite organ-specific.

With cancer on my mind, I was passing through the hospital one evening and saw a sign advertising a lecture by Donald Coffey for the "St. George Society" (slayer of the dragon, in this case cancer) and offering free food. The talk was on the pluripotency of cancer cells and tumor cell heterogeneity, and at the end of his talk, I told him that my work on the slime mold *Dictyostelium* pluripotency was really the same thing that he was talking about in human cancer, that is, there had to be some non-genetic information that was stably inherited but at the same time subject to plasticity. That is when I first became interested in the question of epigenetics, how information might be stored in the nucleus independently of the DNA sequence, and Don suggested I go back to some of my old model building, in this case thinking about chromatin topology, and we wrote a book chapter on DNA loop topology together.

Don also set up the second most important blind date of my life (the most important was with my wife). This one was with Bert Vogelstein, whom Don had recruited to Hopkins, and who at the time was working on DNA replication and loop topology in another slime mold, *Physarum polycephalum*. Bert and I hit it off right away, and I joined his lab, the first person to study cancer there (Fig. 3.2). In addition to experiments testing for the first time for *RAS* mutations in cancer and developing

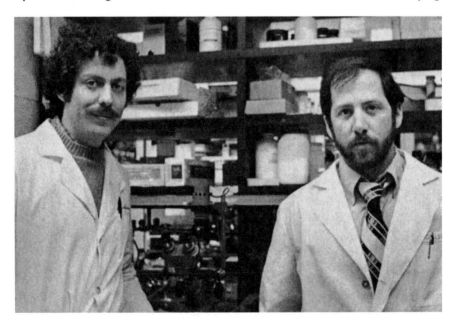

Fig. 3.2 Andy Feinberg (aged 31), Assistant Professor, and Bert Vogelstein (aged 35), Associate Professor, fashionably dressed and hirsute, at Johns Hopkins University School of Medicine. Figure reprinted with permission from The Baltimore Magazine

an assay for tumor clonality, we decided to test the epigenetic hypothesis directly on human cancer cells. I mentioned the wizardry of lab work during my postdoc in California, but Bert was a grand wizard. He's Gandalf himself, a wizard among wizards, and I believe one of the world's greatest living scientist.

And here are the two secrets this sorcerer's apprentice learned from him. First, one must read. Voraciously. And not just in one's own discipline. Most of what we need to know for the next great advance is already in the scientific literature, but is often opaque to the authors of the articles. You have to look at the data themselves, and as much as possible skip the text, at least until you draw your own opinion regarding what's really going on. Second, one must learn how to take methods apart and understand what matters and what doesn't. Often there is something idiotic about the way we do things and one can change it. Or there is a trick from another discipline that one can borrow to make something work.

Random priming arose directly from following these rules. Early on I asked Bert, "Why the hell do we make radioactive probes with DNase in them, which eats the probe?" and he sent me to read decades old literature on every way that DNA has been synthesized in the laboratory, the key here being Mehran Goulian's approach to cDNA synthesis using random primers, which Bert already knew but had me work out for myself. Incidentally, Johns Hopkins University decided that the method had no commercial value and elected not to patent it. I know of one company in particular that grossed $100 million on the kits. But there was one small consolation prize. The first company to market the method did not give us credit. Yet their kit contained a low concentration of Tris and a high concentration of HEPES, which makes no sense except for the historical idiosyncracies of my approach. I had used the Tris to make up nucleotide buffers, and the HEPES at varying pH to swamp the Tris and optimize the pH. So I wrote to the head of that company and complained, citing the plagiarism of their kit. It didn't cost them anything to give Bert and me credit, and they added our reference to their ads. Later, when I was a Hughes investigator at Michigan, Peter Rigby was visiting me. Peter is the inventor of the now displaced nick-translation method, which uses DNase. He is a warm, creative and funny guy, and saw a framed ad from one of the companies selling this, all to their own profit, reading "You'll never nick-translate again," and quoting my paper. Peter looked at me, looked at the ad, looked at me again and said, "I hate you." We had a great laugh, because we both knew, as Bert does, that methods come and go, and nobody really appreciates the inventor except other methods developers. For this reason, most people don't know that Bert previously invented the method for purifying DNA from gels, and more recently the key step in emulsion library generation necessary for second generation sequencing.

Doing genetics in the lab also resonated well with my medical school experience in Victor McKusick's genetics course. The Admissions Director was right, actually, that I really would have lost my mind memorizing incredibly voluminous and boring facts in medical school. But what saved my sanity was Victor's class, and interestingly, Bert had the same recollection of that class I did. It was highly mathematical, with Bayesian problems and gene mapping (even then, based on somatic cell hybrid data). So even after I had finally settled into laboratory genetics, I continued my clinical genetics training on the side, eventually becoming board certified.

My Choice Did Not Make Things Easier

These chapters are intended to focus only on the career choice. However it would not be a complete story if I did not point out how much resistance I encountered to my choice of discipline. Some of the folks who entered the field after I did were quite hostile in reviews and at meetings, although that is uncommon now. But at an early critical point, I was told by powerful people to quit, and I think it took strength of character, or perhaps zealotry, to ignore them. When I continued my work on cancer epigenetics as a Hughes investigator at Michigan, Dr. Z, the Scientific Director of Hughes at the time told me that if I worked in this area my funding would be cut off. This was despite the fact that I had not yet been formally reviewed for renewal. I decided that in response to this remark the *only* thing I would do with his money was cancer epigenetics, which was a difficult decision because I had a paper in *Science* on tumor suppressor genes, a more transparently productive direction to follow. Also, cancer epigenetics was an incredible muddle after our initial discoveries. I had a follow up paper on hypomethylation of oncogenes, but it wasn't for three years after my first report that Bernard Horsthemke first observed epigenetic silencing of a tumor suppressor gene, *RB*. Even then, it was not clear whether cancer epigenetics was causal or consequential to cancer, a point made by a reviewer of the original *Nature* paper with Bert, but also in a devastating quip to me in a lunch line at Cold Spring Harbor by one of my heroes, Harold Varmus, who told me he thought it might be an "epi-phenomenon." Harold was an English major in college, and that was a very clever play on words and also a valid and valuable criticism.

So when Dr. Z threatened to fire me because he didn't like what I did, I decided to go ahead with Hughes money to do an expensive study that could establish a causal relationship for epigenetics in cancer. I drew on my genetics background to recruit patients with the hereditary disorder Beckwith–Wiedemann syndrome (BWS) in order to perform linkage studies and map the gene. I thought that this disorder would be the paradigm for a cancer epigenetic predisposition syndrome, since it is transmitted preferentially through the mother, suggesting imprinting. Thus, BWS could be for cancer epigenetics what Li-Fraumeni syndrome was for conventional cancer genetics, a predisposing alteration proving a causal relationship. Over several years, we mapped the disorder to *IGF2*, showed that it is imprinted, found loss of imprinting (LOI) of *IGF2* in cancers and in BWS patients, and discovered that it is a contiguous gene syndrome involving multiple imprinted genes. Ultimately, with my clinical epidemiology colleague Michael DeBaun, we showed that LOI of *IGF2* is the specific cancer risk factor in BWS, and that through this mechanism, causes expansion of the nephrogenic stem cell compartment. This was the smoking gun that proved that epigenetic changes precede and cause cancer, and it led to the epigenetic progenitor model of common sporadically occurring cancers. So I am grateful to Dr. Z for pushing me down this productive path, even though that was not his intent. And that is because bucking the conventional wisdom and following your own instincts may be the most important prerequisite for a career as a physician scientist. I was so mad at him at the time that I put far more energy into establishing my niche than I would have otherwise. Partly for this reason, I have begun to return to my original question about how the brain works as a computer, even though most of my laboratory is still dedicated to cancer epigenetics. Because epigenetics generates the exact opposite reaction than it did when I started—it's now one of the top priorities of NIH—I have been able to explore whether the plasticity of the mind, whether developmental, pathological, or memory itself, has an epigenetic basis. This idea is largely met with incredulity when I talk about it, but nobody has cut off my funding yet, and time will tell whether I'm right about this. But it is fun to buck the conventional wisdom, and there is a greater chance of making a difference that way.

During the horribly boring second year of medical school, when I thought in my alternate life I could have been studying mathematics or computer science, I complained to my father about his sending in the deposit to Hopkins. He told me that in the long run I would have far more choices as a scientist with a medical background behind me. I don't know how he knew that, as he was a non-scientist civil servant, but time has proved him correct. It is almost impossible to imagine another scientific career that would have fulfilled the breadth of my interests. I don't know if clinical training itself mattered, although on two practical accounts it did. Without it, I would not have been able to use BWS as a model to prove the epigenetic hypothesis of cancer. And without it I would not have been able to get the Hughes job at that time. But I also don't think I would have been able to visualize in a general way the role of epigenetics in human disease, or synthesize this with other disciplines, were it not for my clinical training. My general concept of disrupted developmental plasticity in epigenetic disease—described in a *Nature* paper last year—came from a physician scientist's *Weltanscauung*. That's a philosophy term that just fits here perfectly and refers to a way of seeing the world that is rational but grounded in a set of experiences, in this case having been able to experience biology in a comprehensive way that a medical education provided.

But this is just what I think. I would have to repeat my life twice more going to Hopkins, then three more times staying at Yale, and compare the two sets of outcomes to be sure about this with any degree of statistical significance.

Four
A Delicate Balance: Science, Medicine, and Motherhood

Laurie H. Glimcher

Prologue

The question I'm asked probably more than any other is "How did you get to where you are today?" I think that's because even now, physician-scientists who are also women with children are not as common as they ought to be. Patricia Schroeder, the long time congresswoman from Colorado, in response to a question from a colleague about how she could be both a mother of two young children and a member of Congress at the same time, replied "I have a brain and a uterus and I use them both." Looking back on it, I can see that there were many times during the course of my life when, if it had not been for the right kind of help at the right time and place, I could have gone in another direction. But I'm not sure that I actually thought about it in those terms at the time; I was simply focused on getting the job done. So I'm glad for this opportunity to reflect on the path I've taken, and I hope that my musings may be of value to others who find themselves in similar circumstances. It's a cliché that you should begin at the beginning, but in my case, the circumstances of my childhood had a lot to do with where I am now.

Growing Up: I Was Supposed to Be a Boy

I was the middle of three closely spaced daughters born to parents in their mid-twenties (Figs. 4.1 and 4.2). My father named us each Robert Charles before we actually appeared on the scene. When he suggested to my mother after the birth of my younger sister that they "try again," she told him in no uncertain terms that after three strikes, he was out. As it turned out, it was probably a blessing that we didn't have a brother because my parents then decided that girls could do anything boys could do. Both my parents expected and assumed that my two sisters and I would

L.H. Glimcher (✉)
Department of Immunology, Harvard School of Public Health, Boston, MA 02115, USA;
Department of Medicine, Harvard Medical School, Boston, MA 02115, USA
e-mail: lglimche@hsph.harvard.edu

D.A. Schwartz (ed.), *Medicine Science and Dreams*,
DOI 10.1007/978-90-481-9538-1_4, © Springer Science+Business Media B.V. 2011

Fig. 4.1 Me in 1953

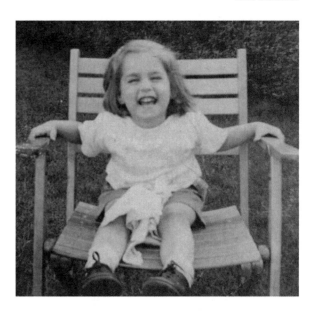

Fig. 4.2 My father with his
three girls—Me, Susan, and
Nancy

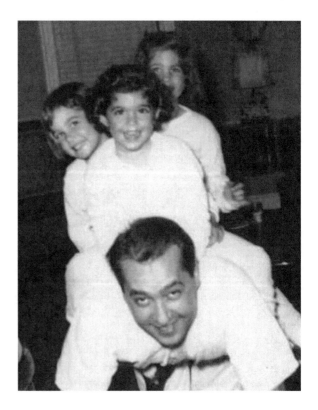

lead independent lives and would have our own careers—there was really never any question about that. We were also expected to provide grandchildren. My mother, who was a homemaker, was at least as ambitious for us as my father, who was a Professor of Orthopedic Surgery at Harvard Medical School and a biophysicist by training. My parents' conviction that there were no limits to what energetic, bright girls could achieve was a persistent theme in our household and was woven into who I was early on. My father is still a Professor at Harvard Medical School, and like me, is a physician-scientist.

When I was growing up, I would trot along by his side to the Massachusetts General Hospital on weekends to visit both his skeletal biology laboratory and his orthopedic surgery patients. I liked to watch all the rat and chicken bones swirling away with magnetic stirrers in the beakers in the cold room, being decalcified, and the amino acid analyzer churning out reams of paper with peaks indicating amino acids. I horrified my sisters at age 6 by dissecting frogs on our front walk during the summer. I was forgiven because of my attempts to rescue dying flowers with various potions I concocted. My sisters hated anything to do with the hospital— they didn't like the smell or the blood or the atmosphere of illness (they both became tax lawyers), so it was up to me to carry on the physician-scientist torch. This began with the usual elementary school science fair projects. I got blue ribbons for building an incubator with a light bulb to house hatching chickens (although sadly, I didn't provide a cover for the bulb so some of the baby chicks scorched themselves to death). The most memorable project was my live display entitled "The moulting cycle of the crayfish." One of my father's colleagues loved marine biology, and she took me out to the river to catch some crayfish early one morning. I brought them home and put them into a nice large container with water in it and went off to bed. When I came down to breakfast the next morning, I was appalled to see crayfish slithering all over the floor—they had piled up on one another during the night and the one on the top of the heap would jump off to escape what they must have sensed was a dismal future. I was paralyzed with horror and had to summon my mother to gather them up. Not a very auspicious start for a budding scientist. But I was only 8 years old.

My Parents

My father, Melvin Glimcher, was an enormous presence in our family—tall, good-looking, dynamic, passionate, extremely articulate and engaging, and a workaholic who only needed four hours of sleep a night (Fig. 4.3). He was what would now be called "a big personality." He did nothing halfway or in moderation. He graduated from Harvard Medical School (HMS) in 1950 after getting degrees from Duke and Purdue in Physics and Mechanical Engineering, did an orthopedic surgery residency at Massachusetts General Hospital (MGH), then trained in biochemistry and biophysics at Massachusetts Institute of Technology. He chaired the clinical orthopedic service and created the Orthopedic Research Laboratories at both MGH and Children's Hospital. I learned several extremely important lessons from him that

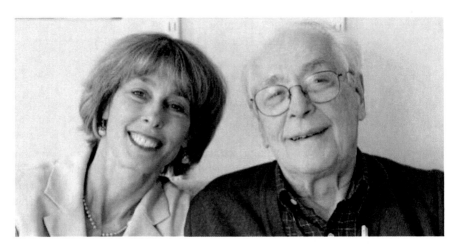

Fig. 4.3 My father and me

have stayed with me and have dramatically influenced my own career: be a risk taker, never fear to try something new, and be as stubborn as a bull. These themes thread through both my career and my personal life and will reappear later in this essay. Life with him could be tumultuous—he had quite a temper—but Lord knows, it was never boring. I loved bringing my friends home to meet him because he would entertain us all with riotous stories about his life as a poor Jewish boy in Chelsea, as a 17-year-old Marine-in-training at the end of World War II, as a surgical resident, and so on. Even in his mid-eighties now and just retired, he is always on the lookout for new adventures. He learned to ski, sail, and speak Russian in his thirties, became adept at ballroom dancing, French cooking, and the French language in his forties, and is a devoted fan of opera and the ballet. We still sing (if you can call it that) our favorite arias together after family dinners, although he and my younger sister are the only ones in the family who can carry a tune.

My mother was just as important an influence on me as my father. She was the rock of the family. Her quiet support, her common sense, and her unshaking belief in the talent of her three daughters gave me the self confidence to move ahead even in painful and difficult times. I remember vividly one example of this. I had decided to go to medical school with some trepidation and not a little uncertainty. My record at Harvard had not been especially brilliant, as I've noted below, and I checked into the Vanderbilt Hall dormitory on a Sunday in 1972, aged 21 and feeling uncertain and insecure. Over the next few hours, I met my fellow students, all of whom seemed to have graduated *summa cum laude* from everywhere and to have done amazing things. My panic slowly grew and finally reached boiling point, and I did what I always did, I called my mother. She undoubtedly remembers my frantic telephone call. "Come get me immediately" I said in a total panic, "I don't belong here—I am surrounded by all these brilliant people who graduated *summa cum laude* and have 4.0 grade point averages and a lot of them are total nerds." She did come and get me and gave me a nice dinner and then promptly ordered me back to the dorm and told me to get on with it. She also said she knew I would do just fine. I believed her. I have been extraordinarily lucky to have both my parents still around and sharp as tacks into their eighties, and perhaps been even luckier that, unlike so many American families today, they have always lived close by. That kind of support, emotional and otherwise, is priceless.

High School and College

I went to a rather stuffy, Boston Brahmin, private girl's school in Boston where I was part of the Jewish "quota" and learned that life is not always fair. This was a good lesson, as I have found subsequently, and one that equipped me well to deal with gender bias later on. At that time, the Jewish girls were usually at the top of the class, since there was no point in admitting a Jewish girl who wasn't smart. I learned that anti-Semitism still existed in the late 1960s and also that I had no intention of putting up with it. My father served as a great example. He had refused to quietly withdraw his name upon the urging of certain senior MGH surgeons as a candidate for Chairman of Orthopedic Surgery at the MGH, and threatened to go to the news media with the story. He became the first Jewish Chair of any surgical department at MGH and then several years later became Chief of Surgery at Children's Hospital, Boston. It was a lesson that I was to remember—and act on—when I was faced with a somewhat similar situation in my late thirties.

The Winsor School might have been rather formal and somewhat socially homogenous, but it gave me an extraordinarily good education, at least in the liberal arts, for which I remain grateful. Math and science in private girls' schools at that time were never very strong, but that was less important than the very firm grounding I received in the English language. The English teachers at Winsor taught me how to write. They were insistent that we learn how to put ideas together in a logical progression, to fashion succinct, clear sentences, and to make a point directly. Every time I write a paper or a grant, I thank them from the bottom of my heart.

The next stop was Radcliffe, where I was in the second class of women who were truly a part of Harvard College. This was the late 1960s to early 1970s, the era of free love, feminism, Gloria Steinem, and Joan Baez, and I embraced it all with enthusiasm. I was a true-blue "hippie" and went around clothed in long serendipity dresses that looked like nightgowns (I still have a fondness for them), demonstrated against the Vietnam War and Henry Kissinger, skipped many classes, indulged my passion for acting, and blew up my "unknown compound" during organic chemistry lab. I majored in biology with a minor in English literature, but in truth, I cared more about and did better in my literature and history classes than my science subjects. Not that I had a particularly distinguished record, but it was good enough to get me accepted to most medical schools I applied to, although hardly phenomenal. I doubt that I would have been accepted at any top tier medical school today. It was at Harvard that I caught the "research bug." I worked in my father's laboratory at

MGH for my senior thesis studying how blood cells differentiate into bone cells. But when I was getting ready to graduate from Harvard, I found that I didn't know whether I wanted to be a doctor or a scientist (or either, since I had vague longings to be an actress but was in touch with reality enough to realize that I would never make it).

It's hard for a young person to know or even to imagine what each of those careers will be like, so at the urging of my parents, I decided to go to medical school rather than graduate school in science because the former path offered the possibility of both. That's one of the great things about getting a medical degree (MD). It opens up so many career paths. One can hang out a shingle and be a family doctor, a specialist in a teaching hospital, a surgeon, a scientist, go into industry, the private sector, be involved in public health, and these days even get a joint MD and Masters of Business Administration (MBA) and get involved in venture capital funding or start biotechnology companies. I thought about taking a year off and teaching English abroad in Italy, but when I was accepted at HMS, my parents advised me not to delay my admission (I think they feared that Harvard would reconsider). Thus, after a holiday traveling in Italy on my own, I found myself enrolled at HMS. A rather nasty member of the admissions committee later made it a point to tell me that I had barely scraped into the bottom of the class. In contrast, my future husband had been, I would discover, at the very top of his class at Yale and had therefore been offered a merit scholarship.

Medical School, Marriage and Residency: The Turning Point

After my initial panic, I settled into medical school quite happily. It didn't take long for me to realize that my parents had been on track. I had made the right choice, and I wanted to be learning all this stuff. I fell in love with medical school. I also fell in love with another first-year medical student, Hugh Auchincloss, who was most decidedly not a nerd, and we got married that summer. We were married for almost 30 years, and it is to him that I owe, in large measure, my success as a physician-scientist. People sometimes underestimate the importance of a supportive partner. Hugh believed in me more than I believed in myself and was always delighted at my successes. He was also a remarkably diplomatic person, while I tended to be overly forthright and candid, and I learned the value of tact from him. In retrospect, it was undoubtedly a huge plus to be married to another physician-scientist who understood what that life was like. It is no coincidence that many female physicians marry their classmates. Although we eventually divorced, we have remained very close friends who delight together in our three children. As I've said, one of the things I've learned over the course of my life is the importance of a supportive partner and a supportive family structure (including, in my case, two dogs). Though my marriage ended after 27 mostly good years, I've been fortunate enough to find another partner, also a scientist, who understands some of the peculiar demands that this profession can make on you.

I loved learning histology and physiology. That first year we went through all the organ systems one by one, and it was fascinating. I thought I would be a practicing physician. And then, we were introduced to immunology by Kurt Bloch. The study of how the immune system, made up of white blood cells that reside in your blood, spleen, thymus, and lymph nodes, fights off pathogens, bacteria, viruses, cancer cells, and allergens while at the same time being able to distinguish foreign proteins from self proteins was riveting. What fascinated me was thinking about diseases like childhood diabetes, rheumatoid arthritis, multiple sclerosis, and systemic lupus, in which the immune system goes awry and starts mistaking self tissues for foreign pathogens. This was a mystery. I found that I had the knack of thinking up experiments that might help shed light on those puzzles. I was hooked. After two years of medical school in the hospital learning how to take care of patients, I spent the last year of medical school in Harvey Cantor's immunology laboratory at the Dana Farber studying natural killer cells. Harvey was one of two mentors that I've had over the course of my career; the other was Bill Paul. Both are giants in the field of immunology, and I was incredibly lucky to have been trained by them. Harvey was and is an unusually innovative scientist and one of the most elegant crafters of the English language I've ever known. One of the very nicest things about being on the faculty at Harvard is that Harvey is there too, and we have continued to work together intermittently over the years. A highlight of the time I spent in Harvey's lab was winning the HMS Soma Weiss research award. That was a very special occasion for two reasons: I was the first female medical student to ever receive it, and this was also the only instance of two generations of one family to have won it—my father had received it 26 years before. This was a theme that would be repeated 13 years later when my father and I became the first father-daughter pair of tenured professors in the history of Harvard Medical School.

But I also really liked clinical medicine, so I did an internship and residency in internal medicine and a subspecialty in rheumatology at MGH while my husband trained in surgery there. We were like ships in the night, often on call on different nights, and we lived right next to the MGH because we were working 120 hours a week. Internship was exhausting but thrilling because the learning curve was incredibly steep. And it felt really good to have acquired that expertise to care for desperately ill people. Even now, when I'm on an airplane and someone asks if there is a doctor on board, I feel obliged to lend whatever expertise I have. A few years ago, I directed the pilot to land the plane in Pittsburgh (we were on our way to San Francisco) because an elderly gentleman was in the middle of having what I thought might be a heart attack (it turned out to be severe pericarditis). I trained at MGH with a spectacular group of fellow residents, many of whom—Rick Klausner, Mark Fishman, Simeon Taylor, Mike Holick, Perry Blackshear, and Joe Bonventre among others, went on to become prominent figures in their fields. It's wonderful to be able to reach out to long standing colleagues and friends from those days for expertise in areas outside my own. But after two years of residency, I found that I was much more interested in thinking about the etiology of disease than in actually treating patients day to day.

Bill Paul and the NIH: A Hotbed of Immunology

So off Hugh and I went to the National Institutes of Health (NIH) to do research. I spent three fantastic years at the Laboratory of Immunology in the National Institute of Allergy and Infectious Diseases headed by Bill Paul, a wonderful scientist and mentor. He urged me to take on a daring and risky project that no one else in the lab was willing to do. The idea was to generate class II major histocompatibility complex (MHC) mutant antigen-presenting cell lines that would allow us to define key epitopes on these molecules for T cell activation. We used chemically induced mutagenesis and two different monoclonal antibodies against a specific MHC class II antigen to select for point mutants in class II MHC genes. This idea was greeted with great skepticism by colleagues, but I decided to give it a try. Remarkably, it worked and garnered quite a lot of attention in the field. This was a really important lesson for me. To be a successful scientist, one has to be a risk taker. Breakthroughs are only made by being willing to dare and to innovate. That fit my personality really well—I always have been a risk taker, I'm the opposite of conservative, somewhat impulsive and impetuous—and, as my knowledge of the field grew, ideas came easily to me. Bill also taught me a lot about running a lab and being an effective mentor. I very much liked his style of individual weekly meetings with each postdoc as well as a weekly group meeting at which one person would present. I've emulated that in my own lab. Another benefit of going to the NIH was getting to know so many spectacular immunologists. At that time, in the late 1970s, it was probably the best collection of immunologists in the country, and therefore it attracted very talented postdoctoral fellows as well. Several of my peer group of postdocs and junior faculty that were at the NIH at that time—Mark Davis, Larry Samelson, Steve Hedrick, Warner Greene, Stan Korsmeyer, Jeff Bluestone, Al and Dinah Singer, Ron Germain, and others later became leading figures in immunology.

Back to Harvard and some very tough years

Our stay at the NIH was a temporary one as Hugh needed to get back to MGH to finish his surgical training, and I wanted to get subspecialty training in rheumatology. Since I had written and been awarded an R01 grant before I left the NIH, I was made an Instructor in Medicine although I was just a first year full time clinical fellow. I simply couldn't bear to take a hiatus from my research on the function of MHC class II antigens and used the funds to hire a technician to help me carry on the work. We had a tiny space with a tissue culture hood and one lab bench. It never really occurred to me to actually undertake a formal job search. We needed to be in Boston and I just assumed I would stay at Harvard Medical School. After a year and a half at MGH as a rheumatology fellow, I relocated to the Longwood area to the Harvard School of Public Health and set up my own laboratory as an Assistant Professor of immunology and of medicine with a dual appointment at Harvard School of Public Health and Harvard Medical School. We never discussed start-up packages, the department gave me $40,000 a year for two years, I had an R01 grant, and I got a salary award from a Foundation. Pretty scary. Suddenly, I was the one running the lab, thinking up all the ideas and experiments, writing up the results for publication, and raising all the money by writing grants to support the research. If I failed at any of those tasks, then my lab would disintegrate. Doing research is really expensive. Even running a small lab with only half a dozen people in it costs half a million dollars a year, and running my current lab of 25 people costs me well over two million a year.

I was 31 then and was trying to combine seeing rheumatologic disease patients at Brigham and Women's Hospital with setting up my own lab, a pretty tall task. I still remember running back and forth between my own laboratory and Jon Seidman's laboratory where I was learning molecular biology, and simultaneously trying to study for the Rheumatology Boards. Most fellows spend hours preparing for these boards, studying the big rheumatology textbooks, but I just did not have the time. I decided all I could do was to try to memorize the key facts in a slim volume called the Rheumatology Primer. I did manage to pass the boards, barely, but only because there happened to be lots of basic immunology questions and straightforward case studies. I had no mentors then, either. There was no senior faculty member who was looking after my intellectual, emotional, or financial welfare other than myself. And on top of this, I had two small children, my toddler daughter and infant son. And my husband was a surgical resident on call all the time, so I was often a single parent. Here is where my most important piece of advice comes in. If you possibly can, live near your parents or your in-laws or family members who will love your children! Even though we had a live-in nanny, my life would have been incomparably more difficult without the constant and tireless support of my mother and father. I remember on weekends, when Hugh was on call from Friday to Monday, packing up the two kids and literally moving into my parents' house. We would get fed, cared for, and I would grab a few hours to run into the lab and get some experiments done while my father took the kids to the playground. Although they must have gotten a little tired of all this childcare at times, I think my parents would say that the close bonds forged with their grandchildren were well worth it. My children certainly would agree. I don't understand why the extended family concept isn't more widely embraced in this country. In many ways, it is the simplest and best solution to the problem of melding family and work.

Children

I think this topic deserves a subheading all its own, because balancing work and family has been such a huge part of my life and is probably the defining issue for many female physician-scientists (Fig. 4.4). The most frequent question I am asked by graduate students and postdoctoral fellows, usually female but not always, is how I managed to make my career work while having three children and a husband who was a surgeon. I always knew that I wanted children, and my husband and I had settled on three as the ideal number. I've talked with many young female scientists who debate the issue with themselves, discuss the pros and cons, and worry about the timing. That's probably a good thing if there is some doubt about the decision. For me, though, it was simple; there was no question in my mind that I wanted

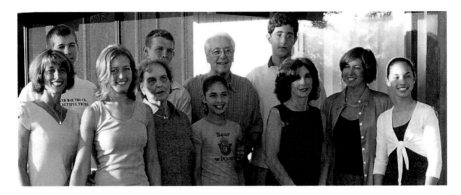

Fig. 4.4 On the Vineyard with extended family in 2005

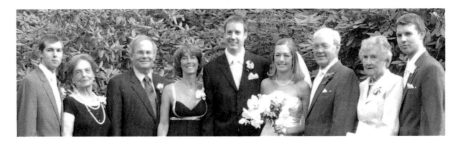

Fig. 4.5 Kalah wedding with Hugh and Greg, my Mother, and Mother-in-law in picture

them and that the best time to start having them was when I finished my medical residency. Clara Auchincloss (Kalah) was born just as I began my postdoctoral fellowship at the NIH in Bill Paul's laboratory. Now 29, she is a lawyer at a law firm in Washington DC where she and her husband Dan Barnes, a PhD student in international relations at Johns Hopkins, live (Fig. 4.5). Hugh Glimcher Auchincloss was born two and a half years later just a few months before I finished my postdoc and returned to MGH to do a rheumatology fellowship. He was the third generation of our family to graduate from Harvard Medical School (Fig. 4.6) and is now a second year surgical resident at MGH, following in his father's and grandfathers' footsteps. Our third child, Jacob Auchincloss had to wait another six years to be born while I was busy running my laboratory and getting promoted through the professorial ranks. He is a senior at Harvard College and is probably headed for law school via the Marines. Much as I adore the kids, I will admit that the rumors spread about my rapid return to work after their births are correct. I managed to stay home for one week after Kalah was born before taking the Internal Medicine Boards and returning to the lab. But when my first son was born, I returned the day after my discharge from the hospital, and when second son appeared on the scene, I asked my husband to drop me off at the lab, take the infant home from the Beth Israel Hospital and come back and pick me up in a few hours. He was understandably annoyed, and I consented grudgingly to delay my return to the lab until the next morning.

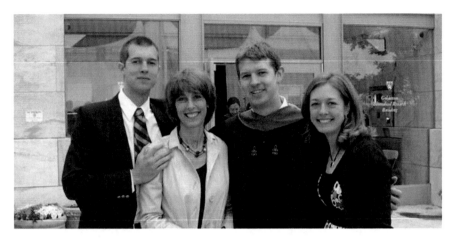

Fig. 4.6 Hugh's graduation from Harvard Medical School, 2008

Prized statements, comments, and reactions about my career from the three of them over the years have included: my daughter at age 5, upon discovering that her best friend's mother was a homemaker: "I thought all mothers were doctors" and at age 12, "I can't imagine what a woman would do if she didn't have a career." My younger son at age 12 after accompanying me to the American Society for Clinical Investigation meeting where I received the Distinguished Investigator Award—"I'm confused. Are you a famous scientist who wins prizes or are you the mom who snuggles us and sings to the dog?" and "Can I buy a motorcycle with your prize money?" My older son at age 5, "I've decided that I would like you to stay home like all my friends' mothers," and bursting into tears when I gently explained why that would not happen. My daughter, aged 14 after I had spent a week at home over Christmas while the babysitter was on holiday: "Mom please go back to work; you're driving us all nuts. I can take care of the boys." My daughter, aged 13 when her father had to do a liver transplant instead of going with her class to the Museum of Science, "It's your fault; you should have foreseen that Dad couldn't go" (I went). My older son, aged 20 upon my 50th birthday, "It's been quite a year for you, Mom. You got elected to the National Academy of Sciences, ran the Boston marathon and got divorced." My daughter, aged 12, when I offered to speak to her class about animal experimentation: "OK, but I'm glad your last name is different from mine so no one will know you're my mother," and afterwards " I have to admit you did a pretty good job." My older son's reply to a caller who asked for Dr. Glimcher, "My grandfather isn't here" followed by horrified chagrin at his sexist response. Finally, all three of them, beaming at me from the audience when I walked on stage to sign the book on my election to the National Academy of Sciences. They are the lights of my life, the absolute best products I've created. I cannot imagine a life without them. Possibly my only worthwhile piece of advice to young women scientists: If you want children, have them. Do not sacrifice family for career. Men don't have to and neither do you. It's not easy, but there is nothing that can compare.

A Very Eclectic Scientific Career: Always Flying by the Seat of My Skirts

I have always felt like an intruder, an outsider who wasn't really a bona fide scientist but just happened upon or strayed into the field, took some risks and got lucky. I certainly didn't have particularly strong scientific credentials: no PhD and not a lot of "quantitative" background. I've discovered that many if not most scientists feel this way at least some of the time, and this is particularly common among female scientists. What I did have was a lot of energy, a passion for immunology, and a willingness to wing it on the basis of incomplete knowledge. I was a master at multitasking and working in the midst of chaos, (a talent I've found usually correlates with the presence of two X chromosomes). Most of my grants and papers were written in the family room of our home, at first on a yellow pad and later on my laptop, surrounded by the kids, their friends, the dogs, and whoever else happened to be around. Venturing out into the unknown was made easier for me because I figured that if all else failed and my lab went up in flames, I could go back to being a doc. And, most important, I woke up every morning to three kids and came back every night to them: reality, balance, and the belief and knowledge that in the long run, if I didn't make a certain discovery, someone else would—I was far from irreplaceable. The reason to be a scientist was because I loved it; it chose me rather than vice versa. I believed as Siddhartha said that "Your work is to discover your world and then with all your heart give yourself to it." What I never wanted to do was continue a research project in incremental steps *ad infinitum* once we had solved a good piece of the puzzle.

My very favorite plan of attack was to ask a simple question (I have a very straightforward brain) —for example, what are the transcription factors that control T helper cell lineage commitment? And then go after it using any technology available. In that particular instance, the right technology was risky. We used a yeast two-hybrid strategy to clone the IL4-specific factor, c-maf, and a yeast one-hybrid strategy to clone the Th1 factor, which turned out to be T-bet. Once we had the new gene in hand, we had to really prove what it did beyond the shadow of a doubt using genetic manipulation in vivo and other strategies. It was always important to me, perhaps because I was a physician, that we test its function in animal models of human disease. Equally important was to understand the biochemical and molecular pathways upstream and downstream of the gene that explained how it worked. Of course this strategy didn't always succeed—we failed more than once. I well remember being totally scooped by another laboratory in our efforts to isolate the master regulator of MHC class II gene transcription—Bernard Mach's laboratory did absolutely gorgeous work in isolating the key genes, including class II major histocompatibility complex transactivator (CIITA), that control that process. I also discovered that predictions about what a particular gene did in vivo from its function in vitro could be dead wrong. A case in point was X-box binding protein 1 (XBP1), which we thought controlled transcription of MHC class II genes. Instead, we found that it was required for the differentiation of B lymphocytes to plasma cells, for reasons we couldn't figure out until other laboratories discovered that it was the long sought-after mammalian homologue of the yeast factor vital in the unfolded protein or endoplasmic reticulum stress response. I liked that outcome because it set us working on a signaling pathway that I knew very little about. I suppose in the end it doesn't really matter that I don't have a PhD, because if I had one, it would have been in the field of cellular immunology, and nowadays, I'm a molecular immunologist, a skeletal biologist, and have ventured most recently into the function of the XBP1 signaling pathway in neurodegenerative diseases and dyslipidemias, again, subjects that are new terrain for me. Most times, but not always, we have been welcomed into these fields by colleagues who share my view that fertilization across disciplines can be very productive. Studying the skeletal system has been particularly fun because my father made his career in that arena, so we have collaborated over the last decade. It's quite lovely to coauthor papers with one's parent.

I wouldn't have been able to do quality work in any of these fields on my own. I have been unbelievably fortunate in attracting gifted graduate students and postdoctoral fellows to my laboratory over the last 25 years. Most of them are a heck of a lot smarter and more knowledgeable than I am, and it has been my privilege, and my most important responsibility, to help mentor them. One of the things I'm proudest of is establishing a pilot program at the NIH that provides technical support to young women postdocs who are also primary caregivers. I have been able to do that for female postdocs in my lab over the years and it really works. Several of my trainees with young children received excellent job offers based on their productive postdoc years working reasonable hours, and went on to have great careers. It's clear to me that giving these overworked young women a boost by providing another pair of hands is an investment well worth making, and something I argued vigorously for as a member of the Summers' Task Force several years ago.

But mostly what I tell them is to have self-confidence and be as stubborn as bulls and persevere during the difficult times. We all know how very tough it can be but also how thrilling. And, really key advice for those of us who must be multitaskers: it isn't necessary to be a perfectionist in everything as long as the data are impeccable.

I'm still as excited about the science as I was 30 years ago, and hope that I have some good years left. Most of all, I look forward to savoring the success of the next generation of female physician-scientists. May they have as much fun as I have.

Dedicated to my parents, Melvin and Geraldine Glimcher

Five
...First Pick Good Parents

Edward J. Benz, Jr.

Someone wise once said "The secret to a happy childhood is to pick good parents."
As I reflect on my career, I would add this variation: "For success in academic
medicine, first pick good mentors." My good fortune in receiving outstanding mentoring and making the best of it has been the single most important reason that my
career has been successful and fulfilling.

The premise of this volume is that the personal histories of successful physician-scientists would be of some heuristic value to those considering a career in academic
medicine. Toward that end, my contribution certainly revolves around the central
theme of the importance of mentoring. In addition, there is a second thread that has
been critical for my development and that of my mentees. Sports analysts continually point out that the outcome of championship games often turns on a very small
number of "key plays" occurring at crucial moments. I am struck by how often
careers have pivoted on analogous key moments. These few key plays and how they
are handled by both mentor and mentee can alter profoundly one's career path. They
are opportunities that must be recognized and seized.

When David Schwartz invited me to contribute to this volume, I was flattered.
I have since come to appreciate why people hire ghost writers to do their autobiographies! The only way I know to share my thoughts with you is to tell you the
basics of my own history, pointing out at the appropriate points in the narrative
where the critical impact of good mentors and those key plays occurred.

My story may be a bit different from that of my co-authors. My circumstances
were such that those key plays and the securing of great mentorship both occurred
very early in my academic life. By the time I was a house officer, my future was
pretty well set and I was already somewhat established as an investigator. Thus, my
narrative focuses on my formative years as a student, and says relatively little about
my life as a faculty member. Though my defining moments occurred earlier, I think
they offer lessons similar to those of my co-authors, who experienced them at later
stages.

E.J. Benz, Jr. (✉)
Department of Medical Oncology, Dana-Farber Cancer Institute, Boston, MA, USA
e-mail: edward_benz@dfci.harvard.edu

D.A. Schwartz (ed.), *Medicine Science and Dreams,*
DOI 10.1007/978-90-481-9538-1_5, © Springer Science+Business Media B.V. 2011

To those of you who read this essay, I extend my thanks for your belief that there might be something here worthy of your attention. I hope that you will find this piece helpful as you embark on your own careers. Most of all, I wish for you a career as fulfilling and gratifying as the one I have been so lucky to enjoy. I also hope that, along the way, you will experience friendships, camaraderie, and inspiration from your colleagues, patients, and mentees like those that have enriched my journey. Finally, may you be sustained, as have I, by knowing as you wake up each day that you are striving to do something truly important and self-transcendent.

Before beginning, I want to thank my wife Peggy for being my partner and sticking with me. A brilliant nurse scientist in her own right, Peggy was my high school sweetheart. We broke up in college. Our first marriages ended in divorce. Fortunately, we met again quite serendipitously more than 20 years after high school and have now been married for 17 years. We each had two children by our first marriages who have turned out to be fabulous kids and successful adults. They are very understanding of the circuitous route we took to our happiness and, so far, have given us three grandchildren. Peggy has shared in and supported me through all the ups and downs, anxieties, and exhilarations of the last 17 years. This part of the journey has been our story, not mine alone, and she has made it the best part.

Early Inclinations Toward Science and Medicine

It has been my good fortune to graduate from, hold professorships at, and fill leadership positions in outstanding academic institutions, including Princeton, Harvard, the National Institutes of Health (NIH), Yale, Pittsburgh, Johns Hopkins and, presently, the Dana-Farber Cancer Institute. I remain a bit mystified as to how this happened. Over the years, I have occasionally bumped into classmates, friends, and acquaintances whom I would have considered more likely to have enjoyed this level of success on the basis of their brains, creativity, and dedication. Yet, I did and many of them didn't. I am too old to deceive myself into believing that this happened because I was any "better" than these other very smart people. Rather, there must have been circumstances and timely opportunities that distinguished their careers and mine. These are the focus of this narrative.

"Picking good parents" was crucial to this good fortune. I was lucky to grow up in a stable family with terrific parents and siblings. While everyone can think of challenges and disadvantages they faced during childhood, mine were few. My circumstances were nurturing and advantageous. Yet, if you had told me at age 10 that I would spend my life in academics, "going to school" every day for the rest of my life, I would have cringed. I hated school. My favorite time of the day was 3:15 p.m.—dismissal time. I would have been quite happy to play football, basketball, or baseball every minute of every day. My first interest in science and medicine germinated quite independently of any school activity. Indeed, the Catholic schools that I attended in Bethlehem, a small Southeastern Pennsylvania steel town, did not teach science until high school. That I had any inkling as to what experimental science meant was due to my home life.

I was born in Pittsburgh, PA. My mother was trained in business administration and my dad was a physician. Because of his residency at the Mayo Clinic and his Army service requirements, we lived in Pittsburgh, Brooklyn, Long Island, Rochester, Minnesota, and two locations in Bethlehem before achieving some degree of permanence. Consequently, I had attended five schools by the time I entered fourth grade. I was also painfully small and thin. Our cohort was the leading edge of the baby boom era; class sizes were frequently 60–100 students, all under the strict disciplinarian and rote memorization teaching style of nuns who were too overwhelmed by sheer numbers to provide much individualized teaching. I was always the new kid and the smallest, constantly bullied, and continually fighting with my bigger tormentors. There was little about this scenario that I found appealing.

The beginnings of my interest in medicine remain unclear to me even now. In one sense, it seemed inevitable that I would become a physician. My dad, paternal grandfather, paternal uncle, and two older cousins were all MDs. I had this notion that I would grow up to be a doctor for as long as I can remember. However, there was no pressure on me or my siblings to enter medicine. Indeed, all of them chose other professions. A few events that deeply impressed me solidified my inclinations to pursue a medical career.

During our years in Rochester, polio epidemics spread across the country every summer. At a kindergarten year-end celebration, my younger brother Tom and I shared a picnic blanket with three other children. Those three contracted polio and ended up in iron lungs, but Tom and I were spared. For years afterwards, my mother would kneel down with us for bedtime prayers each night and we would pray for them. I remember the day that the Salk vaccine was the banner headline on our local newspaper. My mom burst into tears. Within a year or two, nobody worried about polio anymore. Even as a preteen, I thought that it would be great to be able to do something like that; my idea of research was always in the context of medicine, like finding the polio vaccine.

The second event involved one of my worst tormentors, a big kid who would often jump me as I was walking to the ball field. I decided to stand my ground one day and beat him up pretty thoroughly. He didn't bother me after that, but after a few months he wasn't around at all. One night, my dad came home and told me he had died of cancer (he had a retinal melanoma).

His dying affected me deeply. I had feared and hated him passionately, and secretly wished every evil on him. I felt guilty that I had somehow caused his cancer by beating him up and blackening his eye. My parents spent many hours explaining what cancer was and how I could not have caused it, and I got over it. However, from then on the notion of cancer had a haunting aura for me. To me, the ultimate thing you could do as a doctor would be to find a cure for cancer.

Despite my negative attitude toward school, my parents allowed my interest in science to bloom by treating it as recreation. I was always figuring out how things worked and could reason well from an early age, even though I was a terrible memorizer and not very well organized as a pupil. My dad had started his own clinical laboratory. Occasionally, he would take me to the lab with him. It fascinated me that one drop of acid could turn a beaker filled with pink liquid (phenolphthalein) completely colorless, while a drop or two of sodium hydroxide could make it pink again, and that you could blow the cork off a bottle by mixing vinegar and baking soda inside it. Without knowing it, I was probably hooked by the age of nine, thinking that this was fun and had nothing to do with the drudgery and social unpleasantness of school. I retain a vivid memory of wishing for two Christmas presents at age 11: a football helmet with a real face guard and a chemistry set!

In many ways, our parents are our first mentors. This was certainly true for my early interest in science. They did not push the idea that science was an important school subject. In fact, messing around with my chemistry set was no more tolerated as an alternative to homework than staying out too late playing football. There is a valuable lesson here, one too often missed when we encourage young people to pursue academic lives. If we make these pursuits seem too sober, we take the joy out of exploring and learning more. We need to do what my parents did—let young people think of science as a hobby. As I came to the end of elementary school, I was actually looking forward to high school, where science would be a "real subject."

Graduates from our parish school were sent to Central Catholic High School (CCHS) in Allentown, PA. Now a robust magnet school, CCHS was at the time considered good but weak in science. My dad had a part-time faculty appointment at Lehigh University. He learned from colleagues that Lehigh was about to refuse to accept science credits from CCHS. He began to insist that I transfer to prep school, provoking epic verbal battles that only a father and adolescent son can have. This precipitated one of those key plays that I regard as momentous in my own career path.

The school, recognizing its need to improve, had devised a new curriculum with advanced classes into which I was placed. New state-of-the-art textbooks and laboratory manuals were available to us. I showed these to my dad, believing firmly that these would quash further discussion of prep school. Unfortunately, he perused the text and picked up an error: a statement that man had 48 chromosomes. It might only have been a typo, but the nun called on me to answer that very question. When told that my answer, "46" was incorrect, I somewhat recklessly corrected the good Sister, who was disinclined to regard my impudence kindly. To her credit, although I had to endure a few after school detentions, she finally acknowledged that "46" was correct, and actually gave personal attention to my interest in biology.

Until then, I had been a good student but was not especially diligent. However, I was upset enough about being caught between my biology teacher and my dad that I set out to learn more about this chromosome issue. A book caught my eye because of its glossy cover and great pictures. It was a Scientific American monograph about the then brand new concept of DNA as the master repository of genetic information. It told how the pathway of gene expression and the astounding new discovery that some genes regulate the expression of other genes could explain basic life processes. This happened in 1962, only nine years after Watson and Crick's paper on DNA came out. The genetic code, the existence of mRNA, and the whole lactose operon story were all hot off the presses. This was probably the first nonfiction book that I read cover to cover. Suddenly, biology was no longer rote memorization of species and phyla. Instead, here was a way that you could make sense logically out of all of that diversity. I was hooked. My overriding intellectual interest from that point on would be molecular genetics.

This key play was impactful in other ways. I had vaguely assumed that I would end up being a doctor or a scientist, but I had very little idea of what specific things interested me until that moment. From then on, I knew that I wanted to be a physician who did genetic research. Oddly, I never imagined being "just" a scientist. I thought of science as something you needed to be good at to be a doctor.

I became a far more diligent student after this episode. I sensed that I needed to go to a top flight university where I could do independent research. I ended up excelling academically and was accepted at Princeton.

My high school years were transformative socially as well. I gained some self-confidence, made many friendships which last to this day, and became involved in many student activities, including student government. These taught me early lessons in leadership.

Mentoring Makes All the Difference

My first semester in college was one of those "welcome to the NFL" experiences. I entered Princeton in 1964 and immediately suffered academic and culture shock. Everyone else in the class had also been the academic superstar of his high school. The coursework seemed overwhelming. I was assigned to advanced placement courses for which I had inadequate preparation. Moreover, the university in those days provided almost no social support system for freshmen like me, who had no pre-existing network from prep schools.

It took all of my first year for me to realize that I could handle the academic work and even excel. What I lacked was academic and social polish, as well as sufficient self-confidence not to be intimidated by peers. These came slowly but, by the end of freshman year, I had settled in and received sufficient exposure to college level science to confirm my aspirations. During my sophomore year, two more key moments occurred. In each case, a positive outcome depended on making the most of an opportunity, but most especially on good advice from individuals who provided superb mentoring.

Princeton had a combined program in biology and chemistry that required using up sophomore elective slots for upper level science courses. Doing this and still meeting my "distribution requirements" left only one biology course that fit my schedule. It had the rather unpromising title of "Biochemistry and Physiology of Blue-Green Algae," instructed by Mr. George Russell, but I decided to take it. The course, to my pleasant surprise, was brilliantly organized and inspiring. For our laboratory, Russell had us recreate great experiments from the initial era of molecular biology. We were exposed to many of the techniques that had been used by its pioneers. This experience validated my passion for the field. Russell was also instrumental in the second and even more pivotal key play that year by introducing me to Professor Arthur Pardee, a true founder of the entire field of molecular genetics.

Princeton had an undergraduate dissertation requirement. Each student selected a mentor at the beginning of junior year and a senior thesis. This provided the opportunity for a head start on "real" research that I was looking for.

I asked George Russell to be my thesis advisor. To my dismay, he demurred, but suggested instead that Pardee had more to offer for my interests. He took the trouble to arrange an introduction, and gave me a rather generous recommendation. Pardee invited me into his lab, thus beginning an amazing experience, one of the most defining moments of my career. Pardee is a truly brilliant biologist, brilliant at a level I had never imagined. He was demanding but generous with his time and actually worked side by side at the bench with us when we needed help.

Pardee believed, presciently, that the most energy-efficient way for complex organisms to achieve homeostasis was to maintain a small percentage of genes whose expression was inducible or repressible in response to changing external conditions; their net effect would be to provide a constant internal environment in which the majority of genes could be expressed constitutively. My assignment was to learn how the expression of such a constitutive gene could be altered by mutation in *Esherichia coli*. The analysis of these mutations would hopefully identify key elements needed to maintain constancy. In retrospect, the gene expression system we chose turned out to be quite non-ideal for a relatively short-term (20 months) thesis project. Nonetheless, after many failures, I did manage to alter the expression of that gene and to co-author a paper in the *Journal of Biological Chemistry* [1], thus generating my first publishable scientific contribution.

I learned much from this experience. For example, research involves repeated frustrations punctuated by rare but exhilarating eureka moments; results mean nothing without the appropriate positive and negative controls, and macromolecules are quite fragile and require constant care and attention. The true key moments, however, were those spent with Pardee that were focused not on thesis work, but on his reflections on the future of the field. He conveyed to me his firm belief that molecular genetics would be applicable to the study of human disease. This validated my own intuition. He introduced me to many of the now iconic founders of the field (including Pauling, Watson, Crick, Sydney Brenner, and Arthur Nirenburg, among others), and suggested ways to combine an MD with a level of research that he considered worth doing. This working relationship was also my first longitudinal mentoring experience. That Pardee considered me worth as much of his time and wisdom as his graduate students gave me the first glimmer that I might have a shot at succeeding.

On the strength of a strong recommendation from Pardee, I was admitted to all the medical schools to which I applied. I narrowed my choices to the new MD/PhD program at Duke and to Harvard, which had no MD/PhD program at the time. This decision was another key play, and another example of why it helps to pick good parents. The Duke program came with a full scholarship—a free ride. Harvard would be full pay. To their everlasting credit, my parents urged me to select Harvard even though Duke was one of the nation's fastest rising medical schools in 1968. They felt that the odds of my meeting someone who would guide me into this physician-scientist career would be better at Harvard, which back then had the more research-oriented faculty. My three younger siblings, now all highly accomplished in their fields, would also need college and graduate school support. Foregoing the scholarship was an expensive decision. Our family was prosperous but not that wealthy. Nonetheless, my parents made the recommendation they felt was best academically.

I found medical school to be relatively easy. It was like having a curriculum in which everything was your favorite subject. In contrast to my entry into Princeton, where I was the rare student from my kind of scholastic background in a sophisticated elitist university, I arrived at Harvard with several classmates who were good friends. Socially and academically, everything fell into place.

During the second year, a notice was posted announcing a competition for a "Life Insurance Medical Research Fund Scholarship." The winner would be funded to do an MD/PhD. This seemed too good to be true. It would provide at Harvard what I had forgone at Duke. Convinced that this was my first real chance to find a lab and a mentor where I could begin to apply molecular biology to human disease, I visited professors across the medical school. This experience was immensely discouraging, so discouraging that I began to believe that I was dead wrong about what I wanted to do most. Each professor was kind, listening carefully, and complimenting me on my focus and ambitions. But, without exception, they tried to dissuade me from pursuing my aim. "You'll never be able to do molecular biology in man while in medical school" was the repeated refrain. The techniques were only feasible in bacteria and viruses. Unless I wanted to study those, I should focus on something else until the technology was more applicable to mammalian cells.

Fortunately, another key moment and the beginning of a phenomenal mentoring relationship happened just as I was thinking about giving up on the idea of research. A young Assistant Professor, David G. Nathan (Fig. 5.1), a pediatric hematologist, gave the lecture on the hemoglobinopathies in our second year hematology block. He caught my attention when he mentioned that hemoglobinopathies were important as models for the introduction of modern scientific methods to the study of human disease. The accessibility of blood cells and their highly differentiated state made them uniquely suitable. Circulating reticulocytes, which are elevated to very high levels in these disorders, contain remnants of the protein synthetic machinery. Indeed, one could measure the synthesis of hemoglobin in these cells by labeling them with radioactive amino acids. All of this led me to intuit that maybe these were diseases that could be approached at the level of molecular biology.

I approached Nathan at the end of the lecture and explained my plight to him. His response was definitive and immediate: "Grab a copy of your thesis and then meet me for lunch." During that meal, he told me that he knew almost nothing about this new field (then called biochemical genetics), but that he had recently recruited a hematology fellow who did, and that my notion made sense. "If you are going to study gene regulation in humans, you should study genes that produce the most

Fig. 5.1 Dr. David Nathan

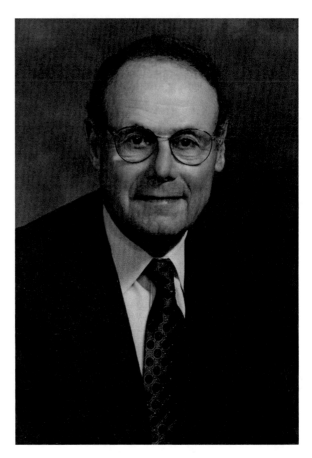

abundant protein in the body. Virtually all of the protein that reticulocytes make is hemoglobin. Mother Nature has almost purified the messenger RNA (mRNA) for you." Two days later, he offered me a spot in his lab working with that new fellow, Bernard Forget (Fig. 5.2). Bernie took me in, marking the beginning of a lifelong mentoring experience and friendship. It was hardly apparent at the time, and many moments of near despair would follow, but my career success was for all practical purposes assured from then on.

These few key plays in college and the first few years of medical school were clearly life changing. I had worked exceedingly hard, and had brought talent, intellect, and perseverance to the table. However, success at each step would have been highly improbable had it not been for those sometimes serendipitous pivotal moments and the care of good parents and mentors. Thinking back, it seems that pursuing them the way that I did was a "no brainer." At the time, however, what I should do seemed much less clear. It was the gentle steerage of mentors nudging me to make the right decision on my own that was so critically important.

Fig. 5.2 Dr. Bernard Forget

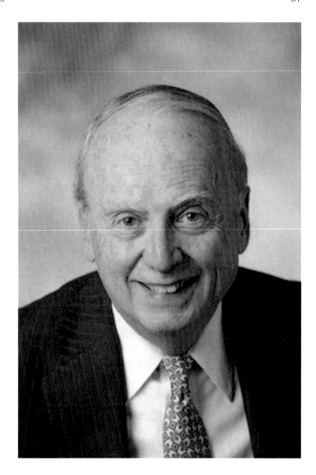

How Do You Help Your Mentee When Nothing Works?

Many of us enter research imagining that there will be steady achievement of results that bring us closer to our goal. Within a few years, we realize that nothing could be further from the truth. Progress is rarely steady. Success is anything but predictable. Most of us have spent many hours staring into the abyss of failure wondering if anything would ever work or if any result would ever tell us what to do next. As energized as I was about having finally found an exciting way to pursue my dreams, I ended up frequently visiting that abyss.

David, Bernie, and I worked out a very ambitious project. We would try to isolate mRNA from human reticulocytes of patients with thalassemia, an inherited anemia in which the individual under-produces one or more of the globin subunits of hemoglobin: the alpha subunit in alpha thalassemia or the beta subunit in beta thalassemia. We would then translate these mRNAs in vitro into their globin products and quantitate the ability of normal versus thalassemic mRNA to code for each chain. Our hypothesis, novel at the time, was that the inherited defect responsible for inadequate globin synthesis would be transmitted by the immediate product of the encoding gene—mRNA. To appreciate how risky this seemed, it is important to note that a species of RNA having the properties of mRNA was believed to exist in mammals only by inference. It was not at all clear that one could isolate mammalian mRNA. In bacteria, it was highly unstable. Bernie's job would be to devise ways to purify human globin mRNA from these patients. Mine would be to develop a "heterologous" cell-free system that could translate the mRNA.

The MD/PhD grant never materialized. Instead, I signed up for an "Honors Tutorial Fellowship," a year off that would pay a modest stipend. In return, I would be expected to write a dissertation and defend it before graduation. My time frame had shrunk to a year. Bernie and I set to work, spending many long days side by side at the bench struggling to capture these molecules and make them behave in ways that had not been done before.

After about eight months, Bernie was perfecting the isolation of human globin mRNA, but I was failing miserably despite having tried just about every manipulation possible to devise my mRNA translation system. Suddenly, there was less than a month left. After that, I would enter a full year and a half of intense clinical rotations. The likelihood of doing any more research before the end of my residency training seemed remote. I despaired, convinced that I simply did not have the brains or talent to succeed in research.

My career in research could easily have ended then were it not for great mentoring insight by David and Bernie. Einstein said that the definition of insanity was to do the same experiment over and over and over again and expect to get a different result. That is exactly what we were doing. We were relentlessly perfecting a system that, no matter how well honed, would not be potent enough to answer the question we were posing. I did not appreciate it at the time, but my experiments were working, not failing. They were just telling me that the answer was "no dice."

Fortunately, Nathan was doing a sabbatical at the Massachusetts Institute of Technology (MIT). He knew a cell biologist, David Housman, who was working with a system that might have more promise. We met at MIT and I learned how to do the prep. As we were driving back to the medical school, I told David of my pessimism. For the first time I verbalized my fears that I could not do this kind of work. Once I got started all my woes came out, including my sense of shame that I was letting Bernie down. After all, this was his first major project and my contribution was essential to his success as well as my own. I believed that I had been wasting everybody's time and should quit.

Nathan slammed on his brakes right on the Massachusetts Avenue Bridge and began lecturing me about not giving up. He told me that he considered me an exceptional prospect. He would not let me quit. This is what happens in research. It wasn't me; it was that this was a very challenging problem. In retrospect, I think I agreed to persevere largely so that he would get off that bridge before we got crushed by a bunch of Boston drivers!

For the next three weeks, Nathan and Bernie rarely let me out of their sight, not to make sure I was working but to be my cheerleaders. I probably worked harder during those weeks than any time before or since. Miraculously, everything fell into place. All of those months of failure had really been preparation. I had learned how to do these experiments just about perfectly. All I needed was the right starting material. During those three weeks, Bernie and I were able to prove that the defect in globin synthesis in patients with thalassemia was indeed due to a deficiency in the appropriate globin mRNA. That work and subsequent experiments that I could now rather easily slip in to free times during my clinical rotations and my fourth year resulted in several well-received papers, high honors, and two student research prizes. My career was launched, and I have never had to look back.

Watching the careers of many peers and mentees unfold has taught me that it is exceedingly rare for someone's scientific interests and career momentum to be firmly established at such an early stage. Most aspiring physician-scientists struggle with the decision to enter the field all the way through residency, fellowship, or even the early faculty years. Few have the chance to get their track records started on a solid footing in the sheltered environment of school, like I did. A fair question, then, is whether my story has any relevance to readers of this volume. I submit that there are lessons worth noting, despite this atypicality.

First, one has to want to do this badly enough to be both aggressive and persistent in finding both opportunities and people willing to help you. Indeed, if it is apparent by your persistence that you do want it that badly, it is more likely that good mentors will be attracted to you. Both Pardee and Nathan would tell you that their commitment to me did not arise from thinking that I was any smarter than other Princeton or Harvard students. It was my focus and doggedness.

Second, failing comes with the territory—but that is ok. Although my story might seem to be of success at an early age, it is also one of many failures during those formative years. In our business, we are too accustomed to getting "A" grades. All too often we have no idea how to deal with failing, particularly repeated failings that defy our best efforts and cleverness. Biological research is hard, and experiments fail more often than they succeed precisely because any project worth doing is at the frontier of the unknown. Great mentors help you learn that failing along the way is normal. They support you enough to accept *failing* without losing faith in yourself, but they won't let you accept *failure*—giving up on yourself or your aspiration just because it is harder than what you have tried before. Many of my peers are reaching that age where one gets roasted and feted as retirement looms. Almost every one of them has a story in which they slogged their way through early failures—a grant triaged, good results that could not get published, or first faculty jobs they did not get. The job of a good mentor is to guide you through these moments of self-doubt and let you know that many illustrious people were once stuck exactly where you are.

Third, it helps to be "coachable." Mentors want to teach and guide you. Your ability to learn and improve is what will impress and motivate them, not constant reminders of how brilliant or clever you are. That doesn't mean accepting that they are always right and you wrong. Rather it means respecting that they are in the position to be your mentor for a reason and that their opinion merits respect and thoughtful reflection before supposing that yours is better. I did not always follow my parents' or mentors' advice, but I never ignored it.

Fourth, it also helps to be alert. It may seem as if those key moments were the only ones that could have gotten me underway, and that they miraculously fell from the sky. I realize now that there likely would have been other opportune moments sooner or later. I was alert and attentive enough to recognize the perfect opportunity when it appeared because I was looking for it. This was because I had conceived in my own mind a sense of what kind of opportunity I needed. Without knowing precisely what that would be, I was able to recognize the chance when I came upon it.

Finally, nothing tops working with people who love what they are doing. I have not stressed this explicitly enough in my narrative, but all of my mentors loved their work and fostered positive working environments. Everyone who tries to do what we do knows that it is hard, anxiety provoking, and often frustrating. It helps greatly if, early in our careers, we are with people who are excited to be on the frontiers of knowledge, who are energized by teaching, mentoring, and caring for patients, and who project that all-important belief that our endeavor is highly important and bigger than our worries about ourselves. In the midst of our early frustrations and anxieties, many of us ask, "Even if I make it, will it be worth all this?" You want to work for people who make it clear by example that the answer is a resounding, "Yes."

After graduation, I joined Peter Bent Brigham Hospital's Research Residency in Internal Medicine. This new program allowed me to devote part of each house staff year to research. I could thus continue my lab work while getting superb clinical training. I loved caring for patients and came to appreciate how complex the interplay of patients, families, and their disease states can be. I then followed that experience with three years of research training at the NIH. These positions allowed me to maintain my research momentum and were, fortunately, also very productive experiences. In 1978, I accepted a hematology fellowship at Yale and joined the faculty as an Assistant Professor a year later. Bernie Forget, who had moved to Yale to become Chief of Hematology, and my NIH mentor, Arthur Nienhuis, were invaluable guides. Having made the transition to independence only a few years before me, they shared their experiences and insights, all of which made my transition very smooth.

There is little more worth recounting about my life as a faculty investigator, clinician and, teacher. I enjoyed having my own research program and loved clinical hematology, teaching, and mentoring my students and fellows. I rose quickly through the ranks, becoming a full professor in 1987. I remain NIH funded; in fact, one of my grants has been funded continuously since I first received it in 1979. Although I am proud of my research record, my contributions as an investigator do not come close to matching those of many co-authors in this volume. What may be of more value, then, is to close by reflecting on some factors that have allowed me to hold some key academic leadership positions, in the hope that these will be instructive to those aspiring to do the same.

Leadership Development

My first leadership experiences occurred in Boy Scouts. I was an Eagle Scout and held most of the leadership jobs one could hold in our troop. These were major confidence boosters in grade school, a time otherwise devoid of confidence-boosting experiences. I was involved in student government and president of some student organizations in high school, but in college and medical school I was completely uninvolved and practically invisible. At Yale, I certainly wasn't looking to lead anything except my lab. Departmental administration and politics were not relevant. It is also true that Yale pretty much left us to ourselves and didn't intrude too much on our daily lives. We were almost like vendors in a bazaar, pretty much self-supporting and largely free to focus on our work. When asked to serve on a committee or pick up an extra class or month on service, I always did, but I was not interested in administration.

As has been the case for many colleagues with whom I have compared notes, my involvement in leadership began gradually. Most of us were noticed initially for the quality of our academic work. However, being tapped to lead thereafter depended on other things: the way that we worked in a group, how we delivered the work we were asked to do, our communication styles, and a belief that we would give some of ourselves to the good of the organization.

This is a lesson for aspiring leaders. Academic excellence may get you noticed; however, it is only necessary and not sufficient. Academic medicine is littered with examples proving over and over again that those chosen to lead *solely* on the basis of brilliance or research or academic stardom often fail as leaders. Leadership depends mostly on who you are. How smart you are and what you have accomplished also matter, but to a lesser extent. At its very core, leadership means guiding others to a desired destination, or at least onto the right path. The best leaders put their time, energy, and talent into getting what or whom they lead to that better place, even if it requires subordinating what interests you most personally. There are examples of brilliant scientists who have led brilliantly as well, but it was not because of their scientific genius alone.

Recognition as a potential leader frequently comes from outside before one gets noticed at home. Partly because of the nice head start that I had, I was being appointed to professional society committees, speaking roles, foundation and NIH study sections, and editorial boards within my first few years at Yale. The recommendations of my mentors certainly helped. By being reasonably articulate, listening carefully and learning, respecting the work, and doing it diligently, I was moved up in the hierarchies of this extramural professional world. My national prominence was greater than my local profile but I was being noticed by the prominent people who were colleagues of my bosses at home. Having heard good things about me from them, my Chair and Dean at Yale began to notice me.

This experience is fairly common. Opportunities for career growth at home often follow recognition from colleagues and "elders" on the outside. Young faculty should thus look for opportunities to be active in their key professional societies. Good mentors will serve as a mentee's "agent" in this context, helping to position him or her on "good" committees, for example, and making sure that he or she gets noticed by prominent leaders.

My first major leadership position at Yale was Chair of the Curriculum Committee and of the Task Force to Reform the Medical School Curriculum. I was newly tenured in 1984 when asked to do this by my Dean. My lab was going great at the time, and I had taken on more clinical and teaching work, but said yes. This would prove to be a daunting job with a high probability of failure. Yale has a sacred curricular icon, "The Yale System," designed in the 1930s to make medical studies more graduate school-like and involve less brute force memorization. A great aspect of this system is a requirement to do dissertation research. There were no grades in the preclinical years. More controversial, especially with basic science faculty, was that there were also no tests. Faculty complained that they had no idea whether students were mastering the material. As many as eight or ten students per year were pulled from third year clinical rotations because they failed Part I of the boards. The lack of accountability was not working for a significant minority of the class.

Naturally, the no test component was embraced by the students as the true essence of the Yale System. The mere suggestion that exams might serve a useful purpose was heretical. Nonetheless, I muddled through a nearly two year long process, convening endless meetings, town halls, one on one visits, and white papers. We were finally able to get agreement that there would be tests, anonymously graded with provisions to help students falling below a "minimum competence" score. We also made several enhancements to the curriculum.

This experience is the one key play in leadership development worth including in this piece, even though it unfolded over a nearly two year period. It created a sharp uptick in my leadership trajectory. The work of our Task Force was at best a partial success. However, it allowed me to learn how to lead faculty, and raised people's opinion of me as a leader. Within a year, I was appointed Division Chief, then in fairly quick succession over the next decade: Vice Chair of the Department, Chair of Medicine at Pitt, and Chair of Medicine at Hopkins. The chance to lead a great cancer center at Harvard came along in 2000. It was an irresistible offer to return to Harvard and, at last, to work on conquering cancer. After all, this is what I had dreamed of doing when I was young. I seized the opportunity, and I am writing this in our downtown Boston condo nine fulfilling years later.

There have been many trying and exhilarating moments along the way, but what I learned during those two years in the mid-1980s formed my basic template for leadership. Sharing a few of the elements of that template might be the best way for me to conclude.

Of all things, the most important element of any success that I have had as a leader is that I respect the work that needs to be done and the people with whom I do it. People can—and sometimes do—lose my respect, but they have it at the outset. Executive leadership is extremely complex and intellectually challenging. I have learned to respect the intelligence, sense of service, and training required to be an exceptional executive, especially in environments like academic medicine, where "administrators" are thought to be idiots by a too large minority of the faculty they support.

Whether in my own jobs, or in looking at what has happened to peers, it has become indubitably clear that we are amateurs at administration. We will never be as good at it as the professionals. Our role is to articulate and actuate our core values, to set the academic vision, and help the organization find and execute the strategies to achieve it. We need the expertise of financial, operations, legal, human resources, communications, and many other professionals. We are much more likely to attract the best people to support us, and to get their best effort, if we respect them and learn from them even as we lead and support them.

Some of the biggest failures I have witnessed have come when colleagues take some business courses or read business books and turn themselves into second rate businesspeople instead of first rate academic leaders. That is not to say one should not strive to learn these things. On the contrary, gaining content knowledge is crucial to success. But, heed what my Chief Financial Officer said to me once as I was leaving for a retreat on hospital finance: "Have a good time but remember that a little knowledge is still a dangerous thing."

Another essential element is often called transparency but is, in reality, simple honesty in its many contexts. Bad stuff will happen no matter how good you and your program are. Without exception, the best outcome of a crisis occurs when one is forthright about what the situation is, how it happened, and what to do next. The worst happens when people try to spin or cover up. Yet, people never learn and all too often do the latter.

Transparency also means that people understand why you are doing what you are doing, especially if it isn't what they want you to do. Trust is critical to successful leadership. People should never wonder what your agenda is or what you are hiding. In an environment of trust, it is more likely that people will accept those times when you must say "I can't tell you everything behind this decision, but this is what I think we must do."

Honesty also means promising only those things you can deliver. I promise very often to try to give people what they need. I promise concrete things far more rarely, doing so only if I am certain that I can deliver.

It is also important to realize that when it comes to decision-making, being decisive isn't the same as being quick or daring. Some think that they must prove their mettle by making dramatic decisions early in their tenures. My colleagues who did do it often got themselves in trouble. Leaders have to make decisions and often need to make them when there is no obvious answer. But leading is a marathon for us, not a sprint. It has been important to me to distinguish the urgency and importance of a decision and to take the time to learn the issue, get input, communicate to stakeholders when nearing a decision, get it as right as possible the first time, and save the "take that hill" decisions for the rare situations when there is true urgency. Projecting calm and coolness under fire is a better way to maintain the confidence of your organization.

Every leader will tell you that you can never communicate enough, and I agree. For faculty in particular, there is no sin greater than leaving someone out of the loop. My only addition to this oft-repeated mantra is that no matter how hard you try, you will invariably fail. Someone you think has been fully briefed and on board will act like the news came out of the blue. In that case, I have learned that it is best just to apologize and ask how you can help. Indeed, in this and many other ways, good leaders understand the power of a real apology and a sincere plea to the offended to help you make it right.

Finally, academics are actually eager to be led, but they hate to be ruled. Efforts to run academic health centers like corporations invariably fail, as they should. We should apply good business practices wherever they make sense. But, we are not at core business. While we must remain solvent, our job as leaders is to create a stimulating and nurturing environment that fosters, supports, and celebrates simultaneously the brilliant, curiosity-driven research of our faculty; the compassion and patient focus of our care; the nurturing, education, and career development of the next generation; and now, the teamwork and collaborative spirit of translational science in all of its forms. Those who make this happen, our faculties and staffs, are extremely bright and already highly accomplished when they start out. They are highly motivated and understandably individualistic. They must buy in to the vision, the strategies, and tactics. Leading them is a process of colloquy and persuasion, of constant iteration and consultation, and not of dictums, orders, or conformity. I have counseled others that leadership in academics is more like being a manager of a baseball team of free agents than it is like managing a company or leading a brigade. They can and will function as a team, but not by being ordered to do so.

Conclusion

I never seriously considered any other career, but I would be amazed if there are many others as absorbing or rewarding. How else can one care for the sick, nurture the next generation, and pursue one's burning scientific interests in a setting that allows great autonomy and independence? For all of our anxieties about funding and tenure, the career of a physician-scientist is also more remunerative and secure than most careers in today's world. While it is always a struggle starting out, it just gets better and better as you stick with it. I highly recommend it to you. If this essay in any way helps you to take the plunge or make your way through those early days, I will regard the effort to write it as very well invested.

Reference

1. Pardee AB, Benz EJ Jr, St Peter DA, Krieger JN, Meuth M, Trieshmann HW Jr (1971) Hyperproduction and purification of nicotinamide deamidase, a microconstitutive enzyme of Escherichia coli. J Biol Chem 246:6792–6796

Six
The Long Way to Somewhere

Moisés Selman

I was born in Chile, the third of four children in an immigrant Palestinian family (Fig. 6.1). My grandparents arrived from Bethlehem at the end of the nineteenth century after having fled from either the declining but powerful Ottoman Empire or the severe cholera epidemic that devastated Palestine in 1902. The journey to Chile was a long and dangerous one for them. First, the Mediterranean, and then the Atlantic Ocean had to be crossed to land in Buenos Aires. After that, an eternal train journey over the Argentinean plains had to be taken before facing the

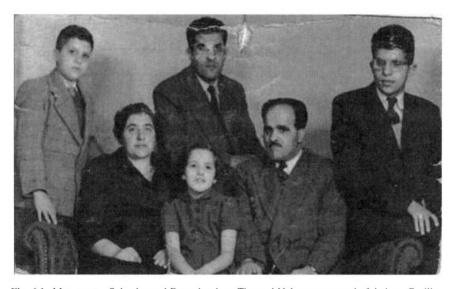

Fig. 6.1 My parents, Salvador and Rosa, brothers Tito and Nelson, my wonderful sister Cecilia, and myself (*left* corner) in our traditional once-a-year photograph

M. Selman (✉)
Instituto Nacional de Enfermedades Respiratorias, Tlalpan 4502, CP 14080, México DF, México
e-mail: mselman@yahoo.com.mx

D.A. Schwartz (ed.), *Medicine Science and Dreams*, 75
DOI 10.1007/978-90-481-9538-1_6, © Springer Science+Business Media B.V. 2011

Andes Mountains. From this point, it was necessary to walk and then ride, hiring mule drivers to guide them across treacherous passes thousands of meters high, and through narrow ravines that led to the thin strip of my grandparents' new Promised Land, Chile.

The exact circumstances surrounding their arrival in Talcahuano, a small seaport located at the end of nowhere, are a mystery. An uncle told me once that one of them arrived at Valparaiso, the main harbor in Chile, but that night a huge earthquake terrified my grandparents, and they took a train to the last possible station and found Talcahuano when they disembarked.

My parents were small business people who opened and developed a small shoe store that gradually grew. Later, they also got involved in toys. Without much formal education, they worked hard from sunrise to sunset, dreaming that their children would have the opportunity to enroll in college and become professionals.

I have fond memories of my childhood in Talcahuano. I remember waking for school surrounded by the tempestuous sea, the air infused with a profound smell of saltwater. I was a normal child (whatever *normal* means), although a bit impetuous and grumpy according to my teachers.

I had so many aunts, uncles, and cousins that family encounters were daily and intense, and I remember well the summer holidays at the seaside, the splendid mixture of Arab and Chilean food, the soccer matches along the beach, the exchange of our favorite comics, and our hopeful dreams for the future (Fig. 6.2).

Then, suddenly, I was thrust into adolescence, and hormones seized my brain, although I was extremely shy in my approach to girls. Every corner of my mind was

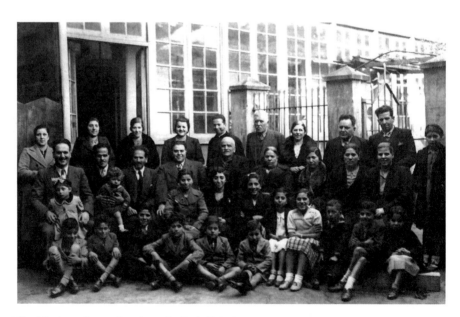

Fig. 6.2 A small part of my large family in Talcahuano

filled with Elvis Presley's song "A Boy Like Me, a Girl Like You" and Paul Anka's "Lonely Boy." My father wanted me to study medicine, but at that time I did not have any clue about my future. Above all, I did not have any academic role model to admire and follow. I just knew that our family doctor was not a very appealing model. And, to tell the truth, I dreamed of being a singer or a soccer player (despite my marginal talent in both of these activities).

The triple catastrophe of 21st and 22nd of May of 1960 changed my life. Two earthquakes and a tidal wave knocked down the country in the middle, left a deep scar in the peoples' spirit, and seriously damaged the nation's economy. In Talcahuano, numerous people perished and most of the houses were fatally damaged, many of them falling or becoming uninhabitable. On the evening of May 22nd, a tsunami raised the level of the beach by ten feet, forcing neighboring populations to leave. At only 14 years of age, witnessing this natural destructive phenomenon was a devastating experience. During those days, our communication with the world was only through the radio and newspaper, so our imagination amplified the tragedy. But the reality was impressive. To walk on the wasteland watching our house, the school, and the only cinema demolished caused a combination of terrifying and dismal feelings. This experience accelerated my maturity. My father lost most of his savings and he decided to move the family to Concepción, a city near Talcahuano that was economically important at the national level. Concepción was well known as the Pearl of the Bío Bío (a river that surrounded the city) and had among its diverse facilities a prestigious university, founded in the year 1919. Within this setting in Concepción, a student atmosphere enveloped my world and influenced my development.

Without any clear idea of what I wanted to be in the future, and to a great extent to give my father personal satisfaction, I enrolled in the School of Medicine in the year 1963. I should say that my time in high school did not particularly steer me toward this area of study. My teachers of biology and chemistry, for example, were not particularly good, and I felt a strong tendency toward the humanities; I enjoyed writing poems and short stories, but my parents did not think it academically acceptable for a son to study such things in a university. According to my father, maybe if I had been a daughter!

My Life at the University

My university life was extremely enriching, not only in the academic sense but also in the political sense, an area in which I had no ideological formation. In a very heated time in Chile, the Revolutionary Leftist Movement (MIR in Spanish) was founded by a union of leftist students groups, primarily in Santiago, in August of 1965. However, this movement grew in the University of Concepción. It was led by great intellectuals such as Miguel Enríquez, Bautista van Schowen, and Luciano Cruz, who studied Medicine when I arrived at the university, and they had a truly deep effect on my beliefs and influenced my future. I must confess, at this point, that my family was highly conservative, and the leftist ideas, moderate or extreme, seemed to them outlandish and misguided. Thus, an abyss opened in our family life, particularly between my father and me, which was irreconcilable for several years (something I now have come to regret).

I enjoyed my college years; I learned medicine (in those times we memorized everything) and read expensive books, many of them from French or German authors that were difficult to obtain. I fleetingly fell in love a couple of times, participated in politics, and was a member of the glorious soccer team of the School of Medicine.

However, there was very little science taught (or learned). As medical students, we superficially and quickly studied physiology and biochemistry, but we lived counting the days until we were allowed to enter the hospitals and diagnose and treat actual patients. We were convinced that the hospital setting was the real place to understand and practice medicine.

I also introduced myself to the works of the formidable Latin American writers who drove my literary pilgrimage. I was delighted in reading Julio Cortazar—*Rayuela had* just been published—and, of course, Gabriel Garcia Marquez' wonderful *One Hundred Years of Solitude*. These and other fantastic writers, like Onetti, Puig, Fuentes, Vargas Llosa, Donoso, and Lezama Lima, among others, were part of the so called "Literary Boom" during the Cold War in Latin America. The "Boom" was in full swing throughout the 1960s and 1970s, although important pioneers, such as Jorge Luis Borges, were known earlier on the internationl scene. The "Boom" brought up a new genre of writing coined "magical realism" because the novels had a propensity to mix together magic and dream-like features with hard-hitting reality. These writers had a keen and rooted impact on my judgment of life. Primarily, they helped me to lose my innocence. The stories opened my mind about the complexity of people and Latin-American reality. Magical realism portrayed a fictional response to the political conditions of disruption and alienation that prevailed in our countries, and in this context this literature represented a transgression just in the time that I was, in some way, contravening the conventionl way of thinking.

The Dawning of a Broken Dream

I graduated in 1969, but in those times the School of Medicine of the University of Concepción was not authorized to grant the degree of Medical Doctor, and consequently, all graduates had to take part in month-long theoretical and practical examinations at the University of Chile in Santiago to receive an MD degree, which I finally obtained in the year of 1970.

In that year, Dr. Salvador Allende campaigned for the fourth consecutive occasion for the Presidency of the Republic of Chile. In a close election, he obtained the majority of the votes and was elected president by the National Congress. Thus, in 1970, he became the first Socialist president in the world to occupy the post democratically. Allende's administration, supported by the Popular Unity—a conglomerate of leftist parties—tried to establish an alternative way toward a socialist society, "the Chilean via to socialism." The coup d'etat led by General Augusto Pinochet on September 11, 1973 and the consequent assassination of Salvador Allende put an end to socialism in the Republic of Chile.

However, the three years of the Popular Unity had a profound effect on my life. I set out in my professional career as a General Physician in a new Hospital located between Concepción and Talcahuano, and then began to explore some specialties and a formal medical residence. Between 1971 and 1972, I traveled to Santiago with a scholarship to make a stay at the Thorax Hospital while I participated, in the heart of the country, in the dreamed construction of a newer and fairer world. Naturally, I was committed to the health care field, absolutely convinced that medical care and services must be free and of high quality in any public hospital. Nobody should be prevented from receiving medical care or university entrance because of economic reasons. Demanding substantive economical support for education in public universities was another personal battle that I fought.

The coup d'etat took me by surprise that day while I was at work in the Thorax Hospital, where my colleagues and I, along with general personnel and patients, saw the airplanes on their way to bomb La Moneda, the President's House where Allende died. Those were frightening moments, and the long months that followed were filled with terror, anxiety, and concern. Mass media were co-opted by military that also imposed a strict curfew during which nobody dared to move, and it was almost impossible to know what was really happening. Many friends and colleagues were detained or simply disappeared. Many of them were not really activists but had cooperated by using their professional knowledge in order make a better country. I moved underground from one place to another until I had the opportunity to escape from Chile.

Arriving in Mexico

On January 1974, I fled to Ecuador, and two months later I obtained the authorization of the Mexican Government to make a formal residence to study Pulmonary Medicine. I arrived in Mexico on April 8, full of frustrations and hopes, accompanied by my girlfriend Marcela and her son Matías, with whom I lived for some years.

México is a splendid and multifaceted country that received the exiled Chileans with open arms. Certainly, this gracious hospitality facilitated our lives, although the adjustment was difficult because the pain and angst of exile were always present.

During my residency, I fell in love with Pulmonary Medicine and had very good training in clinical practice. Nevertheless, as during my medical studies in Chile, scientific research did not play any role in my development; training involved almost exclusively the daily practice of the specialty: to prevent, diagnose, treat, and rehabilitate patients with lung disorders.

When I finished my residence in Mexico, the Director of the Thorax Hospital of the National Medical Center of the Mexican Institute of Social Security offered me a position, but I faced an unexpected problem. To work as a physician in Mexico, I needed a special certification, and to obtain it, the studies I did in Mexico were not enough. It also required some documents left behind when I fled Chile; I certainly did not have them, and it was virtually impossible to obtain them. Chile had since deprived me of my nationality, I did not have a passport, and nobody wanted to run the risk of going to ask for my papers in the middle of the persecutions that the military government had initiated.

Hence, I was unemployed for a couple of years and, to avoid starving, I found myself as a translator of comics, wrote television scripts, and participated in research, though not as a researcher but as the subject of experimentation.

During this hiatus, I frequently examined patients with lung disease from the Chilean colony in exile or my Mexican friends, and I did this at no cost. To relieve the tedium of my daily life, I decided to take basic science courses, particularly immunology. And, for the first time, I became imbued with some theoretical aspects concerning lymphocyte behavior and host defense mechanisms. This was an important step for my future. I was fascinated by the complexity and "intelligence" of the immune cells and the ways by which they process their own data and respond to external challenges. I suddenly understood that it is not possible to probe deeply into the causes and manifestations of a disease if we do not understand the pathogenic mechanisms driving the disease. It may sound a little bit ridiculous now, but 30 years ago this was a real revelation.

At the same time, I was becoming quite desperate for a job and began to consider other opportunities when a sudden stroke of luck changed my destiny. The parents of an asthmatic girl whom I occasionally took care of were appointed to an important position in the Mexican Government, and although my documents were still being processed, these individuals helped me get hired in a hospital of the Secretary of Health. I do not know why, but from several options I chose the Hospital of Huipulco.

My Arrival to the (future) National Institute of Respiratory Diseases

The Institute was a sanatorium for tuberculosis patients, known as the Sanatorium of Huipulco, and was built in 1936 in the midst of a small wood of cedars in the unpopulated outskirts of Mexico City. It was a horizontal construction, consisting of many small one-story buildings with large windows, surrounded by gorgeous and expansive gardens. When I arrived in the year 1978, the setting had retained its original beauty, and the hospital was devoted almost entirely to patients with tuberculosis, along with some minor interest in nontuberculous pathology.

When I began my work in general aspects of respiratory medicine, the academic environment at the Santorium of Huipulco was poorly defined. Nonetheless, I was extremely pleased to be practicing medicine given the difficulties I had faced in the previous few years.

The painful feelings of exile and a melancholy state of mind that plagued me in this new country continued for some time, as I passed from one crisis to the next, until one day I reached the moment of my unique and definitive decision. I decided to become a new man; I opened the suitcases and started to accept my Mexican shelter. I think that this idea was unconsciously running through my head for a long time before the instance of truth. I must say that many of those driven into exile broke up, and after some time, many families split when some members decided to return to Chile while others decided to remain in Mexico. It is impossible to describe a single tear in a dark storm.

My First Ripples and Eddies with Investigation

Six months after my arrival to the Hospital of Huipulco, the General Director passed away and was replaced by a young pulmonologist who resolved to reinvigorate the Institution. One day he called me to his office and said to me, "You surely have noticed that we have a research unit that is empty. I wonder if you would like to make it work." I was surprised and replied, "But I do not know anything about investigation; I am unable to distinguish a pipette from a test tube." "But, how can that be," he said to me, "if you know so much of immunology and of lymphocytes?" On second thought, some days later, I accepted the charge and became the head of an empty building that had been originally designed as a unit of experimental surgery.

Thus, I spent the next 12 months taking care of patients with nontuberculous pathology, taking small but definitive steps toward developing a scientific research program in a hospital virtually devoid of traditional research infrastructure.

I should emphasize that the problems facing my research were not difficulties found only at this hospital. In general, even today it is not easy to do research in developing countries. There are numerous limitations, including scarce government funding and almost zero private investment, an insufficient number of scientists as well as medical and graduate students, and inadequate public policies for research and development. Furthermore, our specialists are not interested in research. Generally speaking, our pulmonologists are primarily interested in assisting patients and tackling clinical problems and do not consider themselves scientists. Thus, the Pulmonary Medicine Divisions in most hospitals provide neither a suitable nor a stimulating environment for the physician-scientist.

My First Approach to the Field of Pulmonary Fibrosis

Several situations that accidentally coincided almost simultaneously led me to the field of pulmonary fibrosis. First, within a few weeks of my arrival at the hospital, two young women with slow progressive respiratory problems were admitted; their biopsies indicated "non-specified fibrosis." In hindsight, I believe that both had chronic hypersensitivity pneumonitis.

One of them, Pily, passed away a few weeks later. After all of these years, I clearly remember her. Pily was the only child of a needy family that worked in a rural area, and her family's desperation was evident. However, Pily was an introverted, quiet young woman that seemed to accept her destiny (our ignorance)

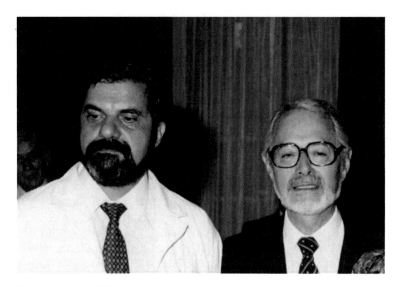

Fig. 6.3 My mentor Ruy Pérez Tamayo

without complaints. For me, our inability to treat her successfully was a devastating experience.

The second circumstance was learning of the elegant work of Ronald Crystal, who was then the Chief of the Pulmonary Branch, National Heart, Lung and Blood Institute, at the National Institutes of Health (NIH), which addressed different clinical and basic aspects of fibrotic lung disorders. At that time, the hot topic in this field was collagen, "the hallmark of the scars." However, in a controversial paper, Crystal asserted that: *"Although biopsies in idiopathic pulmonary fibrosis seem to show increased amounts of fibrotic tissue, biochemical studies suggest that the disease is probably one of collagen rearrangement to rather than collagen increase"*[1].

This was a terrific concept that I could not understand properly. Tormented by my ignorance in basic science, I decided to undertake a Master's in Sciences, and serendipidously chose as my mentor Dr. Ruy Pérez Tamayo (Fig. 6.3).

Ruy Pérez Tamayo

Ruy, an expert on liver fibrosis, was formative in my development as a researcher. He not only guided my steps toward laboratory tasks and experimental animals, but also revealed science as a universal concept that is tied to humankind's culture and progress. Although Ruy's superb research skills enabled him to be prominent in the area of fibrosis, perhaps his greatest legacy will lie in the many pre- and post-graduate students he has mentored over the years. Ruy is also an expert in the philosophy of sciences and wrote numerous books and essays related to epistemological, metaphysical, and ethical issues in the biological and biomedical sciences.

With him, I developed numerous experimental models in search of one that was representative of idiopathic pulmonary fibrosis (IPF), the most common form of pulmonary fibrosis in humans. Eventually, we developed a model that included a complicated combination of paraquat (a pesticide) and hyperoxia (high concentrations of oxygen).

Meanwhile, I wondered how to reconcile Crystal's biochemical findings with the morphological evidence that clearly showed an exaggerated deposition of collagens. I decided to quantify collagen in aliquots of lung tissues from patients with diffuse interstitial fibrosis that we believed was IPF. And, of course, collagen was significantly increased.

We tried fruitlessly to publish these findings in several prestigious journals in the USA. The answer we received from editors was always the same: "*If Crystal says there is no increment of collagen, then there is no increment in collagen.*" So, we published the paper in a little-known journal in Mexico that nobody read, and the results went unnoticed.

However, I continued working on the topic and included aspects related to collagen metabolism, and in 1986 I published in *Thorax* [2], an English journal, my findings that confirmed that collagen was increased in patients with IPF and that this increase was essentially related to a diminution in collagen degradation.

Annie Pardo

If I believed in destiny, I would say that destiny (*whatever it means*) programmed my encounter with Annie. Annie is the eldest daughter of a Bulgarian family who settled in Mexico after fleeing from Hitler's fascist violence during World War II. The invisible lines of understanding resulting from our respective exiles contributed to our cogent, enduring, and amazing affective relationship.

Annie has always safeguarded her Jewish Sephardic memory. She experienced the turbulent times of 1968, when the Mexican Government oppressed the student movement that was fighting for democracy. I am sure that our destinies crossed precisely from this point.

Annie studied Biology and later completed her PhD in Biochemistry, and in short time, she became interested in the connective tissue, mostly in collagen degradation. Annie was leaving Pérez Tamayo's laboratory to accept a head position at the laboratory of Biochemistry of the Faculty of Sciences when I arrived with Pérez Tamayo, and we superficially crossed our sights several times around the interstitial matrix. I confess that I liked her very much and was captivated with her brightness, strength of mind, and character. One evening in 1987, she called me to propose a collaborative project related to lung fibroblasts and collagenase. A year later we started living together, and since then, we have been cultivating extraordinarily strong and wonderful academic and emotional bonds. Together, we have made a fantastic journey through life.

While I developed my course in the National Institute of Respiratory Diseases, Annie, an outstanding mind, became a research leader and devoted faculty mentor

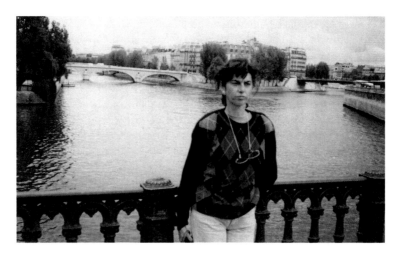

Fig. 6.4 Annie Pardo

at the National Autonomous University of Mexico. I have learned many things from her, particularly the three "C's" of science: curiosity, creativity, and critical thinking (Fig. 6.4). Furthermore, she has a striking sense of honor, and in this context, she is always guided by an astonishing and innate sense of what is and is not right.

When Annie and I started working together, the putative involvement of collagenases in the pathogenesis of lung remodeling was virtually unexplored in the field of interstitial lung diseases. We first began to examine the so-called fibroblast collagenase or matrix metalloproteinase (MMP)-1. Interestingly, we found that in IPF, this enzyme was expressed by epithelial cells, and it was virtually absent in the interstitium, where collagen, the substrate of fibrosis, was accumulating. With these and other findings, we hypothesized that a non-degradative microenvironment was at least partially responsible for the exaggerated collagen deposits in the fibrotic lung. We then explored other MMPs and finally, in collaboration with Naftali Kaminski a fantastic scientific and friend, we revealed using gene expression arrays that most of the members of the MMP family were transcribed in IPF lungs and that the degradome was also active in this disease. The transcriptional signature of IPF brought several surprises; one of them was that several MMPs, including MMP-1, were upregulated. But Annie and I believe that perhaps this is a matter of location and compartmentalization, and for some reason the enzyme did not reach the substrate.

The Challenge of Iasha Sznajder

Iasha is an individual of integrity and generosity without limits. I met him in Barcelona, Spain in 1990, during a hot Catalan autumn, in an Ibero-American meeting of Pulmonary Medicine that was the basis for the present Latin American Association of Thorax. Annie and Elena, Iasha's wife, met at the lobby of the hotel, talked for a while, and arranged a dinner for that same evening. Since then an increasing and deep friendship has developed between us. Iasha being a man of multiple exiles as well, our pasts brought us together.

In 1994, I obtained the John Simon Guggenheim grant, with the commitment to write a book on Interstitial Lung Diseases in Spanish. With this award plus additional support, Annie and I spent a year in Chicago on sabbatical at the Michael Reese Medical Center, at one point renowned, that was at that time in decay. Iasha was the Head of the Pulmonary and Critical Care Division, and with few resources but a bright intelligence he was doing cutting-edge research in the sodium/potassium ATPase field.

That year in Chicago was unforgettable. First of all, Chicago is a pluralistic and cosmopolitan city on the shores of Lake Michigan, which seemed like an ocean. Second, it was my first long-term stay in the USA, where I could for the very first time experience first-hand scientific developments in the front lines. I attended multiple sessions of basic sciences and clinical rounds, where I observed what we today call translational research. I heard the thoughts of the editors of some top journals in which I hoped to publish my own research from the distance of the Third World, and I lived vicariously through several cycles of NIH funding applications, witnessing the long wait for the answer and also experiencing the frustration of rejection when colleagues' grant applications were denied.

But my universe was not just science. Elena actively participated in a Reading Club with diverse Latin American friends of the most varied professions, and there we enjoyed our readings and high-minded discussions.

Years later, in 1999, Iasha called me at home and said—Moisés, as you know, we organize hot topics in pulmonary medicine, and in September this year we will hold the 4th Annual Chicago Conference on Current Issues in Pulmonary & Critical Care Medicine. In this context, we would like to include a debate between you and Jeff Myers (a remarkable pathologist, who I had not met but turned out to be a magnificent person, a great friend, and my preferred consultant for our toughest interstitial lung disease cases). At first, I didn't want to accept this invitation, mainly because of my poor spoken English. But my vanity imposed itself over my prudence and I accepted the challenge. The following week I telephoned and asked him what exactly the topic under debate was, and he answered, —the title is: "IPF is an inflammatory disease," pro side: Jeff Myers, contrary side: Moisés Selman. "But how can this be debated?" I said, "we all know that IPF *is an inflammatory disorder*, so how can I sustain the opposite?" "Well, that's your problem," he replied.

The Whispers of Wisdom

In the third century of our era, a king called Ts'ao decided to send his heir, young prince T'ai, to their holy shrine to meditate under the observation of the honorable master Pan Ku, so he would be worthy of becoming the next king. When young T'ai reached the holy place, the honorable tutor commissioned him to the Ming-Li Forest by himself for a year to detail the voices of the Forest.

After the year Pan Ku inquired young T'ai about all that he could hear from the Forest. "Honorable master," T'ai answered, "I learned songs from cuckoos and hummingbirds, gave my ears to the crickets, and the bees buzzing, and carefully attended the leaves stirring, the grass agitation, and the wind sighs and rage."

Young T'ai was demolished when the learned master shook his head and resolved that he must go back and discern more from the voices of the Forest. The royal heir was shocked. He said to himself, had not I clearly described what dwells in the Forest?

New mornings and sunsets young T'ai spent alone listening again to the Ming-Li Forest, but he was not able to distinguish a new voice from the Forest that he already had perceived. All of a sudden, while the prince meditated down below the trees, he was hooked by mysterious delicate sounds distant from the ones he knew so well. The more keenly he listened, the more audible the accents became. He got enlightened and told himself, "Now I can hear the unrevealed harmony the master cast me to contemplate."

Soon after, the prince met his master at the temple, and was questioned on his experience and he said, "Master, I heard the arcane movements of nature—the sound of flowers opening, the sound of the sun warming the earth, and the sound of the grass drinking the morning dew." The master approved. "To hear the unheard," elucidated Pan Ku, "is a necessary discipline to be a good ruler." (Harvard Business Review, July–August 1992)

In Search of a New Hypothesis About the Pathogenesis of IPF

I think that the ability to hear the unheard and to see the unseen is a key attribute necessary to discover the secrets of nature. Thus, in a very modest capacity, to debate against inflammation as a key element in the pathogenesis of IPF, I began to re-read pertinent papers, to dig deeply into the literature of experimental models, to analyze the morphological slides of early and advanced cases of IPF, and primarily to think in a completely different way, trying to hear the unheard. Surprisingly, three months later, I was convinced that IPF was, in fact, not an inflammation-driven form of fibrosis. The bases for this new hypothesis were simple. For one thing, inflammation is mild or at most moderate, and with the exception of the extent of the lesions and honeycombing, the disease actually looks morphologically the same during early and late stages. Additionally, long-term use of potent anti-inflammatory and immunosuppressive drugs is not effective, and the disease usually progresses until death. Also, some animal models indicate that it is possible to develop fibrosis without inflammation and, finally, there are several human fibrotic diseases in which inflammation is irrelevant.

Nevertheless, the obvious question was, if IPF is not an inflammatory disorder, what is it? Again, to hear the unheard, to see the unseen... I should emphasize here that I had the invaluable help of Annie, and of Talmadge King, a great pulmonologist and marvelous friend who quickly "bought" the idea. After numerous discussions, we postulated that IPF is an epithelial-fibroblastic disorder provoked by a miscommunication between these two cell types. This new hypothesis was a watershed in the knowledge of the pathogenesis of IPF, and I dare say, it has had a profound effect in our experimental and therapeutic approaches to the disease.

The Innocent Birds and Hypersensitivity Pneumonitis

From the beginnings of my academic course, I was intrigued by hypersensitivity pneumonitis (HP), a lung disorder provoked by exposure to a variety of organic particles.

Mexico has an incredible variety of birds. Mexicans love birds, and it is a common hobby to have a few of them as pets. Actually, I think that Mexico has the largest number of songs devoted to birds! Therefore, HP provoked by the exposure to avian proteins from pigeons, canaries, budgerigars, and parakeets, among other birds, is a relatively frequent interstitial lung disease in my country. Importantly, this type of HP, called pigeon (or bird) breeder's (or fancier's) disease is quite peculiar in many ways, and it was shown to be different from farmer's lung, which was the most frequent and studied form of HP when we became involved with this problem. Probably the main difference was the clinical form, usually acute in the case of farmer's lung, and subacute or often chronic in the case of bird-provoked disease, among other reasons because of the type of exposure (intermittent and intense versus continual and low-level) and perhaps because of the type of antigens.

Although difficult to believe, it was nearly impossible to convince the international scientific community that HP could be chronic and evolve to fibrosis even in the absence of antigen exposure. Furthermore, a number of patients with chronic HP could die of progressive fibrosis. After some modest papers published regarding putative pathophysiological mechanisms, in 1993 we published a now seminal paper showing that chronic pigeon breeder's disease had a high rate of mortality, and moreover, we suggested that patients with chronic HP with usual interstitial pneumonia (UIP)-like pattern in the biopsy exhibited a survival rate similar to that of patients with idiopathic pulmonary fibrosis.

It has been also quite difficult to convince people that having birds as pets may be dangerous. *But, how come? They are so cute and innocent; a pigeon is the symbol of peace!*

During the last 15 years, we have tried to understand more fully the different molecular aspects of the pathogenesis of HP. For example, we determined the role of some matrix metalloproteinases in the development of HP-related lung fibrosis, the participation of the major histocompatibility complex in the genetic susceptibility, and the role of newly described chemokines in the migration of lymphocytes to the lung. After a careful review of a number of HP cases, we noticed that we were observing a new clinical/pathological entity that we called airway-centered interstitial fibrosis. The latter showed some similarities in the airway lesions, but lacked the characteristic HP features in the surrounding parenchyma and, importantly, it seemed to have a worse outcome. More recently, we described for the first time the presence of fetal microchimeric cells in HP lungs, and we made a substantial contribution to understanding the phenotypic and functional behavior of the immune response in subacute and chronic cases. Hypersensitivity pneumonitis is a multifaceted disease, and I think it can teach us about many aspects of the inflammatory-driven forms of fibrosis.

The Research Unit at INER, My Other Son

I feel extremely proud of the progressive development and maturation of our Research Unit. From the early 1980s, we incorporated young biologists, chemists, and pulmonologists, encouraging them to accomplish graduate studies by guiding them to think critically about clinical and basic pulmonary research and stimulate them to pursue scientific endeavors. Also, we gradually improved the laboratories' infrastructure, struggling with our administrative authorities—most of whom believed we were wasting our time resolving useless puzzles—and engendered the formation of groups interested in diverse respiratory topics. All of these issues led to the establishment of several productive groups of research not only in fibrotic lung disorders, but also in chronic obstructive pulmonary disease, AIDS, sleep apnea, tuberculosis, and asthma, among others. These groups have made important scientific contributions under suboptimal conditions, including lack of funding and miserable salaries.

Conclusions

Thirty years with continuous changes in direction made me become a physician-scientist, a rare avis in a developing country. This unparalleled experience and dual role gave me, on the one hand, the capacity of assisting patients and resolving human dilemmas, and on the other hand, the chance to bring clinical observations to the laboratory for in-depth study and to translate basic science into medicine, thus contributing findings, almost always modest, to the collective body of knowledge and proposing a better management of the medical issues faced all the time.

My job has given me multiple satisfactions: I have been honored to receive several awards, including the National Prize of Science and Arts, México in 2008, the highest distinction that the Mexican government awards to its intellectuals, artists, and scientists, and the Recognition Award for Scientific Achievement of the American Thoracic Society in 2009.

However, I must emphasize that these accomplishments have been the result of a group work (Fig. 6.5), and many pulmonologists working in the clinical service and PhD scientists working in the lab have made strong contributions to the generation of ideas and to the development of research in the field of interstitial lung diseases.

Unfortunately, the fibrosis field is still full of uncertainty, we ignore much more than we know, and the current treatments for managing these disorders, in general, and idiopathic pulmonary fibrosis, in particular, are far from being optimum.

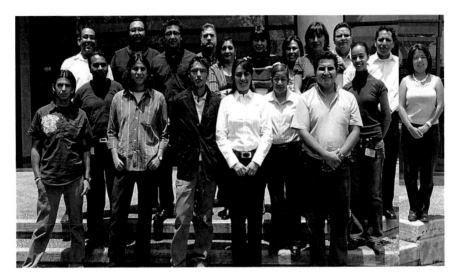

Fig. 6.5 The staff in the National Institute of Respiratory Diseases dedicated to fibrotic lung disorders

Nevertheless, I hope that in the not-too-distant future our knowledge in functional genomics, proteomics, epigenetics, and other basic sciences will open new paths for understanding and healing fibrosis. Hopefully, we will generate powerful new tools for studying the initiation and progression of IPF, enhancing our capacity to reveal the secrets of disease susceptibility and engendering new opportunities for preventive medicine and effective treatment.

References

1. Fulmer JD, Bienkowski RS, Cowan MJ, Breul SD, Bradley KM, Ferrans VJ, Roberts WC, Crystal RG (1980) Collagen concentration and rates of synthesis in idiopathic pulmonary fibrosis. Am Rev Respir Dis 122:289–301
2. Selman M, Montaño M, Ramos C, Concentration CR (1986) biosynthesis and degradation of collagen in idiopathic pulmonary fibrosis. Thorax 41:355–359

Seven
Sputnik, Slime Molds, and Botticelli in the Making of a Physician-Scientist

R. Sanders Williams

Sputnik and *Hemo the Magnificent*

Establishing a clear chain of cause and effect in any person's life is an inherently uncertain business, but I can say with some confidence that my career as a physician-scientist had its origins on my ninth birthday on October 4, 1957, when Sputnik (Fig. 7.1) was launched into orbit by the Soviet Union. I recall noting the event itself with some fascination, but it was the response of our public education system

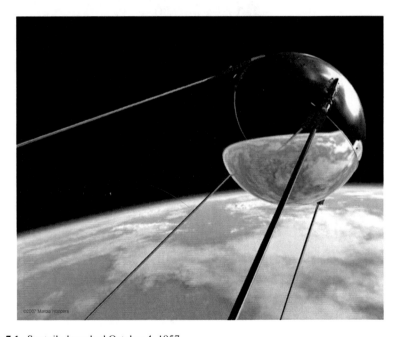

Fig. 7.1 Sputnik, launched October 4, 1957

R.S. Williams (✉)
The J. David Gladstone Institutes, University of California, San Francisco, CA, USA
e-mail: rswilliams@mc.duke.edu

D.A. Schwartz (ed.), *Medicine Science and Dreams*,
DOI 10.1007/978-90-481-9538-1_7, © Springer Science+Business Media B.V. 2011

to the "missile gap" [1] perceived by US policy-makers that really had a formative effect, because, for the next few years at least, my classrooms became filled with a wondrous array of materials for learning science. More important still, and in contrast to the American cultural milieu of more recent decades, being good at science in the 1950s and 1960s was perceived by me and many of my contemporaries as a pretty cool thing to do.

Another recollection from that time was seeing the film *Hemo the Magnificent* (Fig. 7.2), which provided my first introduction to human biology as a science. I can remember nothing at all about the film, except that it portrayed the functions of hemoglobin in a way I found exciting, and it stoked some appetite to understand the mechanisms of how things work in our bodies. Interestingly, *Hemo the Magnificent* was produced by Frank Capra, who also gave us the American classics *Mr. Smith Goes to Washington* and *It's a Wonderful Life*, thus illustrating the positive and meaningful connection between science and mainstream culture at that time. Without the effects of Sputnik on the priorities of the American educational establishment of the late 1950s, along with the perception I gained as a young boy that science is cool, my pathway could have been much different.

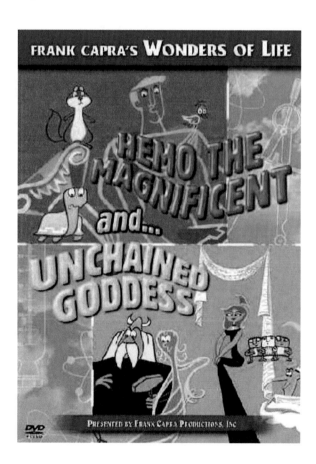

Fig. 7.2 *Hemo the Magnificent*, a film directed by Frank Capra

Saving the World, and Enter the Slime Molds

"Know thyself" [2] is an important maxim for any person, but for me the process of coming to know myself in a way that translated into career choices was a protracted one. My interest in science, kindled in the aftermath of Sputnik, was a thread that ran consistently throughout my high school and college years, but it only led to career choices late in my university experience and even beyond. As my friend Peter Agre noted recently in his introduction as the President of the American Association for the Advancement of Science, almost every successful scientist can look back and recall one or more teachers who inspired a love of scientific reasoning and discovery, and this was true for me. A high school physics teacher, Jack Carter, brought a mischievous wit to the art of experimentation in the classroom. I also had the great advantage during summer vacations in high school of taking college level math from John Christmas in the Georgia Governor's Honors School and chemistry from Mitchell Sienko and Robert Plane at Cornell University in a National Science Foundation program, where I was surrounded by kids from other schools (including some attractive girls) who shared my admiration of science as a cool endeavor. After high school, I attended Princeton, where chemistry professor John Turkevich imparted an irrepressible joy to the understanding of the breaking and forming of chemical bonds, and the whispered allusions among my fellow students to his shadowy but integral role in the Manhattan Project gave him a glamorous aura as well. Hubert Alyea, legendary to generations of Princeton students for his showmanship in illustrating principles of physics in the classroom, was similarly inspiring. The pivotal experience, however, came in a junior year biology course taught at Princeton by John Bonner, and centered on the fascinating story of the slime mold, *Dictyostelium discoideum*. I'll get to that story in a moment, after describing the inefficient but ultimately useful pathway my college experience took in between.

I had exceptional good fortune to have gained a strong background in natural sciences during my high school years and early college years, but my first two years at Princeton also opened other new worlds of knowledge I had not tasted before, at least not at a similarly invigorating level. My first exposure to sophisticated interpretations of literature led to lots of electives on American and European writers (sadly, Western culture dominated almost completely the university canon at that time, of course), and I had a period of fascination with foreign policy that led me into demanding courses in economics, political science, and modern history. I even took a course in American Constitutional Law. At the time I was not at all pre-medical. I reveled in the tutorial method that characterized the Princeton undergraduate experience, where students in small groups had to formulate and defend our ideas to peers, usually with only minimal poking and prodding from the professor. Ever a quietly fierce competitor, I sought entry into the undergraduate program of Princeton's Woodrow Wilson School (WWS) of Public and International Affairs as my major. Admission to the WWS was based on competition for a limited number of undergraduate slots (good preparation for writing grants later), and once enrolled, students participated in structured policy conferences in addition to conventional course work. These exercises involved teamwork with fellow students to divide a major topic into component parts and then put it back together again with policy recommendations in a final report. I recall two of these, focused on "Academic Freedom" and "Public Health in America," for which the final products were forgettable, but the experience was not. My ideas then about where this poly-glot educational background was leading as a career were fuzzy, to be sure, but I suppose I imagined myself grandiosely as a future Secretary of State, wisely and adroitly directing American know-how, magnanimity, and power to bring solutions to trouble spots around the globe, and saving the world from the threat of nuclear winter (since global warming and an end to humanity by fire instead of ice was not yet evident). In more expansive moments, I also imagined myself producing time-less works of masterful literature on the side. My pantheon of heroes (there was a sad paucity of heroines known to me at the time) spanned Faulkner, Melville, Lippman, Kennan, Marshall, Marcuse, Dylan, and Sandy Koufax.

Now let us return to the slime molds. During my junior year of college, though I was well-established within my public policy major, leading a policy conference on academic freedom, and writing a novel (which proved to be quite forgettable in itself but greatly rewarding for the experience), I took biology as an elective. My flirtation with public policy and my fantasies of becoming a famous man of letters were soon to be subsumed by what ultimately was to become the true love of my intellectual and professional life (the true love of my romantic life was yet to appear, but hap-pily she did so later during medical school). Aspects of this biology course remain fresh in my mind today. I recall that I could not stop pondering the way in which the cellular slime molds challenge the distinction between unicellular and multicellu-lar organisms. Living happily as microscopic, unicellular amoebae in the soil when nutrients are plentiful, *Dictyostelia* respond to lean times and food deprivation by merging together, forming a macroscopic, multicellular structure known as a fruit-ing body (Fig. 7.3) by which they reproduce in the form of spores. These long-lived spores can rest dormant until the right conditions promote their maturation to restore the autonomous unicellular lives of slime mold amoebae, as they blissfully resume hunting bacteria among soil particles. While the description of this remarkable bit of arcana from the natural world was interesting in itself, what really caught my atten-tion is that a chemical signal controlling this behavior had been deciphered. What a fabulous accomplishment of human intelligence, and what a definitive and satisfying answer to a question! Within a very short time, my prior interests in nuclear diplo-macy or in understanding the historical dynamics that brought violent revolution to France but not to Britain began to suffer by comparison.

I did not abandon the WWS, but navigated the program successfully for the cer-tificate establishing my credentials in public and international affairs that still adorns my wall today, plus I did complete my novel. However, after meeting the slime molds, I set my course on medical school and molecular biology. This required me to take some extra courses in summer school, and it required some adventurous medical school to be willing to relax some of their requirements for prerequisite science courses and admit me. As great good fortune for me, a few very good ones did.

Fig. 7.3 Fruiting bodies of
the cellular slime mold

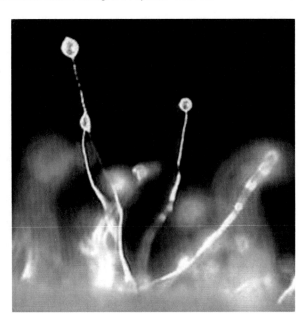

The Ceiling of the Sistine Chapel, in Biochemistry Class

I chose Duke (Fig. 7.4), the youngest of the nation's research-intensive medical schools, primarily because of its unique curriculum that in effect compresses what other schools teach in four years into two, thereby permitting students to pursue individually designed research in the third year and select clinical clerkships tailored to their interests in the fourth. Coming from my public policy major and having steered clear of the pre-med advisory system, I was not well informed or savvy enough yet to understand the potential value of a combined MD–PhD program, but fortunately things worked out quite well anyway, and ultimately I was able to earn what might justifiably be called a PhD equivalent through a series of postdoctoral research experiences.

The first year of medical school at Duke, then as now, required students to run a demanding gauntlet of examinations that seemed to occur continuously, interspersed between lectures and labs that presented the course material at a dizzying pace. My classmates and I, like generations of medical students everywhere I suppose, managed this through comradeship, offbeat humor, and lots of hours in the library. I recall some pride in attaining familiarity with seemingly arcane medical terms and concepts. "Subacute bacterial endocarditis," "right bundle branch block with left anterior hemiblock," "the pores of Zahn," or the "Accessory Duct of Santorini" sound commonplace now, but stood out then as marvels of medical argot. The dominant memory, however, of that first year of medical school for me was an epiphany I experienced in biochemistry class as I first got my mind around the orchestral beauty of intermediary metabolism, and the breathtakingly simple elegance of "how

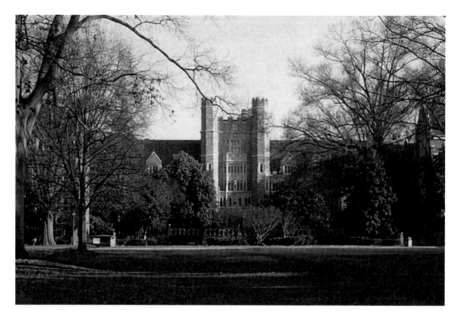

Fig. 7.4 Duke University School of Medicine

DNA makes RNA makes protein." Francis Crick called this the "central dogma of molecular biology," a curious choice of words for a scientist since we are trained to reject dogma and demand evidence, but I think he was sending a message about the provisional nature of the explanations scientists provide about how the natural world works. It's important to recall that knowledge of the genetic code was only 4 years old when I entered medical school in 1970, and my interest in biological science that was sparked by the slime molds in college was brought into full flame by first year biochemistry in medical school.

Physician-Scientist Means Physician First

The curriculum at Duke plunged its students directly out of the first year of classroom and laboratory work into patient care experiences with medical students functioning as integral members of hospital ward teams. I have likened this to learning how to swim. If learned correctly at the start, the basic movements, style, and form of a first-class physician in questioning and examining patients, and in drawing conclusions that guide medical decisions, become imbedded in deep memory and are not forgotten, even if in subsequent years periods of patient care responsibility are sandwiched between months or even years of laboratory work away from daily contact with patients. Factual information in memory must be refreshed and amplified frequently, of course, and sometimes unlearned as medical research corrects fallacious dogmas of the past, but the fundamental thought processes of good doctoring should last a lifetime. I learned first hand how good doctors think and act from Eugene Stead, Sam Katz, Jim Wyngaarden, Bill Kelly, David Sabiston, Bruce Dixon, and many others. It is essential, I believe, for physician-scientists to have intensive clinical training, since for most of our professional lives, we will care for patients as a part-time calling. I had the benefit of such experiences at Duke, and later in my residency at the Massachusetts General Hospital, where master clinicians like Roman DeSanctis, George Thibault, Lloyd Axelrod, Dolph Hutter, Peter Yurchak, and many others engrained in me an approach to patient care that became part of the permanent software of my nervous system.

Botticelli Had It Right

During my year of research at Duke, I decided to purify the regulatory subunit of cyclic adenosine monophosphate (cAMP)-dependent protein kinase (now known as PKA) by synthesizing a covalently linked multimer of cAMP that we hoped would bind its protein target to form a unique complex we could identify and isolate by gel filtration or affinity chromatography. It is cAMP, by the way, that provides the intracellular signal for the clarion call of the cellular slime molds to merge and form the fruiting body in response to food deprivation. Working at Duke with Francis Neelon (who also was a poet given to extemporaneous renditions in the laboratory of Wallace Stevens or Proust) and Hal Leibovitz, I made some interesting progress. Predictably, however, as I can see now, the goal was beyond the scope of a student's capacity in one year. Nevertheless, this early experience with its accompanying coursework in the theory and practice of the molecular biology of that era, which was provided through Duke's innovative Research Training Program, taught me a lot about good laboratory technique and about the daily activities of laboratory-based scientists. I liked what I saw, and I took the first opportunity to return to lab life as a postdoctoral fellow after my medical residency. It was then that I had the most outstanding luck in choosing Bob Lefkowitz as my postdoctoral mentor, working in a cardiology division headed by Andy Wallace.

These two gentlemen became the people of most importance to my destiny as a physician-scientist. When traveling from Boston to interview at Duke, I was immediately enamored of Bob's personal style. Returning sweaty from a midday jog to meet with me, he launched into a cascade of irreverent observations, witticisms, and aphorisms delivered staccato in that New York accent now known so well throughout the scientific world. Bob's love for doing science was immediately infectious, but I had little concept then how well I had chosen in being drawn to Bob as a mentor. Years after graduating from Bob's lab, I could still hear his voice in my mind as I grappled with decisions in the laboratory. It should evoke little wonder that my own path in science was most successful when I listened to that voice, and less so when I rebelliously chose to ignore it. I accomplished a few things in Bob's lab relating to the characterization of adrenergic receptor subtypes in the mammalian heart and the regulation of adrenergic receptor properties by hormonal and physiological stimuli, but that was not what was really important. Bob taught me what serious biomedical science is all about, and he showed me how it is done at the highest level.

Andy Wallace pioneered modern cardiac electrophysiology through his contributions to the understanding of the pathobiology of Wolff–Parkinson–White syndrome in human patients, and to its surgical cure. This was not the scientific area I chose to investigate, but Andy became my role model for how to combine the life of a physician-scientist with leadership roles in academic medicine, and to explore a broad range of serious intellectual, cultural, family, and athletic interests. With Bob Lefkowitz and Andy Wallace as role models, and ultimately lifelong friends, I have been fortunate indeed!

I had much to learn for myself. However, to reach anything close to a satisfying level of achievement as a physician-scientist took years longer than my contact with Bob and Andy as a trainee. I didn't really grasp the most important principle of doing excellent science for almost ten years after my first introduction to laboratory work as a medical student. Most important, I believe, is this: success in research requires that the researcher must fall in love with the question under study. A deep interest in biology, a curiosity about how things work in our bodies, and an affinity for the intellectual environment of a great university with an outstanding medical center—these are necessary but not sufficient. Ambition helps, but yearning for fame, power, and wealth is misplaced (and unlikely). It is true love of the scientific question, I believe, that drives success in science.

I'll explain further what I mean based on my own history in the laboratory. In my initial laboratory experiences at Duke, I relished the environment, and I was interested by the scientific questions that were the focus of my work at every stage, but I was working on questions that belonged primarily to others and not to me. I carried on the research happily enough, drawing great benefit from the experiences, but I had not yet found my own true scientific love from among the questions we were seeking to answer. I did find Jennifer, my real true love romantically and still my bride, at Duke during medical school, but that story would require another chapter, or an entire book, and I will not tell it here. In science, however, I had to look ten years longer for true love. Between 1972 and around 1984, my work as a scientist was productive: I wrote papers that were published in top journals; I wrote grants that were funded; I earned academic promotions. However, I was not in love with the problems I was studying. In large measure they were borrowed as side tracks from the main lines of investigation in Bob Lefkowitz's lab, merged with interests inherited from Andy Wallace in his second incarnation (after WPW) as a leader in preventive cardiology. From this background, however, like Aphrodite's natal emergence from the sea in Botticelli's masterpiece (Fig. 7.5), I found the problem to love, and this sustained me for decades of satisfying work in the lab.

The question I fell in love with is this: How does the body know and remember that it exercised yesterday, or the day before, and convert that experience into molecular, biochemical, and structural changes in cells and tissues in ways that make us fitter and healthier? The question is not unlike the one that John Bonner asked about the slime molds that led to my early interest in molecular biology: How do the slime mold amoebae know that food is scarce and convert that information into

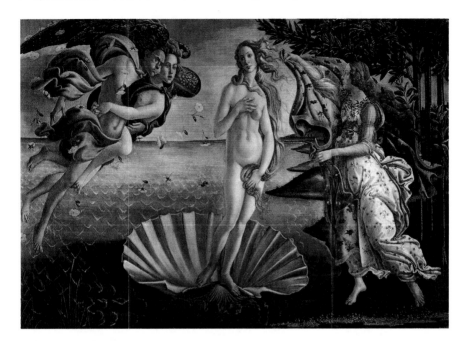

Fig. 7.5 Botticelli: "The Birth of Aphrodite"

such dramatic biological events that ensure their reproduction and survival? I don't know how long Bonner worked to find a satisfying answer, but for me it took 20 years—a wonderful 20 years I would add—and, like most scientific problems, the answers we found led to more questions.

My instincts told me I had found my question, but to truly earn my love, it had to pass three tests that through years of application and repetition to trainees I have dubbed as the "*So what?*", "*Why me?*", and "*What next?*" screens. In my case, a serious effort to elucidate the molecular signaling pathways by which repeated physical activity produces the constellation of cellular adaptations that collectively promote fitness (greater capacity for physical work performance) and health (freedom from disease and greater longevity) seemed clearly to pass the "*So what?*" screen. In almost all cultures, humans have been aware since antiquity that regular exercise produces salutary effects on fitness and health. This can be observed as a feature of everyday personal experience by folks who like to exercise, or through observations of athletes by those who prefer a sedentary existence. Solid epidemiological analyses consistently demonstrate lower rates of heart disease and greater longevity in humans who engage habitually in physical activity as adults through work or recreation. A lucid explanation of the molecular mechanisms of exercise-induced adaptations would be interesting to many, and potentially useful in the development of better strategies to prevent and treat disease.

"*Why me?*" Even if the question that most interested me was unquestionably important, on what basis was I well-suited to study the problem and succeed in advance of competitors? By the mid-1980s, I had acquired a reasonably sophisticated understanding of the physiology and biochemistry of exercise through my clinical experiences in exercise testing and rehabilitation of patients with heart disease. In addition, through my training with Bob Lefkowitz and my early independent work in adrenergic receptor biochemistry, I had an advantage over physiologists with less advanced biochemical training. But the most important insight that gave me the clearest advantage over competitors was to reduce this classical problem of whole body physiology to the level of gene regulation in a single cell type, and to find an appropriate and powerful model system to facilitate the work. Thus, I redefined the question of "How does habitual exercise make us fit and healthy?" to "How does a skeletal muscle fiber sense that it has been actively contracting for sustained periods of time and transmit this information to the genome, thereby regulating the genes that drive the important physiological adaptations to increase work performance and to alter intermediary metabolism in health-promoting ways (e.g., greater insulin sensitivity)?" Although the Jacob–Monod model of gene regulation had been known for years by the mid-1980s, techniques for discovering transcription factors and how they are regulated in mammalian cells were just being developed.

I realized that to define my question in this way, I needed some additional training in recombinant DNA technology and in methods for identification and study of transcription factors to complement what I had already learned about exercise physiology and the biochemistry of signal transduction pathways. My firm belief in the importance of the question I wanted to study (*"So what?"*), and my sense that I could gain competitive advantage on other scientists interested in same question by applying the latest techniques of molecular biology (*"Why me?"*), led me to take an unconventionally bold and risky step, the success of which made all the difference in my subsequent career. I am sure my Department Chairman in 1983, Joe Greenfield, was shocked when I told him that after only three years on the faculty, I wanted to give up my cardiology clinic, my attending and consult rounds, and other clinical duties of an Assistant Professor, as well as to mothball my lab and give back an unfinished NIH grant, in order to pursue this new direction by becoming a postdoc again for a year! To his everlasting credit, he saw the opportunity too, and gave me a year's leave, stipulating only that, "You pay for it yourself!" A fair deal, I thought. So in 1984, with Jennifer and the first two of my three children at my side, I left Duke for the Biochemistry Department at Oxford in the UK (Fig. 7.6), sponsored liberally by both an Established Investigator Award from the American Heart Association and a Fogarty International Fellowship from NIH. Chairman Rodney Porter, a Nobel Laureate, graciously welcomed me to his department and set me up to work at the interface of two labs, one run by Eric Newsholme, a trainee of Hans Krebs and an expert in muscle metabolism, and the other by Alan and Sue Kingsman, rising stars in molecular biology. Up the road from Oxford as well, at Birmingham University, was Stanley Salmons, who had developed an animal model I thought ideal for application to the work I had in mind. My guardian angel proved to be Kingsman postdoc Jane Mellor, whose patience and grace in guiding my first stumbling steps in the manipulation of DNA and RNA was a godsend.

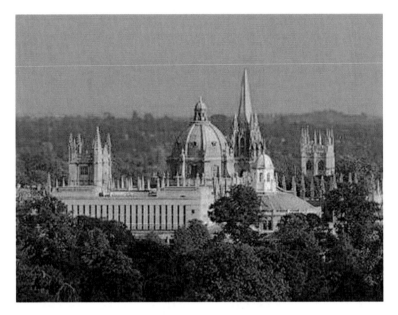

Fig. 7.6 Oxford, UK

By the end of the year in Oxford, I was adept at all the basics of "gene jockeying" and my medical training, I suppose, which had engrained an innate sense of sterile technique, helped to make me rather a local master at preserving the integrity of RNA during complex extractions from adult animal tissues. The intensity of that year, free from committee meetings and patient care duties, led to my first two important papers in my new field. I showed that tonic patterns of motor nerve stimulation innervating skeletal muscles, a surrogate for exercise training, transformed white, glycolytic fibers to red oxidative fibers, and that the mitochondrial biogenesis stimulated as an important feature of this transformation was accompanied by an increased copy number of mitochondrial DNA, along with an increased abundance of mRNA transcripts of both mitochondrial and nuclear genes encoding proteins essential for oxidative metabolism. Thus, activation of mitochondrial biogenesis in an animal model of endurance exercise was reduced to a problem of gene regulation, opening the door to 20 years of identifying the specific first and second messengers, protein kinases, protein phosphatases, transcription factors, scaffold proteins, and pathway modifiers that are engaged in sensing and transducing exercise-induced biochemical signals. Even before returning to Duke, I secured a major NIH grant within the first ever request for application put out by the National Heart, Lung, and Blood Institute to focus on molecular signals in cardiac hypertrophy, which I won out over several more famous labs. I was off and running, and by 1986 the "*Why me?*" question had been answered successfully.

With "*So what?*" and "*Why me?*" in the bag, the "*What next?*" question loomed larger, and led me down a number of interesting scientific and career development pathways. In the conventional parlance of career progression, my lab at Duke was highly productive between 1985 and 1990, largely through the efforts of exceptional postdocs and students who joined my group during that period. Several folks from that period have become scientific and academic leaders in their own right, including: Ivor Benjamin as Chief of Cardiology at the University of Utah and noted expert on heat shock transcription factors; Brian Annex as Chief of Cardiology at the University of Virginia with major accomplishments in angiogenic signaling mechanisms; Ludwig Neyses as head of cardiology at Manchester University Medical Center in the UK; and Bill Kraus who became a leader in the genetics of early onset cardiovascular disease. A reductionist decision I made during this period bore fruit for a long time when we chose the myoglobin gene as our primary readout for signals that promote transformation of white glycolytic myofibers into red oxidative fibers. We extended our studies into the developmental biology of muscle specialization, in addition to continued work on models of muscle subtype transformation induced by changing patterns of neuronal firing in adult animals.

The measure of success I was having at Duke in the 1980s made other schools start to call, and after saying "No thanks" to several interesting opportunities, in 1990 I said "Yes!" to the University of Texas Southwestern (UT) in Dallas, and moved there as Chief of Cardiology and Director of the Ryburn Center for Molecular Cardiology. A decision by a physician-scientist to take on an administrative leadership role is distinctly hazardous, and I suspect an epidemiological analysis would reveal more casualties than successes with respect to an individual's subsequent scientific productivity, especially in procedure-based specialties like cardiology. This is why the Howard Hughes Medical Institute discourages its investigators from taking on leadership roles beyond their own labs. However, the evident primacy of science within the institutional culture of UT Southwestern convinced me that the leadership opportunity there, in contrast to what might prove true elsewhere, would be empowering to my science and not a quagmire of administrative headaches, and this proved true—even more so than I could have wished.

Between 1990, when I arrived in Dallas, and 2001, when I returned to Duke, I hit my stride as a scientist, producing the most important research of my career, working with terrific trainees, and establishing scientific partnerships that were exceptionally rewarding and fun. One step at a time, my colleagues and I developed an efficient engine of discovery that combined a few clever and creative insights with technically sophisticated experimental capabilities ranging from yeast two-hybrid screens and transcriptome profiling to conditional gene knockouts in mice, thereby elucidating features of the biological wiring diagram that determines how patterns of motor neuron activity drive the formation of specialized phenotypes of striated myofibers—a molecular basis for a major feature of the exercise training response that explains why a trained marathon runner can complete a hilly 26 mile race at a mind boggling speed, while others fatigue in ascending one flight of stairs (and why a chicken breast looks different from a duck breast or a chicken leg). We discovered some novel genes and proteins, and we discovered some novel functions for other signaling molecules already known. We also got scooped a few times when other labs were first to discover some of the critical genes and proteins in this system. The work is not finished, by any means, nor have the fundamental discoveries been extended to the point of revealing highly druggable targets within the signaling machinery through which our discoveries could best be translated into new therapeutics. However, that period left fond memories of the high excitement of discovery, and of the pure pleasure of feeling oneself a part of successful team. Virologist Rhonda Bassel-Duby was invaluable in most everything my lab accomplished during this period, and the chance to share ideas freely and collaborate with Eric Olson, one the greatest scientists of our time, was unforgettable. I'm also proud that close colleagues and trainees from this period distinguished themselves. Stephen Johnson, perhaps the first yeast geneticist to hold an endowed Chair in a cardiology division anywhere, was my first senior recruit and he brought intellectual rigor, technological sophistication, incredible creativity, and a maverick spirit to everything we did in our molecular cardiology unit. Tom Kodadek taught us how to use real chemistry to tame our biological systems, and later won a Pioneer Award. Skip Garner was our resident physicist who put his background at General Dynamics to work on computational and engineering innovations that empowered our work. To name only a few of the trainees: Dan Garry is Chief of Cardiology at Minnesota and a leader in stem cell biology, Ralph Shohet leads Cardiology at the University of Hawaii, and Beverly Rothermel has done important work on the RCAN gene family. Paul Rosenberg first moved our focus to the cell membrane with the observation that transient receptor potential (TRP) channels provide a signaling pool of calcium important for driving muscle specialization, and he and my latest K08 mentee Jonathan Stiber are pursuing this work in very interesting ways. Many other trainees are still in the pipeline, with great things yet to come, to be sure.

My growth as scientist at UT Southwestern was greatly abetted by a few others I must mention. Dan Foster, beloved as my Department Chair, did more than anyone else to encourage my scientific development while fulfilling my duties as Clinical Division Chief. David Hillis and later John Rutherford served as Clinical Chiefs to keep me in the lab. I believe such partnerships between a lab-based chief and a master clinician co-chief will be found in the most successful academic divisions of clinical departments. The Texas "giants"—Mike Brown, Joe Goldstein, Al Gilman, and Joe Sambrook—took me under wing, each in a different way, and made me a better thinker about how top science should be done. In 1995 and 1996, I realized a longstanding dream and spent a year working at the Cold Spring Harbor Laboratory (Fig. 7.7) on Long Island, where Director Bruce Stillman graciously gave me an opportunity to return to the bench in postdoc mode. Our work in Dallas had revealed a novel transcription factor that functions to modulate important steps in the transitions of adult myogenic stem cells to and from quiescence during muscle regeneration, and I wished to expand my understanding of cell cycle controls and DNA replication to pursue this lead. Since Cold Spring Harbor is the crossroads of top biological science for the world over, this experience allowed me to meet and share ideas with a cavalcade of the world's best, in addition to participating first hand in Bruce Stillman's brilliant combination of genetics and biochemistry in both yeast and human model systems to elucidate how DNA replication is initiated. The

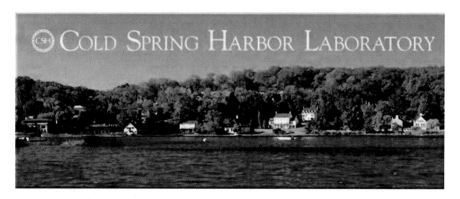

Fig. 7.7 Cold Spring Harbor Laboratory

experience of rubbing shoulders with all of these incredible stars was invaluable to my development, and I only wish I could have done it as well as the standards they set, and as Bob Lefkowitz had taught.

One Life but Three Careers

The year 2000 was perhaps the most productive of my entire scientific career with respect to the number and quality of important papers published from my lab. In addition, we had reached an enviable level of funding from NIH and other sources, and I had outstanding trainees, terrific infrastructure, and the best colleagues imaginable. So what perverse impulse led me to give up such a fine situation to embark on the quite different job I accepted to become Dean of the School of Medicine at Duke in 2001? It clearly was neither that my powers as a scientist (such as they were) were fading, nor was there anything whatsoever negative about the wonderful environment at UT Southwestern. Many of my scientific colleagues were shocked and dismayed that one of their stalwart comrades had gone over to the "dark side" of academic administration. Holly Smith, a greatly admired hero from the University of California, San Francisco, remarked sardonically (though kindly) that "Dean" is only one letter removed from "Dead." My love affair with the scientific life was not over, but, as a distinguished Texas colleague commented, I seemed "to be seized by a moment of reckless idealism" in wanting to become a senior administrator. Idealistic and unselfish, it was indeed, at least to some degree. I had enjoyed the ability to help others prosper in academic medicine, and the prospect of doing that full-time had appeal. In moving directly from the pinnacle of my scientific career into a deanship, I felt the temporal proximity of my laboratory life to my Deanship would give me greater credibility and effectiveness as a school leader. There was, however, a more self-centered aspect to the decision. I have always been a somewhat restless spirit, curious about new things, and eager to avoid falling into repetition of habits. These traits have served me well in becoming a person who has led a most interesting life, although it likely held me back in science, where I too often manifested an unwise tendency to chase interesting new observations into new fields, rather than maintaining the deep and consistent focus, focus, and more focus that the very best scientists exhibit. My tendency to have broad intellectual interests, often a failing in a scientist, became, happily, a strength for Dean. In the final analysis, I became a Dean as a new mountain to climb, to see if I could do it well, and to try to make a different type of contribution to the academic enterprise.

The Basic Unit of Time in Academic Medicine Is the Decade

When students ask about my personal history of career choices in academic medicine, usually in the context of me trying to advise them, I tell them first that my story probably is not one that they, or anyone else, necessarily would want to emulate. My professional history is full of false starts, dead ends narrowly avoided, and far too much good luck to represent a model. However, there is certain logic to the saga that makes sense, at least in retrospect. I had a very fine liberal arts education, which cynics say may make one unfit for 90% of useful work, but in my case gave me rather advanced skills in reading, writing, and in the formulation and presentation of complex thoughts and ideas. These abilities have served me well along a career path I never could have imagined as a student. After college, I spent the next 10 or 15 years primarily learning and then doing the job of a physician caring for sick patients. The science I learned and conducted, though it has dominated what I have written here about the origins of my career as a physician-scientist, actually was in the background to clinical medicine during that period. As I went through the phase transition I described earlier and fell in love with a scientific question in the mid-1980s, I entered the next 15-year period, which truly was dominated by doing science, with clinical medicine moving to the background. I became, one might say, a scientist-physician rather than a physician-scientist during that wonderful period. The third and current phase of my career, which began in 2001, essentially has been spent as an academic executive, with both science and clinical medicine as tasks I do myself on a daily basis moving to the background, replaced by activities intended to make others better able to do those things.

Being an academic executive is less far removed from the skills and traits that work well in clinical medicine and in laboratory science than one might think. In the lab, at least for the kind of molecular biological investigations that were my métier, the goal is to find a solution to a problem, the answer to which is unknown and perhaps unknowable. If it is knowable, the answers likely will be revealed only by years of work involving hundreds of linked steps and many failures. Success and satisfaction come, if at all, in unpredictable spurts amid a long span of difficult and sometimes tedious work. Well, administrative life can be described in much the same way. As for comparing the practice of clinical medicine to administration, the life of a physician is dominated by the great and wondrous diversity of human beings, and by the spectrum of ways individuals are affected by, and respond to,

circumstances wrought by fate or by their own actions. That's not unlike the cavalcade of human behaviors that a Dean observes and must manage as best as possible
through knowledge, judgment, patience, and discipline. I don't mean to press these
similarities too far, but I find some truth in them. A consistent reward of my years
as a physician, scientist, and academic executive has been the enjoyment of continuous learning, and the satisfaction that comes from a sense that one has grown in
capability to deal successfully with whatever a job may require.

I'll conclude these reflections by reference to the yin-yang of life as a physician-
scientist, within which lies its blessing or its curse. Every day presents an interesting
but daunting selection of choices about how to spend one's time and energy, with
every choice potentially opening doors to activities of enjoyment and value to oneself and to others. The blessing of having such options is obvious, and in few
endeavors can a person be so blessed. The curse is that only a small fraction of
the possibilities can be made real, and there is a serious risk of diverting time and
energy in multiple directions so that nothing of real value and fulfillment is achieved.
Fortunately for me, this yin-yang has produced mostly blessings, and for that I am
grateful indeed.

References

1. Snead DL (1999) The Gaither Committee, Eisenhower and the Cold War. Ohio State University
   Press, Columbus, OH
2. Suzanne B Plato and his dialogues. http://plato-dialogues.org/plato.htm (Accessed 24 August,
   2010).

Eight
Success for the Whole Community

Talmadge E. King, Jr.

I grew up in a small coastal town near Savannah, Georgia. Darien, my hometown, was founded in 1736, making it the second oldest city in Georgia. Despite major growth around it, Darien remains a quaint and unspoiled coastal town, with ancient live oaks and beautiful Spanish moss. With its strong sense of community, Darien was a good place for instilling values that would serve anyone well. Many of my friends stayed after high school, and those who left for military service or college often returned to the area to live.

I chose a path less traveled. In many ways, it was not so much a choice, but destiny. I was raised by a "village," and it appeared that my accomplishments were successes for the whole community as well. In fact, my path to becoming a physician-scientist involved several "villages."

Hard Work and Education

I am the oldest of five children. From an early age, it was made clear to me that a lot was expected of me, and I came to accept this role. My parents (Fig. 8.1) were hard workers and they believed in education and did their best to ensure that we achieved the highest level possible. There was never a question that we would all go to college.

My father, who remains fiercely independent to this day, owned a number of small businesses. His main endeavor was a television and radio repair shop. As a solo business owner, my father worked long hours, but he enjoyed his work.

When I was a teenager, he became one of the first African-American police officers in our region. This was more of a community decision than his decision. As a widely-known and respected member of the community, he was a choice that was acceptable to all members of our still very segregated community.

T.E. King, Jr. (✉)
Department of Medicine, University of California, San Francisco, CA, USA
e-mail: tking@medicine.ucsf.edu

D.A. Schwartz (ed.), *Medicine Science and Dreams*,
DOI 10.1007/978-90-481-9538-1_8, © Springer Science+Business Media B.V. 2011

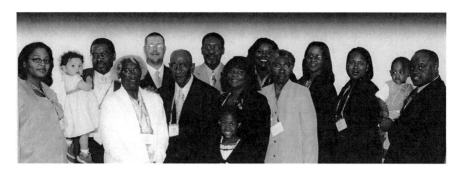

Fig. 8.1 Shown are my parents (front row third and fourth from *left*) with other members of the family

The opportunity to shadow my father as he traveled through our community left an indelible mark on me. It was his self-confidence and ability to connect with a variety of people that interested me. Invariably, his playful spirit made these exchanges pleasant and enjoyable for everyone.

One day, we delivered a repaired television to a customer in a very rural part of our county. As people often do, they started talking about money. My dad told him, "Everybody knows you have a lot of money." The man said, "No, King, I'm a poor man." My dad said, "Everybody knows you bury your money out in the backyard." Hearing this, the guy immediately ran to his backyard, where he dug up a can full of money.

Back in the truck with my dad, I asked him, "How did you know he buried his money in the backyard?" My dad said, "I didn't! I just made that up." Those were the kinds of things my dad understood about people. He could talk with anybody, anywhere, any time. He taught me that people are all basically the same. They have the same needs and desires, and you can connect with them by talking, listening, and sharing common concerns.

My mother has more of a no-nonsense approach, but she also connected with people. She had firm ideas about right and wrong and the way things were supposed to be done. She expected you to treat everyone well. Her mantra was, "Be nice."

My mother's college education was interrupted by marriage and the birth of me and one of my brothers. However, her dream of a college degree never wavered, and she managed to attend college while raising five children. Her college graduation ceremony, an inspiration to all of us, was held one week after I graduated from high school.

My extended family helped make her success possible. Her college was a three hour drive away, and my two grandmothers spent a lot of time taking care of us. They had different personalities: my paternal grandmother was a complete sweetheart and let us do anything, and my maternal grandmother was very strict and "took no prisoners." We loved them both.

I was also very close to my aunts, uncles, and cousins. From an early age, I spent lots of time with them. Often, my brother and I would spend summers with my aunts and uncles in New York City. That was a very good experience, because it took me away from the South and showed me a very different world.

Mrs. Cooper and the *Weekly Reader*

I grew up in an integrated neighborhood but went to segregated schools. That was typical of the South. The neighborhood kids played well together until we were about 12. Then, we went our separate ways. This was also typical of the South, at the time.

Segregated schools were separate but by no means equal. Often, there was disparity between facilities as well as supplies. Books and other materials often arrived at my school after having been discarded by the "white" schools.

Fortunately, even in this environment, there were excellent, caring, and committed teachers at my school. Conditions at our public school improved dramatically as I entered middle school, and a new school, gymnasium, and athletic fields were built. These changes transformed the spirit of our community, and the school became a centerpiece of the region.

Around sixth grade, it became obvious to me that my teachers had deemed me the chosen one. I was a good student, and it was made clear that there were high expectations for me, in particular. The school counselor, Catherine Cooper, took a special interest in my education. She began by tutoring me at her home after school. I distinctly remember our weekly sessions, going through the *Weekly Reader* and other materials together. She wanted me to understand the world around me and to go beyond the outdated books at our school. I was somewhat intimidated by her and certainly did not want to disappoint, so I tried hard to live up to her expectations. My friends would joke that Mrs. Cooper was my other mother. The good-natured ribbing never got to me because my parents were very supportive, and I was also highly motivated.

I attended high school in the early 1960s, when the battle against segregation was heating up and a number of programs were started to improve opportunities for underrepresented minorities, especially African-Americans. Mrs. Cooper heard about a program for high school minority youth called the Summer Studies-Skills Program (SSSP). It was sponsored by the United Presbyterian Church's Educational Counseling Service of the Board of National Missions. The program gave students from small towns and rural areas in the southern USA a structured six-week curriculum of mathematics, communications, and reading. SSSP helped give promising but educationally disadvantaged students the tools to succeed in high school and at competitive colleges. Mrs. Cooper insisted that I apply to SSSP, and then worked hard to make sure that I was accepted. I spent two summers in this program at Knoxville College in Tennessee.

SSSP was a major turning point in my life. It was inspiring to meet other accomplished and highly skilled students, and the program showed me that I could compete on a larger stage than my small high school. The program's director,

Samuel Johnson, was a no-nonsense, lovable person. Much like Mrs. Cooper, he let me know that to succeed I had to step it up a notch or two!

In addition to the academic courses, we were exposed to the college application process and were introduced to many institutions that we would not have ever considered. Many college admissions officers—mostly from small colleges in the Midwest—came to meet and greet us. It was here that I learned of Gustavus Adolphus College in St. Peter, Minnesota, where I later applied and was accepted.

Pursuing the Dream: In the Valley of the Jolly Green Giant

I took the train from Savannah to Minneapolis —it seemed to take forever as we crisscrossed the country. Bruce Gray, an administrator at Gustavus, picked me up at the train station. Immediately, I felt like Dorothy arriving in the Land of Oz. I was definitely not in Georgia any more. Actually, I was in "The Valley of the Jolly Green Giant." On the hour-long drive to Gustavus, one of the first attractions I noticed, poking above the trees heading south on Route 169 toward St. Peter, was an enormous wooden sign of the Jolly Green Giant. Indeed, I was a long way from home, and I saw virtually no one there who looked like me.

Fortunately, there were a number of people in my new "village" who wanted to embrace me. Chief among them were Bruce and his wife, Sue (Fig. 8.2). Similar to Mrs. Cooper, Bruce became a mentor, advisor, supporter, and lifelong friend. I could go into his office and talk with him any time. He steered opportunities in my direction and talked to people on my behalf. Bruce was committed to helping underrepresented minorities, and he made sure we were not overlooked. Bruce and

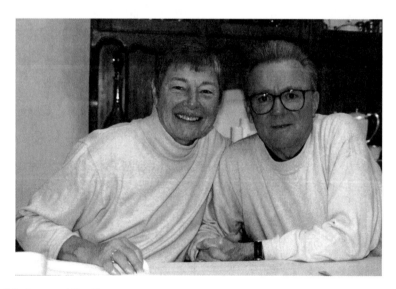

Fig. 8.2 Bruce and Sue Gray

Sue opened their home to my future wife and me, later provided advice on raising our family, helped us find part-time jobs, and much more.

In high school, I had the good fortune of being at the top of my class and helping others. But in college, most of my classmates were much better prepared than I was. My first semester was really difficult. I was struggling to get my grade point average above a 3.0. Several professors were enormously supportive, especially Charles Hamrum and Arthur Glass, my biology professors.

I will never forget the independent study course with my advisor, John Kendall, and several other students. Class was held in his barn. We discussed key issues of the day, read and reviewed classic books, and went on field trips to observe and learn at interesting places, especially in nearby Minneapolis. I learned many valuable lessons in this course. Importantly, despite our apparently very diverse backgrounds (mine by far the most divergent), we discovered that we all shared common concerns, insecurities, desires, and hopes. We weren't that different as human beings.

Despite the major differences I found between Gustavus and my hometown, I soon embraced Gustavus as my own. I ran track and joined a fraternity, where I was surprised to learn that it was common practice to share notes and copies of old exams. I was also active in student government, which was a very educational experience during the era of the Civil Rights Movement and the Vietnam War. I was often a conduit between more radical African-American students and the college administrators.

At Gustavus, I would never allow myself to feel like an outsider. I think this came from my parents. My dad received the Purple Heart during his military service in World War II. He made it clear to all his children that this was our country, and that we had every right to claim its resources, just as any other American. Whether at Gustavus Adolphus College, Harvard Medical School, or anywhere my career took me, I always felt like these were my schools and workplaces, and I took great joy in being part of these institutions.

The Family: The Highest Priority

During my first few weeks of college, I met my future wife, Mozelle Davis (Fig. 8.3). We married during our sophomore year. The combination of marriage and family had a challenging and stabilizing impact on both of us. We complement and support each other.

Mozelle was one of the very few minority students at Gustavus. She was an attractive woman, but more important, she was smart, articulate, and outgoing. Mozelle was also from a small town in the South, Brandon, Mississippi. She had attended Holy Ghost Catholic High School in Jackson, Mississippi.

Mozelle majored in mathematics in college and completed graduate school at Boston College while I attended medical school. She taught mathematics in public schools for many years.

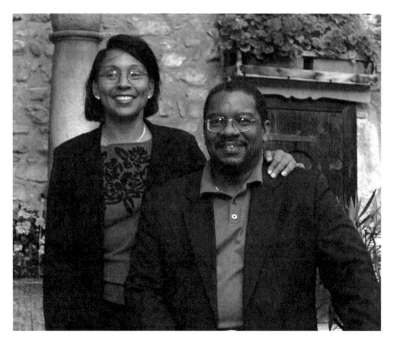

Fig. 8.3 Mozelle and me

Our first child, Consuelo, was born while we were undergraduates at Gustavus. Our second child, Malaika, was born five years later while we were in graduate school. Many people helped us during these early years of our marriage. We both worked, studied, and cared for our daughters.

The successes of our professional careers pale in comparison to watching our daughters' journeys through life and seeing them succeed in their lives. Malaika and her husband Chad have two daughter, Madison and Siena. Our granddaughter's unbridled zest for life brings pure joy to our lives.

Medicine as a Career

The idea of becoming a doctor evolved slowly, rather than being rooted in a sentinel event. I realized that I wanted to pursue some graduate level work but I was not sure in what field. I had a career in medicine in the back of my mind, but I didn't know if I could get accepted to medical school, especially given my limited scientific background in high school.

I was always fairly healthy and had little contact with physicians growing up. However, one of my brothers and my father had really bad asthma. I shared a bedroom with my brother, and I would see him gasping for breath during his asthma attacks. There was not much the doctors could do for either my brother or father, although they did try a number of treatments that I now know were largely ineffective and potentially dangerous. Looking back, I think watching this might have encouraged me in subtle ways to go into pulmonary medicine.

One of my high school summer jobs involved working as a darkroom technician in a radiology department at Lincoln Hospital in the Bronx, NY. There was a lot of excitement there. I spent time around the emergency room, watching the nurses and physicians and sometimes assisting the radiology technicians.

What really jump-started my decision to apply to medical school was participation in the Health Career Summer Program at Harvard Medical School during one of the first years of its existence. A college mentor suggested that I apply for this program, which gave minority students from around the country the opportunity to spend a summer at Harvard taking classes and meeting professors and medical and dental students. That summer, I also met a number of Harvard faculty members who were committed to improving minority participation in the health sciences, particularly Alvin Poussaint, Edwin Furshpan, and David Potter. This experience confirmed that a career in medicine was possible and was something I eagerly wanted to pursue.

I applied to and was accepted to several medical schools. One day, I received a telegram and thought that something bad had happened. Instead, it was a message from Harvard Medical School notifying me that I had been accepted. There was a lot of excitement in the "village" that day!

Harvard required a year of calculus, and I had only taken one semester. As things turned out, the last few weeks of regular classes were cancelled in my senior year because of the protests against the Vietnam War. Therefore, I was able to spend every day at the library, cramming calculus. Fortunately, my wife was a math major; she tutored me and helped me complete the course.

A Wakeup Call: Meeting the Challenge

Like college, the first year at Harvard was a struggle. Although I had made considerable academic progress, I still lagged behind my peers. Some courses were particularly difficult. I managed to make it through the first two years and passed Part I of the medical boards.

However, it was during the "Introduction to the Clinic" course, which introduces students to the examination of the patient, that I had a major life-changing event. This was the period of medical school that I was waiting for—getting a chance to work with patients. However, for the first time in my life, I encountered a professor who felt I did not belong. He thought I wasn't up to Harvard's standards and that I wouldn't accomplish much in my career. Although I felt his comments were mean-spirited and hurtful, this was a wakeup call that I believe spurred me to develop several skills that have been critical to my career in academic medicine.

Although this was an introduction to the clinical phase of medical school, I did not realize what was expected for this course. Being married and living off-campus,

I wasn't talking with other medical students in the dorms, and I missed out on the "informal" curriculum, which was similar to my college experience prior to joining a fraternity and having access to previous years' exams. This taught me that I needed to be more actively involved with my peers, because this was also critical to the learning process.

Another concern was that my patient write-ups were poorly constructed and not well-written. Mortified by this very critical evaluation, I asked for help. My advisor and the Student Affairs Office arranged for a tutor, who turned out to be a walking *Elements of Style* and reminded me of Mrs. Cooper. She gave me tools that I still use today for both reading and writing, and taught me how to organize and condense my thoughts. Although writing can still be laborious and slow, I have been successful in writing and editing books and papers—a critical skill in academic medicine.

The other thing I learned from this experience was that negative feedback can be helpful, even if you think it is unfair. I try to keep my emotions in check, clarify and understand the feedback, think it over, and develop an action plan to improve, if it is warranted. I am absolutely convinced that the best "payback" is to simply do the smart thing and the right thing.

In the end, my clinical years at Harvard were outstanding. I truly enjoyed working with patients and, needless to say, I found the training exceptional. One of my first hospital rotations was on the Internal Medicine wards at Beth Israel Hospital. It was during this rotation that I had my first direct and personal contact with another African-American physician, Donald Henderson. Don was a very smart resident, and wise beyond his years. He was the first person to emphasize that a key to surviving clinical rotations in medical school and residency was to develop a strategy. Treat it as a "game," he advised: Learn the rules, anticipate what will happen, don't get trapped in the craziness, and play to win.

I still remember our preparation for one of my first presentations at attending rounds, where trainees describe the new patients admitted the previous day to the attending physician. Despite being extremely busy with multiple other admissions to the hospital, Don helped me complete a patient write-up. We identified the most significant problems to be addressed in caring for the patient. Then Don said, "Remember, the attending is only going to ask you about what he knows best." Although the patient had many problems, Don advised me that one of the patient's problems was in the attending's area of expertise. Therefore, it was critical that I read as much as I could about that problem and be prepared to answer questions about its management. I did as Don suggested, and my attending was happy with the write-up and the discussion. My presentation was a success.

In very different ways, both the "Introduction to the Clinic" professor and Don taught me several valuable lessons: networking is a way to learn what is expected, organizational and writing skills are vital skills and critical to good communications, and one must learn how to handle feedback—positive or negative.

Approximately 30 years after medical school, I was elected to membership in a prestigious medical society. The professor who had delivered harsh comments when I took Introduction to the Clinic, along with his wife, joined Mozelle and me at our table for the gala event. The professor was gracious and complimented me for my achievements. I am convinced he supported my election to this society. Of course, I thanked him.

Doctoring and Teaching

I decided to do additional training in internal medicine (Fig. 8.4). I entered the residency match and matched at Emory University, which proved to be the right place at the right time. I had a number of inspirational teachers there, in particular J. Willis Hurst and H. Kenneth Walker. Both were deeply committed to "doctoring and teaching," as Dr. Hurst often called it.

I arrived at Emory as they were implementing the "Problem-Oriented Record," introduced by Lawrence L. Weed in the early seventies. They were convinced that Weed's approach could be used by both trainees and practicing doctors to improve thinking, medical care, communications, and the teaching of medicine. The Weed system involved four elements: (1) a *Database*: accurately collecting appropriate and defined data; (2) a *Problem List*: defining key issues that need to be managed; (3) a *Plan*: constructing an action plan for diagnosing and managing each of the problems on the *Problem List*; and (4) *Progress Notes*: following up on each problem to determine whether the plans produced the expected or desired outcomes. Given my earlier problems with recording and communicating the observations I obtained from my patients, the Weed system was perfect for me. I have used its basic principles throughout my career not only in my care of patients, but also as a teaching tool and record for clinical research.

Dr. Walker, the head of the residency training program, was a tough taskmaster, both revered and feared by the housestaff. I was no exception. Dr. Walker led the "morning report," a meeting with housestaff to discuss cases admitted during the previous 24 hours and any problems that had occurred overnight. This was one of

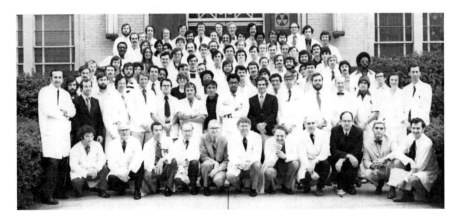

Fig. 8.4 Housestaff photo at Emory University (1975); Drs. Hurst and Walker are in the center of the first row (kneeling sixth and seventh from the *left*)

the critical activities in our training, and it was an opportunity for Dr. Walker to review the medical records prepared by housestaff. I arrived at one of these sessions after another very busy night at Grady Memorial Hospital, the public hospital and main teaching site for the residency. I was armed with all the pertinent charts, save one—this from a patient who had died during the night. Well, Dr. Walker demanded that I get that patient's medical record. Surprised by the request, my mind (and heart) raced as I tried to determine why seeing this chart was so important. I was very concerned that my day of reckoning had come!

Fortunately, the chart had not yet been dismantled and was still on the medical ward. As I scanned the chart on my way back to the conference room, I felt that Don's "rules of the game" were about to be put to the test. First, I knew that Dr. Walker would want to know that I had followed the Weed method for documenting the patient's problems. And, above all, he was a true believer in the adage that "good doctors leave good tracks."

The patient was a young woman in her early twenties with end stage renal failure. She had been extremely sick for many years and was hospitalized numerous times. She had now been refusing all treatments and asked me to let her die. It was an incredibly moving experience for me. We talked for a long time, and I wrote a note detailing the progression of her disease, how many times she had been hospitalized, her previous treatments, and a complete list of all her current problems. I also included quotes from our conversation as well as my discussions with her family. When Dr. Walker got the chart, he read it, closed it, handed it back to me, and said, "Thank you." I believe that on that day, Dr. Walker let me know I belonged, and my confidence soared.

Dr. Hurst, Chair of the Department of Medicine, was the ultimate clinician-educator. He was President Lyndon Johnson's personal cardiologist. I learned two lessons from Dr. Hurst. First, you must care about your patients. Second, every patient teaches you something. I was fortunate to go on rounds with him at Emory Hospital. Even though he was chair of the department and extremely busy, he was never in a hurry with his patients or trainees. He would make the patient feel like they were the only thing on his mind. He would spend five minutes at their bedside, but it felt like 20 minutes. He would hold the patient's hand or sit at the foot of the bed, touching their foot. It turns out that this was part of his physical exam—feeling their pulse and heart rate and observing the patient as he talked with them. A superstar, Dr. Hurst was always a gentleman and he treated everyone with respect—patients, nurses, staff, and his trainees.

The Decision to Become a Subspecialist

Encouraged by Dr. Hurst and others, I decided to specialize. Around the time of this decision, my attending physician was Ralph Haynes, a young pulmonologist who had just become the Chief of Pulmonary Medicine at Grady Hospital. An excellent and enthusiastic teacher, Ralph sparked my interest in critical care and pulmonary

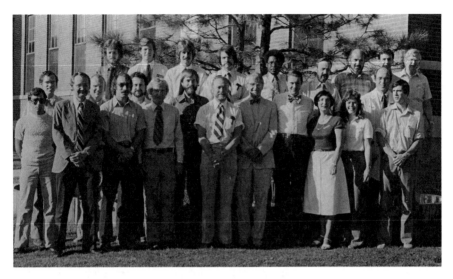

Fig. 8.5 Photo of fellows and faculty member at UCHSC (1979–1980); Drs. Thomas Petty, Roger Mitchell, Reuben Cherniack are on the front row (fourth to sixth from the *right*)

medicine. At the time, there were only a handful of really good fellowship programs in the field. So, I applied to several programs.

On the morning of the match, I received phone calls from the University of California, San Francisco (UCSF) and the University of Colorado Health Sciences Center in Denver (UCHSC). UCSF had the larger and more prominent program, but Mozelle and I decided that Denver might be better suited to our family situation. By then Consuelo was 9 years old, and Malaika was 4. We chose the University of Colorado, and it was a fantastic experience.

Again, I was fortunate to enter a new village with wonderful mentors. Thomas (Tom) Petty was the head of the fellowship program. Like Dr. Hurst, Dr. Petty was a superb clinician, educator, and investigator. Tom was very committed to all of his trainees. Another key figure for me was Dr. Reuben Cherniack. He also had just arrived in Colorado to become the Chair of Medicine at National Jewish Medical and Research Center. Tom and Reuben worked together to make the Colorado program one of the best in the country (Fig. 8.5).

Interstitial Lung Disease: Discovering a Lifelong Passion

I became interested in interstitial lung disease (ILD) during my clinical year as a pulmonary fellow. I cared for a patient, Mrs. Mejía, with systemic lupus erythematosus and ILD. She was a mother of five in her late thirties. She had suffered from systemic lupus for several years but had never been hospitalized. She developed an acute illness with severe lung disease. We had no idea what was wrong with her. She went from well to dead in a few days, and there was nothing we could do. In the last days of her life, I vividly remember seeing all of her children gathered around her bedside. I was very bothered by this outcome and tried to find answers to why she developed this dramatic illness (Lupus pneumonitis) and if we could have done something to help her.

At that time, few researchers were interested in interstitial lung diseases. These diseases were uncommon and few physicians had much experience caring for these patients. I made it my goal to learn everything I could about these processes and to work to find better treatments. At one point, I had five large file cabinets full of almost every paper ever written about these diseases, and I had read them all.

After my year of clinical fellowship, I decided to work with Marvin Schwarz and Robert Dreisin. They were interested in ILD and encouraged me to get training in laboratory research—something I had never done. I worked in the laboratory of Peter Henson and Patsy Giclas, scientists at the National Jewish Medical and Research Center who were interested in inflammation and lung injury. I gained valuable experience in learning how to think about scientific projects, what it took to successfully test your hypotheses, and how to communicate with basic scientists. However, I was not very good at basic research and found the challenges to outweigh the rewards. I also really missed direct contact with patients.

Dr. Schwarz (Fig. 8.6), who was chief of the pulmonary section at the Denver VA hospital, hired me to my first faculty position after my second year of fellowship.

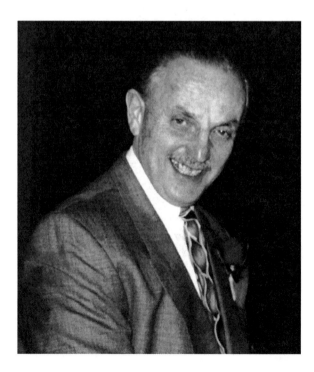

Fig. 8.6 Marvin Schwarz

This was a clinical faculty position, but I made an effort to continue doing research. Fortunately, the National Institutes of Health (NIH) had also become very interested in helping scientists and clinicians discover more about the pathogenesis of interstitial lung disease. Working with Drs. Marvin Schwarz, Peter Henson, Robert Mason, and other scientists at the National Jewish Medical and Research Center, we obtained a Specialized Center of Research grant from the NIH to conduct clinical and basic research into the pathogenesis of lung fibrosis. Marvin and I were responsible for the development of the clinical research program.

"Translational Research": From Bedside to the Bench

We decided to prospectively study patients with ILD, in particular idiopathic pulmonary fibrosis (IPF). IPF is a scarring process in the lung. When the lung scars, the lung tissue thickens and becomes extremely stiff, and it's very difficult to take a big breath. Unlike Mrs. Mejía, my patient with an acute, sudden illness, most patients with IPF have a more prolonged course but with a similarly bleak outcome. On average, patients with IPF delay seeking medical attention for two years after their first symptoms. This is because the disease develops gradually and most commonly manifests initially as breathlessness, which patients often dismiss as aging or deconditioning. Often by the time of diagnosis, the disease had progressed to a stage that was not treatable. We developed a wide array of goals for our studies: improve the classification of this group of diseases, define their natural histories, understand the etiology and pathogenesis, and identify better treatments with the goal of improving the dismal outcomes.

In 1978, just as I was beginning to consider research in ILD, I attended the twenty-first Aspen Lung Conference. The conference topic was "Immunology of the Lung," and Dame Margaret Turner-Warwick was the conference summarizer. The size, location, and structure of this conference allowed participants to interact in ways not possible at most large scientific conferences. I had an opportunity to talk at length with Dr. Turner-Warwick about her research. She was so gracious with her time and knowledge, and her excitement about clinical research was infectious— I was even more excited about pursuing research in ILD. In addition, I met many other key researchers in this field (R. Crystal, G. Davis, G. Hunninghake, C. Kuhn, H. Reynolds, and P. Ward). Most especially, these interactions eventually resulted in several significant research collaborations that were very helpful in our efforts to build an ILD program at Colorado.

A couple of years before this conference, Herbert Reynolds and his team had described the procedure of bronchoalveolar lavage (BAL) and discussed its potential as a diagnostic and research tool. The technique took advantage of the fiberoptic bronchoscope, which had recently been shown to be a safe procedure to sample the lung. It was tremendously exciting, because BAL allowed us to wash living cells from the lung directly at the sites of disease. In addition, for the first time, we could do serial measurements from individuals without having to perform lung biopsies. Given the other laboratory advances that were occurring, this tool allowed us to explore clinical questions in the laboratory ("translational research") where we could bring the bench to the bedside!

There were several presentations at the conference showing data derived from studies of lavage fluid and cells. We decided to use BAL as our main research tool. I was one of the first to volunteer to have this procedure performed at our center. Over time, we helped determine the optimal amount of fluid to inject, which part of the lung was best to sample, and how to adapt the procedure so the patient was as comfortable as possible. We also conducted a multi-center project that characterized BAL constituents in healthy individuals, those with IPF, and selected comparison groups. Using this tool and others, we contributed over the years to understanding the pathogenesis of several interstitial lung diseases.

Building a Clinical Investigation Team

Today, aspiring clinical researchers have access to multiple resources to help them succeed. When I started there were few people trained in clinical and translational research. At this critical juncture in my career, I had the good fortune to work with Dr. Reuben Cherniack, my career mentor. Reuben helped secure the resources and support I needed to build my clinical research program. In addition, he taught me how the world of pulmonary medicine worked: What are the things you need to do? How do you succeed? What do people expect, and how do you exceed those expectations? He was always pushing me to get the work done and think of new research questions. Every time I saw him, he said, "Okay, kid, are you finished with that project yet? Where is the paper?"

Reuben was a very clear thinker and a superb editor. He taught me how to structure my scientific writing. He would eliminate repetition, point out sentences that didn't make sense, and move paragraphs around. Sometimes it would drive me crazy to get drafts back with red ink all over them, but I realized that he cared enough to really read the paper and make specific suggestions. Too often, you ask co-authors or colleagues for feedback on a paper or grant, and they respond with few or no useful comments. Rather than feeling pleased that you must have done a good job, you should be concerned that they did not have time to carefully review your work, especially when this involves looking at early drafts of the document. Reuben helped me see that experts who seriously read a paper will often have differences of opinion or critical suggestions. It does not mean that they are right or that you must accept their changes, but they will at least challenge the way you think.

After deciding that I would be a clinical investigator, I went back to what I was taught by Dr. Hurst, determined that every patient I saw with ILD would teach me something. Using the Weed system, I developed ways to capture data and religiously compiled information about each patient. This was well before we had any electronic medical records.

In the beginning, it was very hard to convince my team to spend the time to fill out all these forms. Sometimes I would fill out the forms for them, seeing the patient

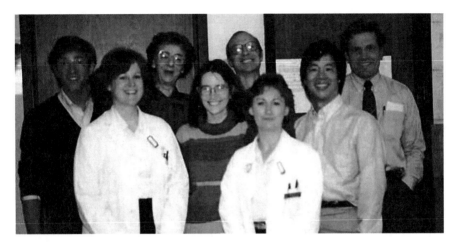

Fig. 8.7 Interstitial Lung Disease group (1986)

they saw, or calling up the patient to fill in missing pieces. Because these were diseases where little was known, this database allowed us to publish data about a number of diffuse lung diseases.

As I have stated throughout, having the help of others is critical to a successful career. Luckily, we hired great people to work with us on our projects and they formed the core of our group for many years [Mary Willcox, Alma (Dolly) Kervitsky, Martin Wallace, and S. Arlene Niccoli] (Fig. 8.7). Mary, a native of my home state of Georgia, was our lab manager. She was a take-charge person with a wealth of experience and contacts. She made things happen. After Mary's retirement, Dolly took over as lab manager and Arlene became the clinical coordinator. Their hard work and dedication was crucial in our achievements.

In those early years, we were also most fortunate to attract outstanding pulmonary fellows to work in our group, in particular, K. L. Christopher, L. C. Watters, T. L. Dunn, A. Shen, L. S. Newman, S. M. Aguayo, R. L. Mortenson, R. J. Shaw, R. J. Panos, and P. Noble. They played key roles in enrolling patients, designing protocols, gathering and analyzing data, and writing manuscripts. Most importantly, because we were trying to build bridges from the bedside to the bench, these fellows often worked with bench scientists to carry out research projects using BAL, blood, and tissue samples derived from our patients.

Referring Physicians and Patients

I believe that one of the keys to my success as a clinical investigator was the ability to work successfully with referring physicians and patients. I have always felt a deep allegiance with community physicians—I believed my research efforts were critical to their success and vice versa. I frequently joked that we were the "R & D" division of the practicing physician's office—trying to find new ways for them to help their patients.

Finally, for those of us involved in translational research, the central people in our village are our patients and their families. My patients were very helpful and willing to allow us to study them. Like my parents, I enjoy working with people, and I made the commitment to spend time with patients and answer their questions. After helping them, I would ask them to help me by enrolling in our clinical trials. It is remarkable that so many people are so willing to help others in this way.

Reflections: Seven Habits of Successful Clinical Investigators

I am an admirer of Stephen Covey's book *The Seven Habits of Highly Effective People*. I have tried to think of the "seven habits" (i.e., internalized principles and patterns of behavior) that have been especially vital in my development and success as a physician, scientist, and teacher:

First, it is important to have high expectations. Mrs. Cooper and many others set these for me. I learned to have high expectations for myself, as well as how to combine hard work and thoroughness to achieve these goals.

Second, develop good people skills. My father, especially, taught me how to connect with people from all different backgrounds, and he showed me what we can accomplish when we work together.

Third, balance persistence and determination with an appreciation for delayed gratification. Nothing worthwhile comes easy, and research takes time. You must be able to celebrate your own successes. I tell those I mentor that they will probably labor in obscurity for the first five years of their careers. Over time, people will come to know them and value their opinion. Also, doing research and writing papers can be very lonely, and sometimes even your best work will be ignored or criticized. If you don't get a warm glow putting the manuscript in the mailbox, or hitting the "send" button on your computer, don't choose this career path—sometimes that warm glow is all the reward you'll get. Also, to avoid burnout, it is imperative for physician-scientists to overcome the feeling that the job is never done.

Fourth, learn to seek and handle feedback (both positive and negative). You should not try to do everything on your own. Mentoring is a critical component of career development. You need to seek feedback and use it to your advantage. Listen carefully to all advice, and then decide what is best for you.

Fifth, keep an open mind and trust the scientific method. The scientific method is not foolproof, but if we study things carefully, we can learn what the truth is. I have learned that some of the things I believed deeply were found to be flat-out wrong when carefully examined.

Sixth, develop a niche and then focus on achieving your goals. It is critical to become an expert in something. However, it can be most difficult to remain focused on your goals because you will be challenged by many opportunities that may be simply enjoyable and thus valuable from that perspective. Others may be too time consuming and detract from your goals. Opportunities will arise in the future, so, it is possible to make careful choices—your colleagues will respect and support your decision.

Seventh, do not be afraid to share freely. A willingness to collaborate and to be a team player have been keys to our success—the more I gave the more I received. I believe in the adage, "It is amazing what you can accomplish if you do not care who gets the credit."

Academic medicine is a noble calling—both fulfilling and rewarding. As physician-scientists, we have the distinct privilege of helping the sick and dying while being engaged in exciting intellectual inquiry.

Acknowledgments   I am grateful to Elizabeth Chur for her many excellent suggestions and help with the writing of this manuscript. Also, I thank my earlier devoted assistants, Mary Peterson, B.J. Burnett, Nancy Esajian, and my present assistants, Amy Bates and Vanessa Dancer, for a level of loyalty and support which is truly uncommon. I feel a deep sense of gratitude to Mozelle, Consuelo, and Malaika for their support. Finally, to my granddaughters, Madison and Siena Kattke, who have inspired me to "keep first things first."

Nine
The Irony of Disease

David A. Schwartz

I was born with club feet. My mother was young and scared; my father was just starting out as an accountant in New York City making $30 a week. They had just moved into a small house in the suburbs of Long Island, and routine health insurance did not exist. They were shocked that I was less than perfect, but there I was. It was 1953.

My mother, who tends to be overly emotional (some would say theatrical) and not particularly good at coping with uncertainty, I am told vacillated from frantic to depressed; while my father, one of the more optimistic people I have ever known, was proud of his first son and looked for a solution. As luck would have it, Dr. Maurice Langsam (Fig. 9.1), a community orthopedist, happened to be in Flushing Hospital, my birthplace, shortly after I was born.

Dr. Langsam was middle aged, but I remember him as older. He had just come into his own as an orthopedist and, I think, mostly took care of children. While I have no memory of him in the hospital, I spent much of the next 10 years in and out of his office and got to know him quite well. He was short, slightly overweight, with gray-black hair and a mustache. Dr. Langsam loved what he did, was extremely supportive, easy to understand, and had a reasonably good sense humor. In hindsight, he reminds me of a Norman Rockwell physician, but Jewish. Imagine getting to step into a Rockwell painting every couple of months; it almost makes you want to see the doctor.

Dr. Langsam was a bit of a risk-taker (a trait he shared with my father and me), and was somewhat ahead of his time. In the early 1950s, the traditional treatment for club feet involved a surgical procedure. However, this procedure, cutting the Achilles' tendon and stretching out the plantar facia, left the patient with a weak foot for his or her entire life. Dr. Langsam and only a handful of other orthopedists at that time had a different view. Their approach was to strengthen the weak portions of

D.A. Schwartz (✉)
Departments of Medicine, Pediatrics and Immunology, Center for Genes, Environment, and Health, National Jewish Health, Denver, CO, USA; Departments of Medicine and Immunology, University of Colorado Denver, Denver, CO, USA
e-mail: schwartzd@NJHealth.org

D.A. Schwartz (ed.), *Medicine Science and Dreams*,
DOI 10.1007/978-90-481-9538-1_9, © Springer Science+Business Media B.V. 2011

Fig. 9.1 Dr. Langsam

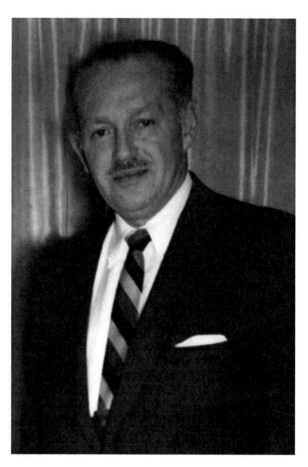

the foot while stretching and exercising the contracted tendons. This meant bracing, casting, orthopedic shoes, and exercise, as well as lots of setbacks. It also involved an ongoing commitment from me and my mother.

Dr. Langsam's expectations were extremely high; he was seeking perfection. The problem was that perfection of my feet rested largely on my rather small shoulders. Despite this pressure, he made me feel responsible and able to achieve his expectations. Every month or two I would walk for Dr. Langsam. It's hard to walk when you have someone watching your every step, especially knowing that a misstep would mean a leg cast or even two leg casts that would make it that much more difficult to play ball or ride my bike. However, walking for Dr. Langsam was easy. His cigar smoke made me feel at home. He encouraged my every step. He held my feet with his big hands and let me know that whatever I did, it was ok, I was ok. In fact, as I think back to those visits, I can still feel him holding my feet. He put on a cast as if he was packing away a valuable piece of art. When he cut off my leg casts (must have happened at least a couple of dozen times), he made me feel like we were opening a gift box, full of surprises. Anything seemed possible.

However, there was a chaotic side to my visits to see Dr. Langsam. His waiting room was always filled with children with all sorts of problems. Kids with missing limbs, cerebral palsy, or very large heads, some in wheelchairs, others appearing physically frozen in time, all brought in by their young, anxious, ever-patient mothers. Nothing seemed to make sense, there was little order, the kids were noisy while the mothers sat in silence; it was all quite hard to understand. I remember sitting in that waiting room for hours, waiting for my turn, looking at all the kids, wondering who would be marred for life, trying to figure out what their unique problems were, and feeling so very fortunate for my own problems, which seemed minor in comparison. I had a sense that my misfortunes would simply fade away, a feeling that I would be made whole again, sometimes even wondering why I was there. It felt almost as if it was just a social visit, some time alone with my mother and my friend, the doctor. The other kids were always of interest to me—had I seen them before? What was their problem? What was Langsam doing for them? Were they going to get better? Their problems were of more interest to me than mine. Thinking about their problems reduced the level of chaos. I spent my waiting time watching, feeling, thinking, and learning.

I rarely viewed my club feet as an impediment. I rode my bike and played as much baseball as I could fit into a day. I never remember being left out. However, I wasn't allowed to wear sneakers or normal shoes. My shoes, even while playing sports, were tight fitting, laced black leather boots that sometimes went as high as my knees. My mother and I purchased these boots in a special store in Manhattan; in fact, the first time I went to Buster Brown's shoe store I felt like the luckiest kid in the world. I remember sitting on a green baseball bench waiting for my time at bat, trying to hide my lower legs under a wooden bench. Although I was occasionally ashamed, I cannot recall a time that my friends ever drew attention to my feet or boots (I think they all lived in fear of my mother). My boots never stopped me. After all, if I wasn't wearing my boots, I was wearing one or two casts. My father, whom I used to go to work with on weekends, shared an office in Jamaica, New York, with several people. Above one of the desks was a framed quote that continued to remind me how fortunate I was—"*I once complained of not having shoes, then I met a man with no feet.*" I learned about relativity at a rather young age.

In fact, having club feet made me special. Every night, my mother and I would spend time with each other, time away from my older sister and younger brother, time when my mother wasn't troubled by the world. I was the center of attention, I did my exercises, and my mother massaged my feet. My wife, Louise, claims that these early experiences have led to unrealistic expectations of our marriage.

While I could regale you with my athletic achievements, that is not the point of this tale. Although our family had to face a setback, this experience made all of us (especially me) much stronger. I was sick; Dr. Langsam and my mother made me feel special. I was crippled; they made me feel whole. I was weak; they made me feel strong. I was ashamed; my doctor, parents, and friends made me feel proud. I learned the importance of persistence and hard work in the face of setbacks, supportive parents and friends, knowledge, and innovation. I also learned about the power of healing and the need to occasionally take risks. These lessons and learned values were worth the price of my club feet. It also turns out that these values are essential to the success of a physician-scientist.

Public School: Dreams, Commitment, and Signs of Confidence

I enjoyed science. I found science easy to learn because it helped make sense of the world. It helped me understand mysteries like my own conception and birth, the beginning and evolution of life, the stars in the sky, and just how difficult it would be to get to the moon. Although much of these "truths" turned out to be wrong, they provided a context to think about the world and to understand nature. While science freed me to think about what could be, it also constantly forced me to think about what is, and what is not. So at an early age, I felt at home with science.

But I loved baseball. In fact, I (like many kids I grew up with) dreamed of becoming a professional baseball player. By age 10, I was firmly entrenched in Little League, had almost gotten Casey Stengel's autograph (actually I had knocked poor Casey Stengel over in the Polo Grounds while trying to get his autograph), had gone to several New York Mets baseball games with my friends, and had a newspaper route that included Choo Choo Coleman, a catcher for the Mets. When we couldn't play on a ball field, we played stickball in the street in front of my home. We painted bases on the street, organized teams, played against other neighborhoods, and contended with annoying traffic. Howard Stall served as the official umpire; he was a few years older than us and wanted to become a Rabbi, so while we frequently argued with his calls, we trusted him. Baseball was part of my daily life, with or without casts on my legs.

Although I'm left-handed, I was able to play every position except catcher (few left-handed catcher mitts were generally available for a good reason). My favorite position was the outfield, where I would play with the flight of the ball before ending its journey. But I loved the quickness of short stop and third base, even though these were nearly impossible for a lefty. Once, I even convinced my coach to let me pitch; however, he only left me in for one batter, which I walked (and nearly beaned). I played on some of the best Little League teams, was occasionally invited to play on the all-star team, and even made it to the county playoffs. One of my trademark plays was to steal home, a mind game between the runner, the pitcher, and the catcher. I must have stolen home at least a dozen times.

The push and pull between science and baseball became evident in my seventh grade biology class. My biology teacher, Mrs. Boyer, was trying to teach us the differences between the theories of evolution proposed by Darwin and Lamarck. I was sitting next to the window, thought I had understood the point of her lecture, and began gazing out the window on a baseball field. The field was empty, but I had fantasized a field of players and several innings of play. In fact, I was just about to catch a high fly ball to left field when I was startled to reality by Mrs. Boyer who was asking me a question about a mouse whose grandfather's tail was removed by Lamarck. I had no idea what she was talking about but was impressed by her anger. She was yelling, her face was red, and her neck veins were engorged. I was one of only a handful of students in her advanced biology course, and she made it abundantly clear to me that if I wanted to stay in her class she expected more of me. A few weeks later, she came by my house, picked me up in her Volkswagen Beetle (vintage 1963), and told me that she believed in me and my abilities but I had to stop daydreaming and become more engaged in class. Although I continue to do some of my best thinking while daydreaming, Mrs. Boyer heightened my commitment to science.

Mrs. Boyer pushed me into science fairs. While my friends completed erector toy type projects (reconstructing the skeleton of a chicken), Mrs. Boyer encouraged me to do experiments. However, no one ever taught me how to do an experiment, and mine were never well-conceived, feasible, conclusive, or won prizes. In seventh grade, I remember being fascinated by the work of Darwin and Mendel, and in one of the science fairs I attempted to extend Mendel's peas to Darwin's theory on evolution. I thought I could do this in one simple experiment in my basement. My plan was to use a stressful environment to select for a mutation that would result in a "more fit" strain of peas. I grew some peas in an aquarium with an ultraviolet light and other peas in an aquarium with a red light source. Soil conditions and water were similar. I used aluminum foil to keep out the sunlight, and kept a log book to record the results. I thought that UV light would result in normal growth and the red bulb would limit the ability of peas to undergo photosynthesis, and then somehow the stressed peas would spontaneously adapt, flourish, and evolve into a new strain of peas in this austere environment. Needless to say, this experiment (as well as many others) did not quite work out. The peas quickly outgrew my 10 gallon aquariums, I ran out of stakes and aluminum foil, the measured effects of growth were too simplistic, I never eliminated the confounding effects of sunlight, I neglected to account for the multi-generation component of the hypothesis in the research plan, and the hypothesis and plan were naïve and unrealistic. But my parents (who may have collectively taken one biology course) became convinced that their son was a budding scientist, encouraged my unbridled passion, and told their friends that I was destined to scientific prominence. It's quite amazing to reflect back on the paradox between the naïvety of these experiments and the support and enthusiasm of my parents. That unrestrained support is an essential element for succeeding in science; how else could we have the confidence to boldly attempt to create new knowledge? But it's also something we, as physicians, are obliged to pass on to our patients; how else could they learn to live with their chronic or untreatable diseases?

Mr. Gerardi was my high school chemistry teacher (Fig. 9.2). We had a very special relationship. Mr. Gerardi made chemistry fun, creating unexpected explosions, and telling stories about his family. The boundaries between work, school, home, and play just did not exist. Everything was fun, engaging, and important. However, because of my scientific curiosity, I had been placed in a more advanced class and was at least two, if not three, years younger than the others in the class. I was also small for my age, so I stood out. Mr. Gerardi kept trying to make class hard enough

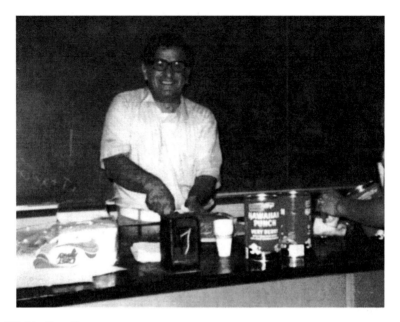

Fig. 9.2 Mr. Gerardi

to challenge me and not push my other classmates too much. While I was doing fine on exams, my fellow classmates were struggling. High school chemistry was just hard. Although I became the class tutor for some of the students, others gave up on the class. One student, John Wilson, was a large senior football player who sat close enough to me to be tempted by the answers on my exam. John would "ask" to look over my homework and tests before turning his in, and shamelessly copied my work verbatim. Luckily the chemistry class room was large, with lots of lab bench space, and Mr. Gerardi found a way to minimize my exposure during exams while not isolating me further or embarrassing the other students. He figured out how to help me fit into this very broad group of kids with different interests, abilities, and backgrounds. Mr. Gerardi taught me how, and maybe even why, it was so important to get along with all sorts of people. He also taught me to have fun with science.

Mr. Gerardi was also the faculty advisor for the student government. Largely as a result of his encouragement, activism, and people skills (that I wanted to emulate), I got involved in the student government and eventually ran for student president. My high school was typical for Long Island, with outstanding education and athletics programs and a large (over 3,000 students), diverse student body. Fortunately, my high school also had a sizeable number of Jewish students, and, as luck would have it, there were three students named David Schwartz in my high school class. So no one really knew which David Schwartz they were voting for. Needless to say, I won the election, and spent the next year engineering change and attempting to address contemporary political issues during the Vietnam War in the wake of the Kent State shootings. While the issues and their solutions seemed crystal clear to my liberal friends and me, many of our classmates (and friends) helped me understand that these issues were not that simple, especially when we tried to lower the American flag in opposition to the war in Vietnam. Although I was friends with many of the jocks (having wrestled on the junior high and high school teams) and led the fight to liberalize school restrictions for all the students, I quickly understood that memories fade quickly and loyalty in politics is short-lived.

Mr. Gerardi was my teacher and friend; in his roles as chemistry teacher and faculty advisor to the student government he was guided by the same principles. His expectations were high, he remained extremely supportive, he helped us realize that there were endless possibilities, and he was not afraid to share his hopes and dreams. I remember walking down the hall on the second floor with him one day. He was wearing his black blazer and gray slacks (with white socks), he was almost as short as me, he put his arm around my shoulder, looked me in the eyes, and said, "You are the future, and I believe in you." How could I not feel empowered?

Larry Grabin: Becoming Inspired

Larry Grabin wasn't my best friend in high school but he was a good friend (Fig. 9.3). We played sports and poker together but most of all we competed academically. But actually, there was no competition; Larry was much smarter than

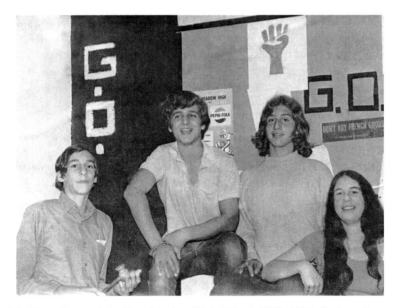

Fig. 9.3 The officers of the East Meadow High School (1970–1971) Student Government Organization (*left to right*): Larry Grabin (*Treasurer*), David Schwartz (*President*), Jesse Reece (*Vice-President*), and Deborah Rose (*Secretary*)

me. In fact, he is one of the brightest people I have ever known. His innate intellect is hard to describe. It was Zen-like. It just was. He never seemed to study but always knew the answers. Larry graduated first in the class, had perfect SAT scores, and was admitted to MIT early decision.

During Larry's freshman year, I spent more time with him than I had in high school, even though we were at different universities. Both of us were good at science (he was much better) and both of us were interested in medicine (though not committed). In the spring of our freshman year, Larry discovered a lump in his right testicle. This was eventually diagnosed as testicular cancer. Unfortunately, the year was 1972 and oncologists had not yet discovered that cisplatin could cure testicular cancer. Repeated unsuccessful surgeries scarred his stomach and removed his emerging manhood. The cancer spread, Larry continued to lose weight, and eventually he wasn't able to keep up. I frequently visited him in Boston, at his parent's home on Long Island, or at the Memorial Sloan-Kettering Hospital. What kept drawing me back to Larry was his will to live, his intellectual clarity, and his emotional honesty. Toward the end though, even he admitted that the cancer was going to take his life.

A few days before his death, I was visiting him in the hospital, Larry's older brother was doing some Hare Krishna mantra in the corner of the room, and Larry looked at me in a very dreamy state. Then suddenly, he focused like a beam of light shooting through a lens and told me that he was going to die very soon and feared that his life was going to be wasted. He knew that science was going to explode and would have profound effects on medicine. Larry wanted to be part of that explosion. He told me how much he believed in me, how much we meant to each other, and how much he wanted to do but simply could not; then his confabulated dreamy state returned.

Larry always wanted to do research in medicine, but he couldn't. However, on his deathbed he passed that vision on to me. He wanted me to think about disease in different ways, to understand the causes of disease to minimize suffering. He wanted me to venture out into the unknown and create new knowledge. In one brief instant, Larry inspired me and gave my life purpose. While I felt sorry for all the things in life that Larry would not be able to do, I felt privileged to have been a part of his life, and I felt that much more responsible. It's interesting how someone you respect can so profoundly affect your life with a few insightful comments. I listened and still listen carefully to the conversations I have had with Larry.

Fanny P.: Why Medicine and Science?

Fanny P. was one of the patients I inherited when my wife, Louise Sparks, and I began our internships at Boston City Hospital in 1980. Fanny was about 75 years old, the daughter of a southern slave, poor all her life, no family around, and losing weight daily. Although several of her physicians had already attempted to figure out what was wrong with her, she had been in the hospital for two months yet still eluded a diagnosis. Fanny was signed out to me as someone who was going to die and required little attention. As a new intern, I thought of Fanny as a challenge, something that I might be able to figure out, and a case that would prove my worth as an intern, almost a rite of passage. However, I was also emotionally hooked. Fanny made me sad; a vital woman whose life was far more challenging than mine was wasting away in silence and isolation. I also fell in love with her; she was engaging in her simplicity and the matter-of-fact way she responded to life and death decisions. Her life story was strange and unfamiliar to me.

Fanny had a very small infiltrate, maybe the size of a silver dollar, in one of the upper lobes of her lung. This was seen on chest X-ray, and in 1980 at Boston City Hospital we didn't have access to chest CT scans. Fanny had been worked up by the previous intern, the pulmonary medicine service, and had a bronchoscopy but still had no diagnosis. Most of the physicians suspected an occult neoplasm and had predicted that this "tumor" was eventually going to take her life through some poorly defined paraneoplastic process.

However, given the weight loss, absence of a smoking history, location of the chest lesion, and lack of apparent growth of the lung lesion or metastases, I was convinced that she had an indolent infection, like tuberculosis. I think I also wanted Fanny to have an indolent infection, so that we would have something to treat. So every morning I would arrive especially early and induce Fanny to produce a sputum specimen by snaking a tube down the back of her throat. At Boston City Hospital, interns analyzed most of the specimens we obtained from our patients. And each morning before rounds I would obtain a sputum specimen, and perform a Gram stain for bacteria, a silver stain for fungi, and an acid-fast bacillus smear for tuberculosis. Two weeks into these early morning sputum inductions, I found a single acid-fast organism but could not convince anyone that this represented tuberculosis. Rather than become discouraged, I became more resolved that Fanny had a treatable infection, and only worked harder to confirm the diagnosis. Finally, after about three weeks of this morning ritual, I obtained a sputum specimen that had enough organisms to convince everyone (including Don Craven, my rather meticulous infectious disease attending) that Fanny had tuberculosis.

I could not have felt better. Persistence, hard work, and instinct had paid off, and better yet, we were going to cure Fanny of her illness. I still remember the words I used at Fanny's bedside. "Fanny I have some great news for you. The reason that you don't feel well and that you're losing weight is that you have tuberculosis. We have drugs to treat tuberculosis and I'm sure you're going to get better." However, as soon as I mentioned tuberculosis, Fanny looked at me with the most despair and anxiety that I have ever seen on anyone's face. Her eyes were deep set, nearly black holes from her malnutrition, and the words came from behind her head. In a deep, low-pitched voice she responded, "That means I'm going to die." While I tried to dissuade her from this belief, she held on and tried to convince me that tuberculosis was a death sentence. Despite treating her with all of the appropriate medications and nutrients, her tuberculosis spread and she died two weeks later.

The lessons of humility, limitations of medical knowledge, effect of cultural beliefs on human health, and the will to live (or die) could not have been stronger.

Although now a physician, I felt the same helplessness that I felt watching Larry Grabin die of testicular cancer. Moreover, diagnosing Fanny P. with tuberculosis and watching her die anyway made me realize how little we understood about medicine, how much we could learn from our patients, and the essential role science would play in understanding disease. In fact, the disease, hardship, and uncertainty faced by my patients and their families continue to inspire my work as a scientist. For me, without this intellectual, emotional, and practical balance between medicine and science, I fear that my dedication might suffer and neither endeavor would be quite as fulfilling.

Learning to Think Scientifically

Undergraduate education was a turning point. Ironically, little thought went into choosing the University of Rochester. Although my parents pledged their support, they had little knowledge of undergraduate schools and entrusted me to make the decision. My guidance counselor told me I could go most anywhere, made a few random suggestions, and was generally unhelpful. The decision to attend the University of Rochester was based on passion. I visited Rochester in the early fall of my senior year with my friend, Richard Hempling, only because his sister, Linda, was a student at the university. However, as we approached the university, my heart began to pound (similar to the heart throbs I felt when meeting my first and last sweethearts), I looked out of the car window as we rounded Campus Drive (now Wilson Boulevard), peered down the quadrangle, and literally felt my destiny. I applied early decision, received a Bausch and Lomb science scholarship, and never looked back.

Although public education taught me how to learn, it did little to foster my creativity. For me (as with most others I suspect), my college education resulted in a quantum leap in my cognitive skills. I quickly realized that my professors were expecting me to solve problems, something I preferred to memorizing lists of information. Moreover, at Rochester, I had the opportunity to work directly with outstanding problem solvers—Jules Cohen (determinants of myocardial ischemia) and Fred Sherman (transcription regulation in yeast). While my own research projects were rather limited, I felt humbled by the challenges and opportunities of biomedical research, inspired by the discoveries of others in these labs, excited to contribute to the camaraderie of my fellow labbies, and privileged to be included in this quest for knowledge. Although my decision to attend the University of Rochester was poorly conceived, my four years at Rochester taught me to view ideas from different vantage points, to think broadly across academic disciplines, and to begin to think scientifically.

As a medical student, I wanted to do research but thought that my family background (lower middle class, public schooling, and lacking any connections to medicine or research) precluded me from this rarified club. I had no idea that science is one of the most egalitarian professions—you live and die by your wits, hard work, persistence, and collaborations. Abraham Braude, the chief of infectious diseases at

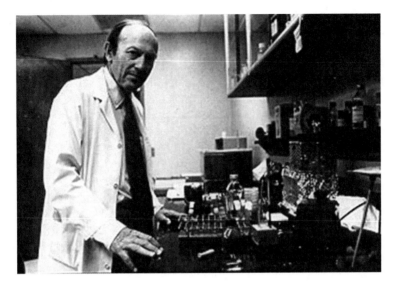

Fig. 9.4   Abraham Braude

the University of California, San Diego, my first scientific mentor, proved that to me (Fig. 9.4). Fortunately, my medical school required a student research project, and Dr. Braude wanted me to work with him. Braude was bright, tough, hard working, and brutally honest. However, Dr. Braude could be vicious (and he used to take pride that his name rhymed with rowdy). He was known for tearing medical students and house staff apart, asking them complicated questions that tested their medical knowledge or basic intelligence. If you answered one question correctly, he would ask a tougher question. A sign that he had given up all hope on a student was his standard final question, "So please tell us which high school you attended." While he terrified many students, house staff, and some faculty, I got along with him. His lofty expectations only made me work harder, and his insults were no different than those I experienced growing up in a Jewish home where most forms of communication are often argumentative or insulting.

In 1978, Dr. Braude, a few other physicians, and I were in the middle of infectious disease rounds, looking at organisms cultured from patients, and trying to decide which antibiotics to recommend. Suddenly, Dr. Benirschke burst into the lab and told Braude that his colony of Probosis monkeys in the San Diego Zoo was dying from *Cryptococcosis*, a fungus (Dr. Benirschke was a professor at the medical school but because of his interest in twinning was also a consultant at the San Diego Zoo). After hearing the story, Dr. Braude looked at me with his one good eye (one eye had been infected with herpes virus from a laboratory accident) and said "Schwartz, go out to the zoo and figure out what the hell's going on." Wow—I jumped at this opportunity. After learning how to anesthetize monkeys, draw blood, obtain lymph nodes, and measure lymphocyte function, Dr. Braude and I discovered that these monkeys had developed an acquired T helper cell deficiency, that their lymph nodes were depleted of mature T helper cells, and that the few remaining lymphocytes responded poorly to lymphocyte mitogens (phytohemoglutinnen and conconavalen A). Unfortunately, we had no real explanation for their acquired immunodeficiency and never thought to culture their lymph nodes for viruses. The title of our paper was something like "Acquired Immunodeficiency in the Probosis Monkeys Leads to Overwhelming Fungal Infection." Our paper was rejected from several journals, and Dr. Braude decided not to pursue the publication. Neither Dr. Braude nor I had any idea that a virus might be causing the immunodeficient state or that humans would develop a similar type of illness that would eventually be linked to human HIV (human immunodeficiency virus) infection. Years later he and I tried to resurrect this research, but we were both going in different directions and never found the needed time to devote to this work. However, to this day, I feel certain that we missed a huge opportunity, because the Probosis monkey probably had a simian form of HIV. This experience taught me how important it is to keep asking questions, not to settle for a superficial explanation, and to get ready to be surprised by new developments in medicine and science.

Following four years of clinical training after medical school and a year at the Harvard School of Public Health, I knew I wanted to focus on the interface between the host and the environment. While I joined a fairly elite research training program based at the University of Washington, I quickly realized that the mentors in the program did not have the expertise to help me study this problem. Although I made the most of the program, I also looked for other opportunities. While the University of Washington has a huge pool of talented investigators, few were doing the type of work that I wanted to pursue. After several weeks of knocking on doors (and thinking that my research career was going to end before it had began), I met Joan Clark (Fig. 9.5). Joan was a young assistant professor who had just moved from Washington University at St. Louis to the University of Washington. Joan had done some work in pulmonary fibrosis and was willing to take me into her lab so that I could begin to study asbestos-induced lung disease. However, since she was somewhat suspicious of my abilities and dedication, she asked me to write a research proposal, outlining my ideas and describing the proposed experiments. Before devoting any of her time or effort to my career, she wanted to make sure that I was able to put my thoughts into words and my words into actions. After agreeing to let me work with her, Joan and I decided to submit the proposal that I had written for her to the NIH. I thought the proposal was terrific. I also thought that the proposed experiments would establish the basic mechanisms to understand why some who were exposed to asbestos developed lung disease while others remained healthy. Joan knew better (and again, I think she was out to teach me a lesson). When I finally got my score back from the study section, I had received a 499 (at that time grants were scored from 100 to 500). I remember bursting into Joan's office to tell her the *great news* that I had received a near perfect score on my proposal. Joan looked at me, quietly asked me to sit down, and told me that the NIH scoring system was like golf, the lower the score the better. Although I was disappointed that I did so poorly on that application, I was amazed that strangers would take the time to seriously consider and critique my ideas, and I loved the way Joan took care of me.

Fig. 9.5 Joan Clark

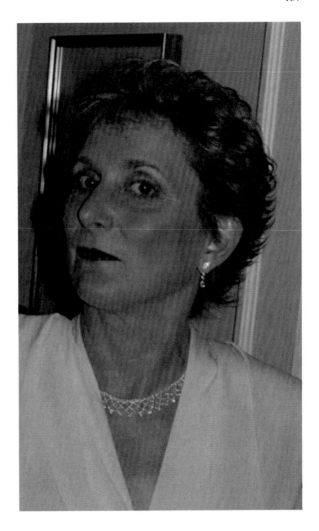

I think Joan felt worse than I did. She also helped me to understand that the lung was an ideal organ to study the interface between the host and the environment, and that if I was serious about my research I had to learn more about the lung. She was right (and I did).

Gil Omenn is almost as bright as Larry Grabin. Gil has a memory that is unsurpassed, and he is able to think very clearly across traditional disciplines. When I met Gil, he was the Dean of the School of Public Health at the University of Washington. Gil and I got along well; both of us were interested in the interface between the host and the environment and knew that genetics would play an important role in explaining how and under what circumstances environmental exposures caused or exacerbated disease in humans. Gil and I also had similar personality flaws. Both of us did not (and still do not) see brick walls, and both were sometimes a bit too persistent in our quest for an answer when we didn't understand. While these traits may seem like necessary attributes for success, they are dangerous and can and have derailed the best intentions.

Gil has always provided perspective for me. When I first started working with Joan, Gil would occasionally meet with us to help us understand the relative importance of our work and the opportunities in the field. He was always thinking five years ahead and helped me to understand the importance of vision as a way of taking bold steps forward. Gil has continued to be a sounding board for me over the past 20 years. I remain awed by his energy, intellect, and high standards.

Nine years after graduating from medical school, I got my first job at the University of Iowa. It could not have been a more perfect place for me to develop my career. I was supported, my time was protected, and everyone wanted me to succeed. Most importantly, I had a clear niche. While there were lots of physician-scientists doing clinical research and many outstanding physician-scientists doing basic research, few individuals were interested in integrating these disciplines to understand human disease. This was especially true for environmental lung disease. Ironically, I did not choose to go to the University of Iowa—this was my wife, Louise's, choice. Louise was also a young physician-scientist and wanted to work in a strong academic program where we could raise our children in a rural environment. Louise made the decision; I followed, and fell into an ideal situation.

However, my problem was that I was not fully equipped to investigate the interface between the environment and the host. Two very wise people, Gary Hunninghake and Frank Abboud, recognized that I needed more training. While other universities were trying to recruit me to take on administrative positions, Gary and Frank encouraged me to do a sabbatical in a molecular genetics lab so that I could begin to understand why only certain individuals developed disease when challenged with environmental agents while others remained healthy. This turned out to be a critical step in my career but would not have happened if not for the support and guidance of Gary and Frank.

Fortunately for me, I ended up doing my sabbatical with Jeff Murray (Fig. 9.6), a faculty member at the University of Iowa. Jeff is someone who stands out in a crowd. He consistently has been one of the best funded investigators at the university and was far from traditional, shaving once or twice a week, and wearing flip-flops with shorts or jeans most of the year. I found him bright, broad thinking, and scientifically creative. Jeff had over 30 people working in his lab ranging in age from 16 to 50. He had a knack for giving everyone enough space and support to move their work along. When you needed him he was usually there, but for the most part, everyone was on his or her own. We were all responsible for our own work, which made us that much more responsible, interactive, and independent.

I had previously discovered that endotoxin, a toxin released by bacteria, was important in the development of airway disease in agricultural workers. However, some people appeared to be more susceptible than others. To identify the gene or genes involved in the response to endotoxin, Jeff and I decided to focus on a strain of mice that was genetically resistant to endotoxin. While the gene responsible for this effect (Toll-like receptor 4) was eventually discovered by a competing group of

Fig. 9.6 Jeff Murray

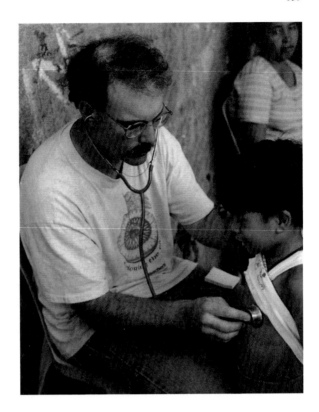

investigators, we were the first to clone this gene in humans and discover a variant in this gene that explained the differential response to endotoxin in the environment. Moreover, this discovery opened an entirely new area of research that has allowed us to understand how people defend themselves against microorganisms and how these genetic variants protect or enhance the risk of developing inflammatory and infectious diseases in humans. This extended sabbatical provided me with the skills needed to more rigorously explore the interface between the environment and the host. Jeff also taught me how to think programmatically without losing focus. Since leaving Jeff's lab, I have strived to create a laboratory environment that approximates the combination of chaos, creativity, friendly competition, productivity, and diversity I experienced during my sabbatical.

I continue to rely on my mentors for advice and encouragement. Mostly, I value their honesty, perspective, and unwavering belief in science and in me. In fact, this past year I spent time with Gil Omenn at the University of Michigan, and he again provided the kind of support and encouragement that has helped me figure out how to move forward with my career. It's important to realize that while all of us struggle, and part of moving forward is balancing our successes with our failures, our mentors, families, and friends often provide the unconditional support that is needed to keep us whole.

Reflections and Lessons Learned

These personal encounters were all somewhat serendipitous, yet each had a profound effect on my life. In part, this was because each involved both a strong emotional and intellectual connection. In part, it was because each of these individuals took an interest in me and in helping me figure out how to take the next step in my life. In part, it was because I was at a point in my life where I was malleable and receptive. While these individuals made it clear that I had lots to look forward to, they also made it clear that the success or failure of these ventures were in my hands. These very special people empowered me to chart my future without imposing their choices on me.

My growth and development as a physician-scientist has been guided by several values and approaches that have been important to me and may prove helpful to others. These elements for success include:

1. Vision: I make important decisions in my career when I can clearly visualize a five-year horizon. Sometimes these visions are so crystal clear it is almost like peering into the future. Other times, there's a general outline with enough surrounding support to assure success. This helps me think more conceptually and programmatically, and not get hung up in the details of a particular decision.
2. Confidence: This is not easy and does not come naturally but is a necessary ingredient of a physician-scientist. All of us have sweaty palms before speaking in front of large audiences or are uncomfortable when proposing novel approaches to science or medicine. However, being at the leading edge of knowledge is what we do, and this takes courage and guts.
3. Dedication: While some may limit this value to hard work, I believe that the dedication of a physician-scientist also requires the ability to accept failure and continue to believe in our work and ourselves. Physician-scientists need to learn to be strengthened, rather than limited, by our failures.
4. Integrity and Character: At a very early age, the Talmud taught me to look inside myself and develop a sense of fairness that would guide my judgment. Being a physician-scientist has allowed me to exercise these values and beliefs in the interactions I have had with my patients and my colleagues.
5. Insight: My view is that the only way to look forward is to know where you have come from, what your strengths and weaknesses are, and what motivates you in your career. This requires thoughtful reflection and conversations with brutally honest colleagues, family, and friends.
6. Celebrate our Accomplishments: All too often, we forget to enjoy our few successes and to reward those who are responsible for our accomplishments. Given the delayed gratification of the biomedical enterprise, this is absolutely essential, pulls everyone together, and makes it all feel worthwhile.

While I feel privileged to be able to care for patients and contribute to science, this expansive sense of opportunity is something that only emerges over time. The life of a physician-scientist is steeped in delayed gratification, many failures, and

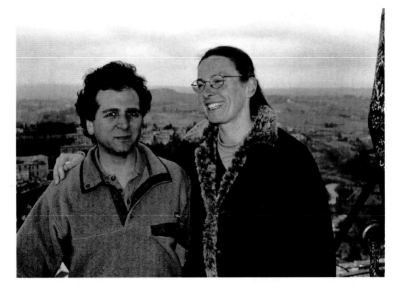

Fig. 9.7 Me and Louise

few successes. A good friend of mine, Dean Sheppard, once said that physician-scientists should only be allowed to give talks at national meetings every two to three years, since it takes that long to develop something substantial. While I agree with him, I think that physician-scientists have the capacity to create new knowledge every day by integrating the experiences and accomplishments of our patients, trainees, and our emerging science with the real limitations exerted by societal priorities and the needs of our families and communities. Fortunately, my wife of 30 years (Fig. 9.7) has never wavered from supporting my hopes and dreams.

Ten
Serendipity and Stamina: Staying the Course

Barton F. Haynes

During my career as a physician-scientist and my time as a mentor to young physician-scientists, I have been impressed that for success, one needs intellectual curiosity, good mentoring throughout one's career, the opportunity to work on important problems where little is known, the good fortune to find astute clinical partners, and the ability to work collaboratively in teams. My professional journey has been greatly enriched not only by insightful teachers and selfless mentors, some whom I have sought out and some who have found me, but also by learning early on in my career the benefits of hard work and a bit of good luck. I have followed a somewhat winding educational path to develop the skills, focus the motivation, and establish the contacts and collaborations that have contributed to my career.

First Glimpses of Curiosity

I grew up as the son of a cotton farmer and a homemaker in rural Tennessee, a less than likely prospect for a career as a physician-scientist. My father was a farmer in Collierville, Tennessee, a small farming town of approximately 2,000 people located 25 miles from Memphis.

From age 3 onwards, I was excited by the kitchen in my house more than any other area. Each Saturday morning, my mother would let me come in the kitchen and take anything off the shelf "to experiment." Flour, spices, eggs, milk, food coloring, oils, you name it—whatever was in the kitchen was used for "discoveries." While I enjoyed cooking, the rigor of following someone else's recipe was not nearly as exhilarating as "experimenting." Experimenting in the kitchen was so much fun that when I was sad or upset, I would go to the pantry and "experiment" to see what I could make. I had my own counter area where I could go to whenever I wanted. I can remember the feeling of joy and excitement from going to "experiment."

B.F. Haynes (✉)
Department of Medicine, Duke Human Vaccine Institute, Duke University, Durham, NC, USA
e-mail: hayne002@mc.duke.edu

D.A. Schwartz (ed.), *Medicine Science and Dreams*,
DOI 10.1007/978-90-481-9538-1_10, © Springer Science+Business Media B.V. 2011

I was the second of three children, and had a traditional southern rural childhood—helping on the farm, spending summer vacations at the lake, riding horses, going to church revivals, playing baseball, and drinking lemonade on the porch in the heat. As a child, much of my time was spent with friends and with nature. I had considerable time to be creative. I built model planes and boats and spent hours with my friends trying to make parachutes that worked when we tried to jump off our garage. There were few scheduled activities, particularly in the summer, so my friends and I had plenty of time to explore. It was particularly exciting to explore empty houses on our farm and see if we could find treasures in them from times past. Only occasionally did I get into mischief, such as the time I was so enthralled by the flight of hand-made airplanes that a friend and I covered the tops of trees by launching nearly a whole ream of paper planes from the top of a fire tower.

Seeing the birth of calves on our farm was a remarkable event for me when I was 6 years old. I particularly remember a difficult birth of a calf with a breech delivery and the heroic but unsuccessful attempts of the farmhands and veterinarian to save the calf and mother. After witnessing the attempted birth and feeling the pain of seeing animals die, I remember thinking for the first time, "I want to grow up and be able to figure out how to prevent bad things from happening." These times on the farm and in the kitchen "experimenting" were important in cultivating my curiosity and creative efforts, and in the simplest of ways, this first got me thinking about medicine and research.

Though I spent much of my early youth in a rural agrarian culture, by the time I was in high school, my father had gone back to graduate school to obtain a doctorate in education and then spent 20 years as a professor of education at Memphis State University. The respect with which he was treated in our community when he became "Doctor Haynes" made a profound impression on me, and for the first time, the idea of doing something that would garner that kind of respect occurred to me. My mother, who had done her best to instill academic values in me early on but who herself had left college to get married, later returned to college at age 60 and eventually became an accomplished scholar on the work of William Faulkner.

Early Mentors

While I was pushed to achieve in early years in school, much of the encouragement I received was harsh and ended with the admonition to "straighten up and fly right" when I underperformed. Once in high school, I came in contact with several remarkable teachers that were supportive, believed in me, and helped me to succeed. Coming from a very small rural school, I was not well prepared for the academic demands of high school or college. I was ambitious and persistent, though, and fortunately, a succession of mentors in high school and college saw that in me and chose to help me along—a theme of my later education and professional career.

Mrs. Ethel Thompson, my high school English teacher, was the wife of a Harvard graduate and local banker (Fig. 10.1). She was short, stocky, and always wore her

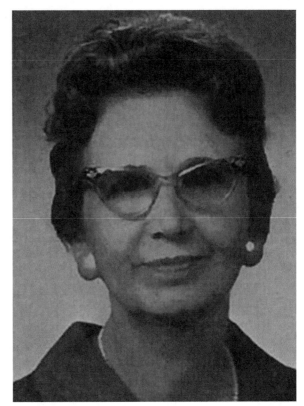

Fig. 10.1 Ethel Thompson in 1965

hair in a French bun. She was precise in her speech, serious about learning, and wonderfully enthusiastic about English studies. Her definition of English studies, however, was broad. She encouraged her students to get out of our small community and go to Memphis to see Shakespearean plays and other cultural events that came to town. She picked me out early in the ninth grade as someone she would guide, push, lead, and cajole to be the best that I could be and to take my education seriously. Amazingly, our school had no book store until she used her own money to start one so that her students could get interested in reading and have access to classic and contemporary literature. Ours was a conservative town and school, and Mrs. Thompson was questioned for bringing J.D. Salinger's *Catcher in the Rye* and other controversial books to the bookstore for sale. In response to this, she came to my home and brought me copies of *Catch-22, Lord of the Flies*, and *Catcher in the Rye*, and told me, "These all rank highly in college discussion circles, and you had better read them." Because she treated me as if I was going to college, I never doubted that I would.

Mrs. Thompson never spoke sharply to me but rather seemed to enjoy my work and discussions, and she even enjoyed my pranks and endured my talking in class. Collierville High School was a difficult school at times, with frequent fights in the halls and sports fields and intimidating behavior by some of the older boys. Being a boy and a good student was difficult. However, Ethel Thompson was somewhat of a rebel and worked hard to recruit some of the boys as well as cultivate the girls who were good students to do their best and to stretch themselves intellectually.

For example, to get me to stop using contractions in my writing, she had an art student make a cardboard albatross with a box with "N'T" in its beak and hung it around my neck in class, and then proceeded to have a discussion of how the phrase "albatross around one's neck" came from Coleridge's *Rime of the Ancient Mariner*. She sent supportive notes to my parents, encouraging them to be proud of me, and told them that I was special, even though in high school, my grades were only in the top 25% of the class. According to a note she sent to my parents, however, I was the top boy student in my English class. I think Mrs. Thompson was simply grateful for a male student that listened to her. In retrospect, if Ethel Thompson had not taken an interest in me and committed herself to getting me into the world, I might neither have learned what was needed to succeed, nor had the self esteem to pursue a scientific career.

When I was looking at colleges, Mrs. Thompson suggested I apply to Harvard; Mr. Thompson was the local Harvard graduate that interviewed me. I did not think that I had the grades to be competitive at Harvard, but I went ahead and applied for her sake. I did not get in, but she was pleased that I gave it a try. I did get in to Emory University in Atlanta, but I ended up at the University of Tennessee in Knoxville (UT) because that was the only school my family could afford. At UT there were excellent and caring people, and I was fortunate to find another supporter in Dr. Samuel Tipton, the Head of the UT Department of Zoology.

When I went to UT as a freshman in the fall of 1965, I went as a good student from my rural high school, but I was woefully unprepared for college calculus, chemistry, and language classes. I was well prepared in English, as well as for other courses such as history that required reading for content and writing essays. However, I struggled in the sciences and language and made poor grades in these studies. These were large classes, often with 300 students in each class, and I rapidly fell behind in this impersonal setting of learning. Most importantly, I did not know how to study effectively, process the volume of information needed to be successful in college, and master the subjects on my own. By all accounts, I was not destined to be a doctor or scientist.

Once faced with multiple bad grades in these courses and realizing that if I wanted to go to medical school things would have to change, I sought out Samuel Tipton in the Zoology Department and asked what I should do. He saw something in my earnestness and he said, "You need to try to take honors courses. They are smaller, and they will challenge you more, but you will have more personal attention from the teacher. If you have what it takes to be a doctor, and if you work hard, then you will do well in these courses. If you do not have what it takes, then you will find out. Why not start by taking my Honors Biology course?" In retrospect, this was a remarkable offer, and was pivotal in my development as a successful student. Samuel Tipton had a capacity for predicting what students are capable of, and must have cared that I was given a chance to learn to work hard and succeed. Seeking him out when I was near failing was one of the best things I did to get on a track toward my goals.

I took Tipton's honors course, worked as hard as I have ever worked in a class, and easily made an A, but more importantly, I became enthralled with the mysteries of science and biology. After that success, that grade qualified me for more Honors courses, and I took honors calculus, economics, and psychology. The teaching and experience in the honors biology course taught me how to study effectively in difficult courses and succeed, and I repeated this effort in other Honors classes, and scored well in all of these courses. For the first time, I finally understood how to study and rapidly grasp and learn new material.

Pleased with my work in his class, Samuel Tipton asked me to take a research elective in his laboratory and to work on the effect of thyroid hormone on induction of fetal hemoglobin in rats. This was my first research experience, and I was hooked! Tipton and his staff taught me to run electrophoresis gels and to use all the instruments in his laboratory. He gave me the key to his laboratory, and I could go and work any hour of the day or night. I completed the independent study elective course and then continued to work in his lab throughout the rest of my time at UT. This was a critically important time for me to have a gratifying first research experience, because this experience showed me how exciting and fun it was to work in the laboratory and perform real experiments. Had Samuel Tipton initially treated me with indifference when I had asked for help, I likely would have continued to flounder in college and would never have applied to medical school.

Having little money for college, I worked many jobs in college, the best of which was as the night watchman of the UT Student Center, for which I received room and board. To save money, I took extra classes, graduated six months early, and worked as a laboratory technician at the nearby UT hospital and research laboratories. There I learned how to work with rats and mice and how to process tissues for in vitro functional assays. While still not very good with my hands, nonetheless, this first laboratory job experience built on my UT college research experience and added to my enthusiasm for the possibility of a career in research, and it also showed me I could actually be paid for research!

My junior year at UT, Samuel Tipton came to me and said "You have shown you can do the work, and you need to go to medical school." He suggested Baylor College of Medicine in Houston, Texas as a good school for me. He must have written me a good letter, because in the spring of 1969, I received a telegram from the Baylor Dean, J.R. Schofield, saying that I was accepted. In this manner, Samuel Tipton handed me off to Baylor.

Medical School Mentors

Going to Baylor was similarly providential for me, in that I met there some of the finest teachers and mentors I could imagine. Clinical teaching was a priority at Baylor, and I was enthralled by the specialties of medicine, surgery, pediatrics, and obstetrics and gynecology. I had the opportunity to deliver over 80 babies in a few months in the public obstetrics hospital in Houston. The Baylor clinical departments competed with each other to see which department could teach the best, such that the medical students would score the highest on their national board tests. Surgery was exciting, because I was chosen to spend the entire surgery rotation on the service of Drs. Michael DeBakey and George Noon. By the end of my rotation, I was assisting residents placing patients on heart bypass, and had the chance to scrub in on over 70 open heart operations. On the cardiology rotation at the Texas Heart Institute, we were able to round with the team of Dr. Denton Cooley and see his huge hands operate so deftly on children's tiny hearts. It was during Dr. Cooley's operations that I first saw the human thymus as it was removed to expose a walnut-sized infant heart.

While on pediatrics, I rounded with Mary Ann South at Texas Children's Hospital on the immunodeficiency patients and helped with the care of the "bubble boy" with severe combined immunodeficiency disease (SCID), who was reared in an isolation chamber because of his lack of a functional immune system. I became interested in SCID and signed on with Don Singer the pediatric pathologist at Texas Children's Hospital to work with him and Mary Ann South to categorize SCID thymuses by histologic slide analysis. I learned about the thymus and human immunology, and this time served me well when I later began my own work on the human thymus. Mary Ann South and Don Singer said to me, "You need to spend time with Roger Rossen and Bill Butler in the Baylor Immunology Department," so Mary Ann and Don introduced me to Drs. Rossen and Butler.

I went to Rossen and Butler's research seminars, reviewed my research data with them, and went to their immunology journal club. They introduced me to all of the immunologists that came to visit Baylor. One especially fond memory is being invited to a dinner at Roger Rossen's house with the great English transplant immunologist, Rupert Billingham. Another is meeting the pediatric immunologist, Max Cooper, and learning about his concepts of separation of the T and B lineages of lymphocytes. In the beginning of my junior year, Bill Butler said, "You need to go to the National Institutes of Health (NIH) to become an immunologist. Let me arrange for you to meet and talk to Vernon Knight." Knight had taught us microbiology in the second year of medical school and was one of my favorite teachers. A tall and distinguished man, he spoke with a soft country accent and was very interested in students.

Vernon Knight at that time was a world-renowned virologist, who had come to Baylor from the NIH, where he was Director of the Laboratory of Clinical Investigation in the National Institute of Allergy and Infectious Diseases (NIAID). There, Knight had performed experimental infections with various viral agents on volunteers and worked out the virology and clinical immunology of viral respiratory infections. I went to his office and sat across from his chairman's desk. He asked what I wanted to do and I said, "I want to be an infectious disease doctor and study the interaction of the human immune system with infectious agents." He said, "Well then, there is only one place for you, and that is to go work with Sheldon Wolff at the NIAID in the Laboratory of Clinical Investigation." I did not know it then, but

Sheldon Wolff was Vernon Knight's protégé and had taken over for Knight at the NIAID when Knight came to Baylor. I immediately applied to the Public Health Service to work with Wolff in NIAID, and soon after interviewing at the NIH with Wolff and others, I received a phone call from Wolff, who said, "You are accepted to come to the NIAID after your first year of residency." I was so thrilled by this handoff to Dr. Wolff, I could hardly contain myself. First of all, the Vietnam War was still ongoing in 1972, and the Army was drafting medical students to serve in field hospitals. Second, the work in the Laboratory of Clinical Investigation was precisely what I was interested in, and third, the Public Health Service paid me a $12,000 salary for my last year in medical school. For the first time since UT, I didn't have to work to make ends meet while in school. Vernon Knight had handed me off to Sheldon Wolff, and with a salary to boot.

I chose medicine for my internship. Henry McIntosh, Baylor's current Chair of Medicine, was sent to Baylor by the great Duke cardiologist and future Duke Chief of Medicine, Eugene Stead. McIntosh said in my senior year interview, "You need to go to Duke, and I will get you in." I had heard that Duke had one of the most difficult internal medicine programs in the country, and most of my classmates were afraid to apply there. I said, "Dr. McIntosh, I had rather not go to Duke. I would rather end up at some northeast hospital." McIntosh said, "Well, just listen to me. You need to apply to Duke anyway, just in case." Henry McIntosh indeed was intent on handing me off against my wishes to the Duke medicine department.

I matched for medical internship at Duke—sometimes you just have to go where you are told and have faith it will work out—and it turned out to be the best program for me that I could have imagined. Baylor and Duke had similar philosophies about teaching and letting students and housestaff have considerable experience in patient care, and the clinical faculty at both schools were superb teachers. While at Duke, I learned to take care of virtually any patient with any disease that came to the emergency room or clinic. By the time I left Duke, I was ready for the NIH and to begin my research experience.

NIH Mentors

When I arrived at the NIH in 1975 as a Clinical Associate, I soon realized that the first year was clinical, spent rounding primarily with Sheldon Wolff (Fig. 10.2) and his protégé and new senior staff member, Anthony Fauci (Fig. 10.3). Fauci came to the Laboratory of Clinical Investigation from a medicine residency at Cornell, completed his NIAID clinical associate time, and then undertook a chief residency in medicine at Cornell before returning to NIAID as a Senior Investigator.

Sheldon Wolff's clinical interest was fevers of unknown origin. This paired well with his laboratory research interest of the biology of fever. Charles Dinarello and Sheldon Wolff isolated and characterized human leukocytic pyrogen (a molecule that causes fever) that came to be called interleukin-1. Wolff's paired clinical and basic research interests were common at the NIH for most investigators at that

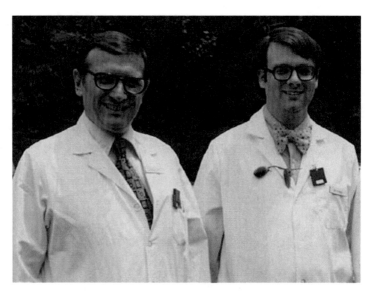

Fig. 10.2 Sheldon Wolff, Director of the Laboratory of Clinical Investigation (LCI) at the National Institutes of Health (*left*), in 1976. I had just finished my first year as a Clinical Associate and was beginning my year in Anthony Fauci's laboratory. I was also beginning my year as Chief Clinical Associate to help Wolff and Fauci manage the clinical service of the LCI. I have no idea why I was wearing a rose

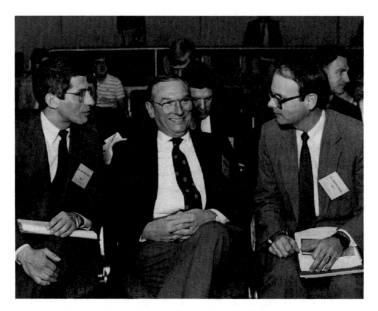

Fig. 10.3 Anthony Fauci (*left*) and Sheldon Wolff (*center*) during a visit to Duke in 1989 for a research symposium. Wolff took great pride in his trainees, and was especially pleased to be reunited with many of his former fellows at the conference

time. The NIH Clinical Center was originally designed with two parallel halls, one with patient rooms, and then a second hallway with research laboratories that were connected by short hallways to the patient corridor, so that the physician-scientist could easily go from bench to bedside and back. Wolff's broad interest in fevers of unknown origin led him to study a number of previously uncharacterized syndromes, and before I came to NIAID, Wolff's team performed classic studies on familial Mediterranean fever, Chediak-Higashi Syndrome, sarcoidosis and granulomatous hepatitis, and various forms of vasculitis. I was working on a paper that I had started at Duke about a form of recurrent meningitis. It was rambling and not publishable. I took it to Wolff and he helped me rewrite the paper to make it concise and to the point. I offered him authorship and he said "No, I just helped you do what you were already doing. That doesn't constitute authorship." While we subsequently published several papers together, that first discussion on authorship with Wolff taught me the importance of making sure one has contributed to a paper before allowing one's name to be placed on it.

In the late 1970s, Anthony Fauci's clinical interests were in various forms of systemic necrotizing vasculitis, and in particular, a form of vasculitis that affects the lungs, sinuses, and kidneys, called Wegener's granulomatosis. His basic research interest was the study of human immune responses in the setting of immune diseases and in response to infections. When I arrived at the NIAID in 1975, Fauci was just finishing up his classic studies on the mechanism of action of corticosteroids on the human immune system, and was beginning his second body of classic work on regulation of human B cell function.

Rounding on the wards of NIAID with the outstanding clinicians in the Laboratory of Clinical Investigation was the most exciting clinical time in my career (Fig. 10.4). In addition to Wolff and Fauci, investigators that admitted patients included Charles Kirkpatrick (immunodeficiency diseases), Michael Frank (immune complex diseases and complement deficiencies), Ray Dolin (viral diseases), Allen Kaplan and Mike Kaliner (allergic diseases), Charles Dinarello (pediatric fevers of unknown origin), John Gallin (neutrophil deficiency diseases), Frank Neva and Eric Ottesen (parasitic diseases), and John Bennett (fungal diseases). Their discussion on every patient was intense, not only about clinical aspects of the disease, but also about how the basic research laboratory techniques could be brought to bear to work out what the pathophysiology of the disease was, and then how to treat the disease. I was amazed that each investigator was also a superb clinician, and each had an encyclopedic knowledge of their particular types of disease.

At this time in 1975 through 1980 at the NIH, there was no intensive care unit (ICU) or coronary care unit (CCU), so if a patient became critically ill, the clinical associate had to wheel a monitor or a respirator into the room and convert the room to a more intensive care environment. My intense training at Duke served me well, since I had considerable CCU and ICU experience in spite of skipping my senior residency year, and unlike some of my colleagues on the NIH wards, I had neither any difficulty with the very sick patients, nor did I mind staying around the wards for long hours. However long we stayed at work at the NIH Clinical Center, it was never as long as we worked at Duke! I do not remember being particularly tired or

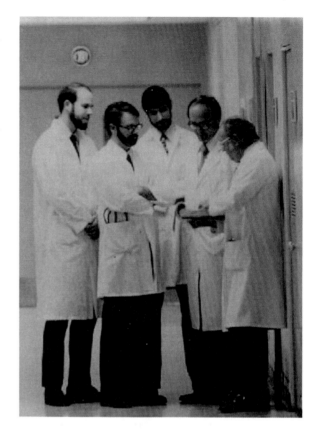

Fig. 10.4 Rounding at the NIH Clinical Center in 1978. Griff Ross (*right*), Chief of the Endocrinology and Reproduction Research Branch was the attending physician. Second from the left is myself, and third from the left is Lynn Loriaux, now chair of medicine at Oregon Health and Science University

sleepy during either the Duke or NIH training experiences. I was simply delighted to be doing what I was doing. What I do remember, however, was the ability to follow patients from the time they were admitted to the time we made the diagnosis and instituted treatment—a critical sequence of events on each patient for appropriate training of a physician.

Rounding with Anthony Fauci was particularly remarkable. While I had superb residents and teachers at Duke, to this day, I have never met such an enthusiastic, knowledgeable, and engaging clinician as Fauci. His clarity of thinking and high principles made me rethink all my patterns of reasoning about patients and clinical problems, and his joy at taking care of patients was an inspiration. No matter what hour of the day or night, he was fascinated and delighted at new clinical data and with making insightful diagnoses. Many of the patients I helped Anthony Fauci care for had obscure diseases with no known diagnosis, and during my five years at the NIH, we struggled to figure out what the pathophysiology was for them, even if we could not determine a named diagnosis, always with the ultimate goal of finding a treatment. When he would decide what he thought should be done for the patient,

I would often reply, "Ok, I will flog it!" These ward rounds taught me lessons in clinical investigation that I have never forgotten, such as, "If you cannot diagnose the disease, that is less important than studying the patient and figuring out the pathophysiology in order to treat the patient" and "Learn to see opportunity and excitement in what is not known" [1].

Midway into our first year at NIH as clinical associates, we applied to laboratories, and I was chosen to enter Anthony Fauci's laboratory. Already in the Fauci laboratory in 1976 were Jim Balow, Joe Parillo, and Gary Hunninghake, who were working on steroid biology, eosinophil biology, and antibody-dependent cellular cytotoxicity, respectively. My initial work centered on the effect of steroids on T cell subsets, the regulation of human B cell responses, and treatment studies with Wolff and Fauci of various vasculitis syndromes. Fauci was a tireless mentor, and we met every day to go over data, talk about patients, and plan future experiments. I thought by this time in my career that I was a hard worker. I had no idea what hard work was really like until I met Fauci. He is not only the hardest worker I have ever met, but he is also one of the smartest scientists I have ever worked with. Tony Fauci taught me that being smart and working very hard went hand in hand, and that both traits were essential for success as a physician-scientist. I was so grateful to be at NIH and so excited about the work that I would come in at 4 or 5 a.m. many days and work until 8 or 9 p.m. to get in two days' work in one day. In the last years of my time at the NIH, Fauci and I worked with George Eisenbarth in Marshall Niremberg's laboratory to make some of the first mouse monoclonal antibodies at the NIH. Some of these antibodies were against human T cells, and from this work came phenotypic panels for diagnosis of T cell malignancies and phylogeny studies of shared T cell molecules of humans and primates.

After five years in the Laboratory of Clinical Investigation at NIH, I was recruited to the faculty at Duke by James Wyngaarden, the Chair of medicine. I had received allergy and immunology as well as infectious disease board training at NIH, and I chose to join the Duke division of rheumatology. There I set up a laboratory to study human B cells, since my work at the NIH had been on B cell regulation. However, soon after arriving at Duke, Richard Metzgar in Immunology came to me and said, " To make anti-thymocyte globulin to treat kidney transplant rejection, we have been receiving human thymus from pediatric cardiac surgery cases where the surgeon has to trim the thymus away from the heart to correct infant congenital heart defects. We now get commercial anti-thymocyte globulin and do not need the thymus tissue. Do you want to study this tissue?" Remembering the thymus from watching Denton Cooley operate and from my work on SCID with Mary Ann South and Don Singer, I said "Absolutely!" and started to receive these discarded tissues. I quickly converted my laboratory over to studying the human thymus in health and disease. We worked out the ontogeny of the human thymus, and we learned how to grow postnatal human thymus under the kidney capsule in immune deficient mice. Working in an area completely different from that of my post-doctoral fellowship turned out to be a good decision, and taught me the lesson of "go where they ain't" to study areas that are not currently popular to find new opportunities [1].

Working in Collaboration with Astute Clinicians

A final lesson in my development as a physician-scientist was to learn to team with clinician-scientists in the study of difficult-to-treat diseases.

In 1993, Louise Markert was a young pediatric immunologist who was taking care of children with primary immunodeficiencies. She had just received a phone call from a physician asking for help for a baby born with DiGeorge anomaly, a congenital absence of the thymus. Hearing about my work with transplantation of human postnatal thymus into immune deficient mice, she asked for help in growing thymus grafts in tissue culture that could be transplanted into children with DiGeorge anomaly so that their normal bone marrow stem cells could colonize this thymus graft. The hope was that the new graft would "teach" the new developing thymus-derived lymphocytes (T cells) to be tolerant to the baby and to the graft. After much trial and error, Louise grew thymus that looked normal to me in histologic sections but had very few carry-over mature T cells that could harm the baby. Although the initial baby died before it was possible to perform thymus transplantation, Louise wrote an Institutional Review Board protocol and was ready when the next baby with complete DiGeorge anomaly who had no T cells was referred the following year. Louise had a surgeon implant the thymus stromal grafts into the thigh muscle of this patient, who would have died soon without treatment. To our amazement, when the graft was biopsied several weeks later, it showed that the baby's bone marrow stem cells had colonized the grafts. Soon thereafter, the baby had normal T cells in the blood. Now, nearly 15 years later, that baby and many others treated by Louise are alive, going to school, and have functional T cells having been cured by the regimen of cultured postnatal thymus transplantation.

Joseph Moore is an oncologist at Duke with whom I have collaborated to study several patients. We were referred a Japanese patient from Florida who was 14 years old in 1945 when the atomic bomb was dropped on Nagasaki. She survived the blast, married an American sailor, and immigrated to the USA with him after the war. In 1980, she came to Duke to see us, because at that time I was studying the origin of malignant cells in a spectrum of T cell malignancies, from acute leukemia to chronic malignant T cell syndromes such as cutaneous T cell lymphoma. The patient had a unique syndrome of ulcerating skin lesions and painful arthritis. Having read Robert Gallo and Bernard Poiez's recent paper on a new virus, the Human T Cell Lymphotrophic Virus Type I (HTLV-I) that causes Adult T Cell Leukemia syndrome, and realizing that the patient did not match other known disease patterns, I took cells from the patient's blood and joints and put them in tissue culture under conditions that would grow a retrovirus if it was present. We isolated HTLV-1 from her blood and demonstrated that the virus in her joints was the cause of her severe arthritis. She was the second patient described with HTLV-1 and the first patient in whom the syndrome of HTLV-1 associated arthritis was identified. This form of arthritis is now recognized to be common where HTLV-1 is endemic, but it was previously diagnosed as rheumatoid arthritis.

With Nancy Allen and Rex McCallum at Duke, I cared for and studied a group of complex patients with Cogan's syndrome, which is characterized by corneal inflammation, autoimmune hearing loss, and in some cases, various forms of blood vessel inflammation. Several of these patients had life-threatening forms of inflammation, requiring us to devise novel treatment regimens to keep them alive. One young boy came to me at age 12 with Cogan's syndrome and eye and inner ear inflammation. We successfully treated this disease with steroids and immunosuppressive agents, but as one autoimmune disease went into remission, he developed another autoimmune disease and then another. Over the next 20 years, it became clear that once activated, he had some type of defect of being unable to shut off his immune system, and this was manifested by recurring autoimmune disease syndromes involving the eyes, joints, and muscles. We developed multiple novel treatment regimens for each life-threatening autoimmune syndrome that for many years controlled each inflammatory event (Fig. 10.5). In spite of these multiple illnesses, the patient went to medical school and completed a pulmonary fellowship. However, after 20 years with uncontrolled immune activation, a malignant T cell clone emerged, resulting in the clinical syndrome of a progressive T cell lymphoma that ultimately led to his death. I grew very close to this patient and became a father figure to him. Before he died, he wrote to me, "You are the reason I wanted to be a doctor." This patient showed extraordinary courage to move his life forward in spite of his disease, and as well, had a remarkable trust in the physician-scientists who performed the laboratory work to decide on his best treatment. I learned an enormous amount from him about how to deal with an incurable and difficult-to-diagnose disease.

On another occasion, Joseph Moore called me to see a young 14-year-old boy with what was thought to be acute lymphoblastic leukemia (ALL). When he was treated with an experimental drug, however, his supposedly lymphocytic leukemia

(a)   (b)

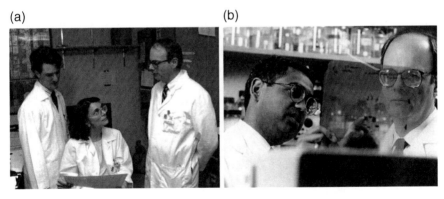

Fig. 10.5 Trainees in the Haynes laboratory in the 1990s. Panel A. Todd Barry (*left*), a MD-PhD student at Duke, worked on the pathogenesis of the young Cogan's syndrome patient described in the text and helped to demonstrate the gradual emergence of a malignant clone of T cells, a finding that helped guide the patient's treatment. Karen Rendt-Zagar (*center*) was a rheumatology fellow at Duke and learned to transplant synovial tissue into immunodeficient mice to study the pathogenesis of rheumatoid arthritis. Panel B. Dhaval Patel (*left*) a Duke MD-PhD graduate and rheumatology fellow who also worked on Cogan's syndrome patients as well as on other inflammatory disease patients we studied in the 1990s

cells differentiated into red cells, polymorphonuclear cells and other hematopoietic cells nearly overnight. After years of study, Joanne Kurtzburg, Michael Hershfield, and I showed that this patient was the first case of what is now known as stem cell leukemia, and that the experimental drug had caused the sudden differentiation of stem cells into multiple cell types.

From these experiences, I learned to listen to astute clinicians when they asked for help, and to always quickly come see their patients that did not fit the current diagnostic categories or for whom no treatment was available. It is important for the physician-scientist to value each patient on research protocols and work to attain and honor each patient's trust.

AIDS Research

My current work is focused on development of an AIDS vaccine. Bob Gallo called me one day in 1982 and asked me to move to Frederick, Maryland and help him determine the cause of this then newly identified disease. He said, "You are an immunologist, a clinician, and have isolated a human retrovirus. You have a combination of unique qualifications and we need you." I was hesitant to commit my research to this new disease. When I told Gallo this, he then said, "You *have* to work on this disease, it will become the greatest pandemic of our time!" [1]. This exhortation by Gallo again turned out to be critical for my career, and to be such sound advice. I had hesitated and come close to not responding to a challenge, for fear of failing and for fear of the unknown [1].

In 1982, Dani Bolognesi at Duke and I joined the National Cancer Institute AIDS Task Force lead by Gallo, and my job was to study Gilbert White's University of North Carolina at Chapel Hill (UNC) hemophilia cohort for those that might be infected with an as yet undiagnosed infectious agent that could be the cause of AIDS. In 1982, we did not know how infectious the new agent was, so we took advantage of the biosafety level 4 (BSL-4) facility built at Duke in the 1970s by the National Cancer Institute for cancer virus work, called the Cancer Center Isolation Facility (CCIF). There we set up a BSL-4 containment laboratory and a sensitive but not specific radioassay to screen for antibodies to retroviruses using HTVL-1 proteins. From this work came the identification of several patients from whom Gallo's team isolated what came to be called HIV-1 in 1984. Gallo's work paralleled that of Luc Montanier and Francois Barre-Sinoussi at the Pasteur Institute, and the lymphadenopathy-associated virus (LAV) they isolated in 1983 turned out to be the first isolate of HIV-1.

As soon as HIV-1 was confirmed to be the cause of AIDS in 1984, Bolognesi and I set out to work on an AIDS vaccine. In 1985, we thought that the best strategy was to identify the principle neutralizing determinant on the HIV-1 gp160 envelope and to use either the whole envelope or a part of the envelope to induce HIV-1 neutralizing antibodies. With Scott Putney and his team at Repligen, Bolognesi's and my groups identified and characterized the third variable loop of gp120 Env as the main target for neutralizing antibodies using the first laboratory-grown strains of HIV-1 identified in the epidemic.

However, soon after this work the extraordinary complexity of the problem of HIV-1 vaccine development began to emerge, initially with the realization that HIV-1 integrates into the host genome, HIV-1 rapidly mutates and exists in a near infinite number of quasispecies, and that HIV-1 strains frequently recombine. Particularly devastating was the realization that the early HIV-1 strains grown continuously in T cell lines in the laboratory were markedly different from those HIV-1 strains that are passed from person to person. Specifically, all the antibodies we learned to induce from 1985 through 1992 against T cell line-adapted HIV-1 strains were generally ineffective against HIV-1 strains directly isolated from patients.

After failure of two initial HIV-1 vaccine efficacy trials, the AIDS vaccine field has gone back to basic research to work on roadblocks that are standing in the way of vaccine development. The US military has now carried out an AIDS vaccine trial in Thailand and the vaccine tested was partially effective in prevention of HIV-1 transmission. While these results were not sufficient to indicate that this particular vaccine would be clinically useful, they did indicate that indeed a successful and clinically useful HIV-1 vaccine can be made. Although many roadblocks remain, I plan to work on this problem either until it is solved or I can no longer help the field to overcome the remaining barriers to a successful vaccine.

Lessons Learned on the Journey of Becoming a Physician-Scientist

What are the lessons from this brief reminiscence? Certainly the main point is that one cannot make the journey to become a physician-scientist alone. Without any one of my mentors, Ethel Thompson, Samuel Tipton, Mary Ann South, Don Singer, Roger Rossen, Bill Butler, Vernon Knight, Sheldon Wolff, and Anthony Fauci, the chain of "hand-offs" would have been broken, and my physician-scientist story could have been quite different from what it is today. Second, it is important to learn that when one senses aversion to a problem because little is known, then it is important to recognize the opportunity, and to "go where they ain't," that is, to go study a problem that is important but where few others are concentrating. Third, it is important to learn to work in teams and to partner with master clinical investigators to be most effective as a physician-scientist. Teamwork is especially important today in science because of the complex nature of technologies and the necessity to work with large datasets in order to solve complex problems. And lastly, it is critical to be proactive and take some risks. Had I not sought out Samuel Tipton, applied to the Public Health Service, taken a risk in working with an unknown disease, and had the stubbornness to persist despite obstacles, I would have missed the opportunity to do work that I now absolutely love.

Now more than ever, it is imperative for current physician-scientists to nurture the next generation of physician-scientists. A word of encouragement or mentoring for young students who show interest in science, a place in the lab for high school or college students who are curious and eager, patience with a well-motivated trainee who needs help in developing critical skills—all these are necessary to develop our successors. In this time of turmoil regarding the future of health care and ever increasing encroachment on physicians' time to see and evaluate complex patients, the need for thoughtful physician-scientists is greater than ever before. We as a profession are in jeopardy of losing caring and curious physicians who can see patients, go back to the laboratory and figure out what the pathophysiology of the disease is, even without a diagnosis, and can devise a treatment. There is certainly no greater joy in medicine than to study a patient, solve an enigma, and then from those studies be able to develop a successful treatment.

Natural gifts and drive are necessary, but curiosity, willingness to take risks and forge new paths, and joy in one's work need the deliberate cultivation and support of those of us who have already found their paths to satisfying careers as physician-scientists.

Acknowledgements I am grateful to my parents, mentors, and scientific collaborators for their work and support over the years. My wife, Caroline, has been especially supportive and a wonderful life partner, and made many helpful comments and edits to this manuscript.

Reference

1. Haynes BF (1997) Mentoring physician-scientists: Fear of the unknown and scientific opportunity. Pharos Alpha Omega Alpha Honor Med Soc 60:10–12

Eleven
Twists and Turns on the Road to Becoming a Physician-Scientist

Stephen I. Katz

Classic Sibling Rivalry with My Ultimate Hero

In retrospect, it was a plain and simple case of sibling rivalry. My brother Robert (Bob) is three and a half years older than me, but he was a full seven years ahead of me in school. So as not to even try to compete, I took a different path. While Bob attained honors everywhere he turned, I barely finished high school, and when I did it was without an academic diploma. While Bob was in medical school at age 19, I finished high school and, at age 17, decided to join the US Coast Guard with my high school buddies. While Bob was the exemplary academic, I was the social butterfly. While Bob was the serious one, I had few cares growing up except for when and where the next party would take place.

Despite this intense rivalry, my brother became and remains my hero (Fig. 11.1). Bob helped open my eyes to the world. He encouraged my academic awakening during college. He strongly influenced my going to medical school. His excitement and enthusiasm for dermatology infected me, and his choice of a research-oriented residency program and his encouraging my visits to his program during medical school certainly influenced my own choice of a residency program. This choice transformed me, and it made me realize that there was more to medicine than seeing patients all day.

My Early Years

My first eleven years were spent in Brooklyn, NY. There is little doubt that the death of my mother at age 31, when I was 5, has had a lasting effect on me. Having recently viewed 8 mm family movies from the 1940s (I was born in 1941), I see

S.I. Katz (✉)
National Institute of Arthritis and Musculoskeletal and Skin Diseases, National Institutes of Health, Bethesda, MD, USA
e-mail: katzs@od.niams.nih.gov

D.A. Schwartz (ed.), *Medicine Science and Dreams*,
DOI 10.1007/978-90-481-9538-1_11, © Springer Science+Business Media B.V. 2011

Fig. 11.1 Brother Bob and me

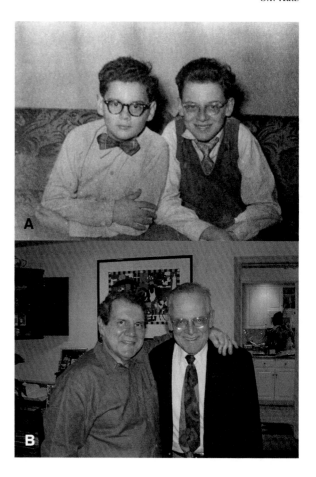

myself as a pretty happy kid, probably because of my father's dual-parent role and the tremendous support of both my father's and mother's families. Shortly after my mother's death, my father, brother, and I moved to an apartment opposite that of my paternal grandparents. These grandparents spoke to us in Yiddish and we responded in English. Their influence has lasted throughout my life and was particularly helpful to me in meeting my foreign language (German) requirement for medical school. (I had failed French in high school and did not want to attempt that again.)

Growing up with only one older brother (one child was born between us but died from an Rh incompatibility) and without a mother drew Bob and me together—a closeness whose importance was constantly reinforced by my grandmother. Bob and I and almost all of my many cousins attended a Yeshiva (Jewish parochial school) in the Crown Heights section of Brooklyn. Memories abound of our bus and trolley trips to school that drew all of us together. We maintained this closeness even after our family moved away from Brooklyn when I was 11.

When my father remarried, we moved to Washington, DC, where he bought an optometry practice, and I attended elementary school for the last half of sixth grade and then went on to junior high school in DC. Although I was a fairly good student at the Yeshiva, I stopped studying anything at all when I moved into junior high school and beyond, until I attended college.

My singular focus in high school was on my social life. My ability to dance certainly enhanced my social success. I was very active in a high school fraternity that was outlawed in Montgomery County, where I attended Bethesda-Chevy Chase High School, which is about one mile from the National Institutes of Health (NIH). Needless to say, I never heard of the NIH during high school, although I must have passed it a thousand times!

I finished high school in the top 80% of my very large class. At the time I did not realize that there were only 20% below me in academic standing. My diploma was a general, rather than an academic one. Thankfully, it was not a vocational one, also offered by my high school. I was mainly concerned with passing my senior classes since I was anxious to graduate and join the US Coast Guard. My friends and I decided that we would get our military service out of the way by serving for six months in the Coast Guard and then staying in the reserves. This seemed to be a good idea for me since I had no thoughts about going to college or even what I would do after my stint in the Coast Guard. All of these ideas were shattered when my father refused to sign for me (I was only 17, whereas my friends needed no parental consent since they were 18). The only alternative to working then became going to college.

My Awakening: The Discovery of Books

Fortunately for me, my state school, the University of Maryland, had very low entrance requirements in the late 1950s. My Scholastic Aptitude Test (SAT) scores (yes, they had SAT exams in those days!) were abysmal, in part (I hope), because I was drunk the night before I took this test. I have often been asked what motivated me to turn things around academically. My answer has always been that fear was my major motivating force. If I failed I would need to work or go into the Army, two very unattractive alternatives. The fear factor is only half true; the other factor was the revelation that learning new things can be a joy.

Before entering college, I began to think that the future is now and that I had better think about what I was going to study and to set a goal. In this regard my father was very helpful. He, his brother, several of his uncles, and two of my cousins were all optometrists, so he suggested that I follow this path. This seemed reasonable to me, so I became a pre-optometry student. The critical course to take and to do well in was physics, one of the courses that I, for reasons I still do not know, almost failed in high school. So, I took liberal arts courses and physics. I loved it all! This was a revelation to me, since I had never read a book before attending college.

Not only did I like learning, but also enjoyed studying. Despite getting "*As*" in physics, which I needed for entrance into optometry school, I decided to get tutored in physics so that I could really understand the basics. Little did I know that I would be the tutor the next year. My confidence was further buoyed when Dr. Sternberg, my physics professor, tried to get me to major in physics, an offer I declined. I majored in history, with a split focus on American and European history. I became intensely interested in history because of the personalities I encountered in reading biographies of our many great statesmen and all of our presidents.

I did very well academically in college—usually making the Dean's list except for the two semesters that I failed ROTC (Reserve Officer Training Corp), which was a requirement at the University of Maryland. My social life, however, suffered tremendously in college. The only social skill that I attained was the ability to play the guitar. My roommate had taught himself, and I thought that he could teach me, which he did. This ability has persisted for the past 50 years, and the repertoire has remained focused on popular music of the 1950s and 1960s and Jewish music of the 1970s.

My summers were spent in the Catskill Mountains, otherwise known as the Borscht Belt, because at that time, it catered to an almost exclusively Jewish clientele. At first I worked as a busboy helping my brother, the waiter. My brother was in medical school at the time and had a knack for calling some of our guests by their real names and others by made-up names. I almost never addressed the guest by name except for the one time that I asked "Mr. Parkinson, what would you like for dessert?" Unfortunately, I did not know that "Mr. Parkinson's" halting movements and flat affect reflected his physical infirmity rather than being his name! Consider the tumult caused by my naivety.

Going to Medical School: A Chance Choice

In my senior year of college, as my father's secretary was sending off requests for applications to optometry schools, my brother asked if I really wanted to go to optometry school. He suggested that since I already took the required courses for medical school admission (they were the same as for optometry school), I should go to medical school and examine eyes as an ophthalmologist. I liked the idea, although I had *never* contemplated going to medical school.

I chose Tulane Medical School because it was far from home, in a fun place and lastly, because it was supposed to be a good school, although I did not know anyone who attended Tulane Med. During my first weeks in New Orleans, second thoughts and frustrations began what has become an extraordinary journey in medicine and research.

The second thoughts? I nearly fainted twice during my first visit to the hospital, once while witnessing the passing of a nasogastric tube into a patient who had overdosed, and again while watching a delivery. The frustrations? September in New Orleans is very hot and muggy and replete with very large hungry mosquitoes. Additionally, a waterfall of rain would come on a moment's notice (I never took to umbrellas).

I was one of those who loved medical school. The long hours during the first two years provided me with a wealth of information about basic human biology. At first I felt woefully unprepared—I had taken the minimum prerequisites—nothing more than anatomy (of frogs), physics, and chemistry. After a month, I overcame the feelings of inadequacy and caught up with my classmates, a handful of whom remain close friends 48 years later.

Dermatology: What a Joke!

During my third year of medical school, my brother moved to the University of Miami where, after two years of medical residency in DC, he decided to become a dermatologist. This was inexplicable to me. He said that internal medicine was not specialized enough for him. Well, I could not imagine anyone going through all this training and then becoming a dermatologist, a specialty to which I had absolutely no exposure.

During my vacation trips when I visited my brother and his wife, Elaine, I began to understand my brother's choice. I spent at least one of my vacation days visiting Miami's dermatology department and greatly appreciated the high-level academic atmosphere that was generated by Dr. Harvey Blank and his outstanding faculty. It was because I wanted to at least be versed in my brother's specialty that I took a 12-week elective course in dermatology. Dr. Vincent Derbes headed the Allergy and Dermatology Division at Tulane. His course was not only very interesting, but he was also the most dynamic speaker and teacher I ever had. Others in my class felt the same—we chose him to be our graduation speaker.

A Summer Break During Medical School: A Life-Altering Experience

I decided that although lucrative, being a waiter in the Catskills would not broaden my medical experiences, so I decided to join the Public Health Service (PHS) and take my chances on where they would send me during the summer. The only good thing about my summer in Columbia, MO, in the PHS Heart Disease Control Program was that it made my application for a fellowship the next summer that much stronger.

It was after my junior year in medical school that I had the summer of my life. I wanted to do some type of research in England, so I went to my British-accented medical attending and asked if he could introduce me to someone in England. I was surprised when he told me that he knew no one in England but thought that Dr. Grace Goldsmith might be able to help. It turns out that Dr. Goldsmith was a world-renowned physician, a nutritionist who was unknown to all of my classmates. When I visited her, she was very welcoming and told me that although she had no connections to England, she knew many people who had been doing interesting work in East Africa. East Africa? Yikes—where was that?

Dr. Goldsmith then put me in touch with Professor Derrick Jelliffe, a renowned pediatrician, who was leading a large research effort in Kampala, Uganda.

My research project was to investigate the effect of urbanization on marginal malnutrition, a problem that was evolving because of demands on the mothers to work to meet increased monetary demands on families that moved from the country to the city. At that time, condensed evaporated milk was the "great blessing" that was a nursing substitute. The only problem was that these people did not know and were not instructed on how to dilute the milk. They ended up diluting the formula to a point that it was no longer nutritious.

Dr. Goldsmith, the person none of us ever heard of, helped me secure a grant that paid for my travel and subsistence in Kampala for the summer. The grant came from the American Medical Association (AMA) Council on Foods and Nutrition, and just happened to be given in her honor in 1965. How lucky for me!

Against my father's wishes, I accepted the fellowship and learned much about the world and about myself that summer. My father was fearful that I would be eaten by the cannibals if I went to Africa, but when I told him about the synagogue that I visited during a sojourn to Nairobi, somehow his fears were allayed.

This experience was my first outside the USA (Fig. 11.2). Arriving in Kampala after spending a week visiting Rome and Athens, I had tremendous feelings of excitement and anxiety. I stayed in the dormitory at Makerere University, where I met many of their medical students. This was a special time, for all of East Africa. Uganda, Kenya, and Tanzania had achieved independence in the early 1960s and had many reciprocal arrangements. Their postal system, airlines, and educational systems were all totally integrated. Makerere University was responsible for the

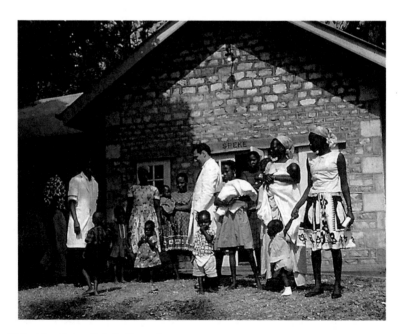

Fig. 11.2 Attending a clinic in Kampala

basic science education for medical students from all three countries. Clinical experiences were obtained in the major cities of these countries, Kampala, Nairobi, and Dar es Salaam. All these collaborations were shattered when Idi Amin took power in Uganda in the early 1970s.

I had many first experiences—scientific, medical, and social. Professor Jelliffe gave me the project described above and provided me with a full-time interpreter, as well as transportation. Professor Whitehead provided me with laboratory space where I could perform biochemical and microbiological studies. I rented a Vespa motor scooter to go into communities where there was no access for the van that was provided. Socially, my experiences were unforgettable: walking into the dining hall while holding hands with my male colleagues, eating foods that I had never heard of, being the only white person in a totally African community, and even falling in love for the first time in my life.

My three months in Uganda changed my life because of the experiences cited above, because I had a modicum of success, and because I became interested in research. I felt that I could actually make a difference in the world by exploring new avenues of research. My research demonstrated that there were clear biochemical and microbiological changes seen in children who came to the city as opposed to those who continued to have a rural existence. The work was published, and it was cited as one of the reasons that I was chosen to graduate with honors from Tulane.

During my senior year of medical school I had to decide where to go for internship, and of course, on a specialty to pursue. I thought long and hard about doing international (now known as global) pediatrics. I loved the concept of having a life like my mentor, Professor Jelliffe, but I could not face spending most of my life in developing countries. I thought, and still think, that in order to talk the talk one needs to walk the walk, and I was not prepared to do so. During medical school I contemplated going into many specialties. Perhaps the only one I excluded was psychiatry, because I thought I would surely fall asleep while listening to patients. Although I was also very interested in internal medicine, I did not want to practice as an internist because I felt that I could never really become expert in all those organ systems.

During the first part of my medical internship at Los Angeles County Hospital, my father died. I felt very alone. My father and I were very close. In fact, we had earlier planned our partnership in optometric practice. His death may have played into my decision to do dermatology since not only was I interested in it, but I also thought it would draw my brother and me even closer. Indeed, it did!

Dermatology: A Specialty That Suited Me

So, dermatology seemed perfect: I could do some medicine, some pathology, and some surgery, and become an expert in a specialty that was beginning to have a scientific base and was becoming respectable. When I chose dermatology as a specialty, it was with the idea that I would have a clinical practice. I interviewed at three residency programs and was delighted when Dr. Harvey Blank ended our Friday afternoon interview by saying, "Steve, we'd love to have you do your residency here [in Miami]. Let me know by Monday if you want to come here." To those vying for a dermatology residency these days, this must seem marvelous. I guess that Dr. Blank was impressed with my brother, who was just finishing his training, and thought that I shared some of his "smart" DNA.

Dr. Blank had an unusual way of teaching and encouraging research. With regard to teaching, there was no obvious didactic program. When I began, it was as if the program proceeded without noticing me or any of the other first-year residents. Because of this unusual approach, one that, despite my familiarity with the program, I did not anticipate, I decided to try to move to the New York University (NYU) Dermatology Residency. The program Chair at NYU, Dr. Rudolf Baer, was ready to accept my transfer but wanted to talk with Dr. Blank about me. By this time, however, I realized that I could thrive on the educational program at Miami. Curiosity and homework were the elements of thrust in this environment. So, I decided to remain at Miami, which suited my wife, Linda, who was pursuing her PhD at the University of Miami.

Dr. Blank encouraged (forced might be a better word) all residents to do a research project. There was a critical mass of dermatologist clinician scientists as well as basic scientists in the program, so it was not hard to attach oneself to an ongoing project. Dr. Blank's great talent for encouraging research among the residents was to send us research articles that were related to our patients. During my first year of residency, I had the misfortune of taking care of two patients who died, one from toxic epidermal necrolysis, and the other from pemphigus. About two years earlier it had been discovered that the sera of patients with pemphigus had antibodies that bound to the surface of stratified squamous epithelia, the precise site of immunopathology. Furthermore, the skin of these patients had antibody bound in vivo to the epidermal cell membranes. This intrigued me because it made so much sense from a biological standpoint.

Although the only immunology I learned in medical school was how to read an ouchterloney plate, I was intrigued by the notion of autoimmune diseases and spent the rest of my residency studying patients with pemphigus, bullous pemphigoid, and other blistering skin diseases. I was indeed lucky that I had wonderful mentors, most notably Dr. Blank and Dr. Ken Halprin, a dermatologist and biochemist who provided space and money for me to pursue laboratory studies on these patients. More importantly, although he was not an immunologist, he taught me how to approach science and how to learn new techniques.

During residency I tried to become as good a clinician as possible, realizing all along that this is a lifetime endeavor. I was also excited about taking new scientific approaches to patient-related problems. My research was also greatly enhanced by the arrival of Dr. Theo Inderbitzen, a German immunologist, to the Miami area. He helped me to focus on very specific scientific questions relating to these blistering skin diseases.

Because of my interest in immunology, Dr. Blank nominated me for a scholarship to attend an annual skin biology meeting in Salishan, Oregon. The meeting in

Fig. 11.3 Proceedings from a "Montagna" meeting in 1969

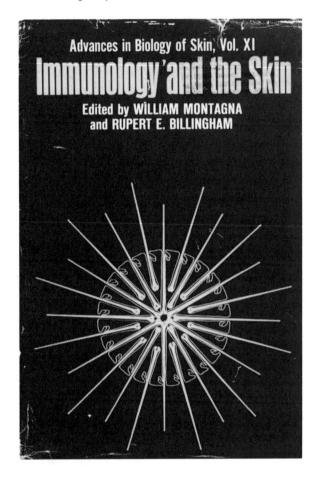

1969 was entitled, "Immunology and the Skin" (Fig. 11.3). This meeting opened up a whole new world to me. I realized that autoimmune blistering diseases represented only a small piece of the potential importance of the immune system in skin diseases. It was at this meeting that I met Professor John Turk, a dynamic outspoken British immunopathologist with whom I would work about three years later.

My residency program was another important turning point in my development as a physician-scientist. The clear mantra of the program was a critical approach to medicine and the importance of research in eliminating dogma. This was clearly imprinted on me in those three years in Miami.

During those three years, my private life also flourished. I had met my wife-to-be at Tulane and we were married 42 years ago, shortly after we moved to Miami. She was actually from Miami and did her PhD in Spanish literature at the University of Miami while I did my residency. Our eldest son, Mark, was born just weeks before we were to leave Miami.

What Next?—"You're in the Army Now"

During my internship I signed up for the Army's Berry Program. This allowed me to avoid being drafted before or during residency, so I agreed to spend two years in the Army after my residency. I had the great fortune to be assigned to the Walter Reed Army Medical Center (WRAMC) for my tour of duty (Fig. 11.4). I was given this assignment because the WRAMC Dermatology Program had been criticized by the Residency Review Committee for being too inbred. My arrival at WRAMC was greeted with some cynicism and jealousy by some of the WRAMC residents, since I was given "free time" to pursue research studies in addition to being in charge of the very busy clinic two days a week. It was wonderful for me that Dr. Mark Dahl

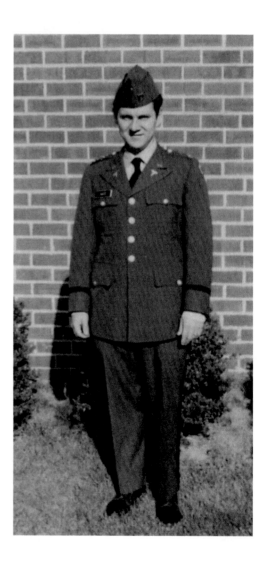

Fig. 11.4 Me in the Army, 1971

was also assigned to the program to assist me in academic pursuits. The Army did not know what to do with Mark since he had done a year of dermatology research in Europe, but did not do any residency. So he was labeled as a partially trained dermatologist but would be of no use in the clinic. He did, however, help me set up a laboratory. The Army was a great learning experience for me, as I explored teaching, doing research, organizing clinics, interacting with many VIP's including some in the White House, as well as beginning my mentoring career. Of course, we did not call it mentoring in those days, but Dr. Dahl (destined to private practice before coming into the Army), had an illustrious career as an academic dermatologist and became, at a very young age, President of the American Academy of Dermatology. Our research was very productive. Most notable was the collaboration with Drs. Warren Strober and Nick Rogentine at NIH on the identification of the association of dermatitis herpetiformis with HLA-B8, an association that had been previously identified with celiac disease.

Decision Time: Should I Pursue an Academic Career?

During my time at WRAMC, I met many basic and clinical immunologists, all of whom had completed formal fellowship training in immunology. I decided that if I were to become a successful academic dermatologist, I needed to do a proper fellowship. My specific area of pursuit was not in question. I had become well-versed in humoral immunity, but I was not knowledgeable at all in cell-mediated immunity. I decided that if I were to do a fellowship, I would work in that area of research. All along I thought that if I did not like doing research, I would be very happy practicing dermatology, since I loved the subject matter and very much enjoyed interacting with patients. So, I was not totally committed to academic and research dermatology. I felt that I had a very good fallback position in private practice. My other potential option was to join the staff at the University of Miami. I eliminated this option early in my decision-making.

My decision to pursue a fellowship in immunology was not really difficult because my wife was very supportive, I was not in debt, I was in no rush to make a lot of money, and my private practice fallback position was also attractive. My next decision was where to go. It had to be an English-speaking country, because I was not fluent in any other language. Additionally, I have always felt that humor is an important part of daily life. Even if I were fluent in another language, humor would be hard to grasp in that language. After speaking with many immunologists, I decided on three options: Av Michison or John Turk, both in London, or Gus Nossal in Melbourne. Each of these laboratories accepted me as a potential fellow. After realizing how far Australia was from the USA, and in view of the fact that we now had two sons, Mark and Ken, the only grandchildren of my in-laws, I decided to go to London.

Since Dr. Michison could not accommodate me until the following February (1973) and the subject that he proposed (finding the thy antigen in the rat) was not attractive to me, I decided to work with John Turk. Funding then became the challenge, but this was not an issue for long since Dr. Blank offered me fellowship support from the Miami Dermatology Foundation with no strings attached. That is, I would not be obliged to return to Miami after my fellowship. Of course, Dr. Blank knew of my wife's family connections in Miami, so he knew that Miami would be attractive to me. Fortunately for me, the National Dermatology Foundation also began offering research fellowship support in 1971, so I applied and received financial aid for two years beginning July 1972—$12,500 per year. I was also eligible for the Government Issue (GI) Bill, but only if I matriculated for a PhD degree at the University of London, of which John Turk's Institute of Basic Sciences, at the Royal College of Surgeons, was a part. This added about $4,000 per year to my income. When I decided to do the fellowship, I began moonlighting in the evenings and on Saturdays to add a financial cushion for our London adventure.

Changing Countries and Refocusing

Moving to London seemed easy at first. My family unit, wife and two boys, aged two years and nine months, was together. Finding an apartment was simplified because John Turk's wife was a matriarch of a northern London community, where she was the senior member of a large community practice of family physicians. Our four bedroom, two bath house had been vacated by a patient of Dr. T. Turk some months earlier. We were very welcomed into lovely Oakwood, a middle class white collar community.

The Turk Laboratory was very active from the early 1960s to the late 1980s. I was charged with studying the mechanisms through which cyclophosphamide, an alkylating agent, would modulate certain types of delayed-type hypersensitivity responses in guinea pigs. At that time it was thought (because of the work of the Dvoraks of Boston) that basophils may be critical modulators of these so-called Jones–Mote reactions. Jones (the resident) and Mote (the intern) had described a fleeting delayed-type hypersensitivity in humans in response to foreign serum, and this reaction was being simulated in guinea pigs. During my first months, I mainly did complete blood counts in guinea pigs in response to various doses of cyclophosphamide. I also spent many hours wondering why in the world I was doing this when I had such a strong knowledge base in dermatology. I now realize that this thought often occurs to clinicians when they immerse themselves in subject matter far afield from their comfort zone. Gradually, I began working with various lymphoid populations, doing passive transfer studies and cell separations, and felt that something might actually come out of this fellowship. I worked closely with Dr. Darien Parker, who taught me how to organize the laboratory, securing adequate reagents and the correct number of guinea pigs for the experiments that were planned, scheduling my time appropriately, and correctly handling the guinea pigs and the reagents. When results started rolling in and were validated, my self-questioning was no longer an issue. The conclusions of my research strongly suggested that in Jones–Mote hypersensitivity, T cell reactivity was modulated by B cells or B cell products. In contemporary immunological parlance I would interpret the Jones–Mote hpersensitivity reaction to be a Type 2 T cell reaction mediated by IFN-γ and IL-4 and IL-10 rather than a Type 1 T cell reaction mediated by IFN-α and IL-2 and IL-12. The results of these studies were published as two papers in *Nature*, two in *Cellular Immunity*, and one in the *Journal of Immunology*.

During my time in London, I actively participated in the Thursday evening meetings at the St. John's Hospital for Skin Disease or at the Royal Society of Medicine (Dermatology). I also regularly attended the Saturday morning Senior Registrars' meeting at St. John's. These meetings enabled me to maintain some of my clinical skills and, as importantly, to learn about how dermatology was practiced in another country. The experience was also broadening in that I saw patients with diseases I had never seen and some that I had never even heard of. Also, I met many people who have become lifelong friends.

John Turk was an excellent mentor (Fig. 11.5). We met regularly, and there was never a "failed" experiment, in that we learned something from everything we did unless the controls did not work. He was always encouraging and he was always able to identify a source for information that was vital to our experimental designs. During those years, there was also a critical mass of investigators in his Pathology Department so that my immunological experiences were not limited to my own studies. In addition, to my great fortune, in my second fellowship year, Dr. Morris Reichlin, an expert rheumatologist/immunochemist came to the lab on sabbatical.

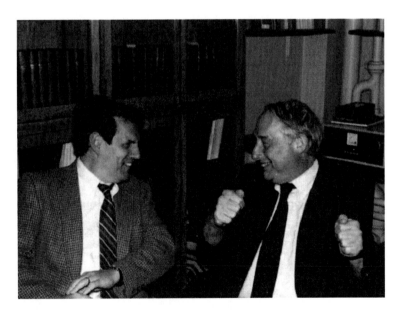

Fig. 11.5   Me with John Turk

He added considerable depth and an important dimension to my knowledge base, and has remained a resource and close friend for more than the past 35 years.

I had many wonderful family and social experiences during my stay in London: new friends, new hobbies (collecting antique earthenware and furniture), becoming a part of a community and most importantly, having our third child, Karen. As my two years of fellowship were coming to an end, John Turk wanted me to finish my PhD dissertation. I had been too busy doing experiments and writing papers to concentrate on the thesis. With Dr. Turk's help, I obtained three months of support from the Dunhill Foundation of England in order to write my thesis, which I returned to defend about one month after leaving London.

Choices Abound for Career Options

After 18 months in London, I knew that I wanted to try my hand at academic dermatology. Although I was not seeing my own patients, I was reading voraciously and had many ideas for experiments that I wanted to do, which involved both laboratory- and clinically-based research. In December 1973, we decided to return to the USA for a vacation and for a job search. There were six offers on the table—two I discarded because they were in New York, and I had no interest in raising my family in New York even though the offers always came with "most of our staff live in Connecticut" or "in New Jersey or in Westchester County." My comfort zone was the University of Miami, where I knew the staff and trusted the Chairman, Dr. Blank. The only other potentially serious option was the Dermatology Branch of the National Cancer Institute (NCI). The salary offer from the Branch Chief was only $25,000 per year, a figure that I felt was impossible to live on in the DC area at that time. On our way to Miami, I visited the NIH and met many notable and very encouraging scientists who embraced my joining the NIH. I was unimpressed with the activities of the Dermatology Branch, but both Dr. Warren Strober, a collaborator from my time in the Army, and Dr. Ira Green, an internationally renowned immunologist, assured me that collaborative potential was extraordinary across the intramural research program at the NIH. Much to my surprise, when I met the Scientific Director of the NCI, he told me that they very much wanted me to join the Branch and asked me how much money it would take to "get me." I hesitatingly said "30, 31, 32, 33" and he said that this would not be a problem. Wow! (I was amazed that one could "negotiate" with the government. One lesson I have learned is to be prepared to negotiate for any position that you are considering.) DC was my home; lots of childhood friends and my brother and his family were all additional attractions. In the back of my mind, I thought that if I were not successful in science, I would always enjoy my fallback position of going into practice on my own or with my brother.

I next visited the University of Miami, where they and I expected that I would go. This did not happen for a number of reasons, most important of which was my attraction to the potential of an NIH experience to determine my ability to work as an independent scientist. Other reasons entered into this decision not to go to Miami, including my being viewed as a very junior faculty person (former resident), not having enough protected time for doing research, and being told about how costly research was going to be, particularly the cost of guinea pigs that were my experimental animals of choice. Bottom line, my decision was based on the enormous potential of the NIH. It seemed like a candy store where one could choose from a myriad of possible research pursuits. The only down-side of going to the NIH, according to Morris Reichlin who was working in the Turk laboratory during this decision-making time, was the lack of students and residents at the NIH. Teaching was something that I enjoyed during residency and knew I would miss as a staff person, but I thought that this would come in three or four years, after I left the NIH when I would, if successful at NIH, move to join an academic health center.

The NIH: The Possibilities Are Limitless

I decided to accept the NIH offer and began my supposedly three or four year adventure in the fall of 1974. Unfortunately, the Dermatology Branch Chief, Dr. Marvin Lutzner, failed to tell the current occupant of my future lab that he had to move. After considerable consternation during which time I needed to return to London to defend my thesis, I finally had a laboratory of 330 square feet; this included desk space for me, a technician, and a fellow.

On my first day at NIH I was greeted by a very personable fellow named Kenneth Hertz. He introduced himself and told me that he was to be my fellow. This was a surprise to me, but I was pleased. Ken helped me set up the lab—I was planning to continue my studies of the modulation of T cell reactions using various animal models, particularly an experimental autoimmune encephalomyelitis guinea pig model, as well as to continue pursuing my interests in autoimmune blistering diseases.

Another personnel surprise came about two months later when I very uncharacteristically went to the cafeteria for lunch. I saw a Japanese doctor who I recognized as an attendee at our weekly Dermatology Grand Rounds. When I asked him what he was working on, he told me about something trivial that he was doing but then followed with "but I am supposed to work with you." Imagine my surprise. Dr. Hideo Yaoita and I worked together for four years and began a collaboration and cooperation with the dermatology Department of Tokyo University that has lasted for these past 35 years (Fig. 11.6). This cooperation expanded to many other Japanese dermatology departments and has been mutually beneficial. I have learned that if collaborations are not mutually beneficial, they do not last. To date, seven fellows who worked directly with me and eleven who worked in the Dermatology Branch are or have been professors and Chairs of Dermatology Departments in Japan. Most important and gratifying is that most continue to lead productive research programs. More about mentoring later.

Fig. 11.6 Me with Hideo
Yaoita

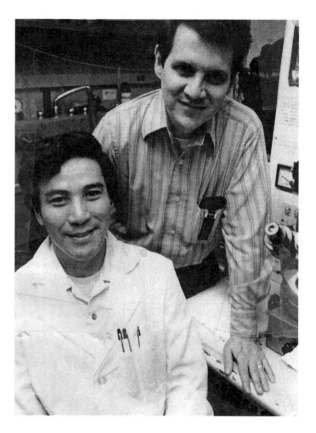

About one month after I started at the NIH, my brother referred to me a patient
with herpes gestationis, a blistering skin disease of pregnant women, now known as
pemphigoid gestationis. Clinically and histologically, the lesions appeared as those
of bullous pemphigoid (BP), but we found that rather than having in vivo bound
IgG and C3 at the basement-membrane zone, as in BP, the patient had only C3
bound in vivo at the site of primary immunopathology. The only way we could
study this patient was with the cooperation of people in other NIH institutes (I was
in the National Cancer Institute) who lent me reagents, a cryostat, and a fluorescence
microscope. The joy of this discovery was shared with those who provided me with
what I needed, led to many collaborations that followed in the ensuing years, and
further propelled my interest in clinical research.

During my first years at the NIH, I actively pursued my clinical interests in
autoimmune blistering diseases and helped oversee the dermatology clinical consultation service at the NIH Clinical Center. I also actively participated in the
Washington, DC Dermatological Society, whose members became my primary
referral sources. I maintain that, in order to maintain an active referral base, it is
critical to provide regular feedback to referring physicians.

My clinical acumen was tested when a 6-year-old was referred to our infectious disease service with "neutropenia and a rash" that had persisted for four years. After obtaining several skin biopsies, I thought this patient had a disease that was so rare that I had questioned its existence. I diagnosed the patient as having erythema elevatum diutinum and suggested that we treat her with dapsone. The infectious disease fellow shrugged me off with a pejorative statement that dermatologists always come up with weird ideas. I then went to his Chief of the Laboratory of Clinical Investigation, Dr. Sheldon Woolf, and presented the case for proceeding with my suggestion. Dr. Woolf agreed to treat the patient with dapsone and, in three days, the patient was 95% improved. This patient is still, 34 years later, dependent on dapsone therapy to keep her skin clear. It was because of this patient that I decided to study this disease in depth. The beauty of NIH is that we could bring in patients from around the country, and we were able to study six such patients. This clinical diagnosis established my role for many other interesting clinical consultations at the NIH for many years.

Establishing a Laboratory Program

The focus of my early laboratory pursuits was in two areas: (1) determining the immunopathological and inflammatory basis for autoimmune and inflammatory diseases, and (2) studying the modulation of T cell-mediated diseases in guinea pigs. The latter focus was on mechanisms involved in delayed-type hypersensitivity and contact hypersensitivity.

Because of my modicum of success and, I believe, because of my continued interest and enthusiasm for clinical dermatology, I was able to attract many very bright fellows to the NIH Dermatology Branch. Some of these, like Thomas J. Lawley (current Dean of Emory University School of Medicine) had never performed any research before coming to the NIH, while others, like Georg Stingl (now Professor of Dermatology at the University of Vienna) already had considerable laboratory experience before coming to the NIH (Fig. 11.7). It was Georg, who came to me with his in press paper about immune-related receptors of Langerhans cells (LC), who propelled me to move to mouse models because there were many more reagents available for mouse studies. During Georg's time and thereafter, we demonstrated the important functional role of LC in immunological reactions in skin and also demonstrated that LC were derived from bone marrow precursor cells.

For many years, my laboratory studies have continued to focus on all aspects of the skin immune system. The model system that we have been using utilizes a transgenic mouse model that expresses membrane-bound or soluble ovalbumin (OVA) in the epidermis and other stratified epithelia. In this adoptive transfer model, we utilize T cells from transgenic mice that have a T cell receptor that recognizes OVA peptides in association with Class I or Class II MHC molecules. Maintaining an active laboratory continues to remind me how difficult research can be, and how exciting it can be to overturn dogma.

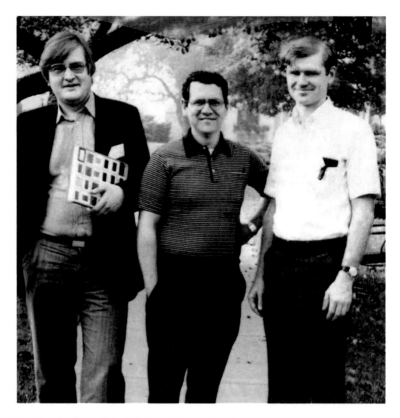

Fig. 11.7 Me with Georg Stingl (*left*) and Thomas Lawley

Becoming Branch Chief at an Early Age

About two years after I started working at the NIH (1977) my Branch Chief, Marvin Lutzner, took a year of sabbatical. Although he had designated someone else to be "Acting" in his absence, his direct supervisor, Dr. Alan Rabson (NCI Scientific Director), asked me if I would like to be the Acting Branch Chief. I decided to do this because I thought I could be an articulate and convincing advocate for our Branch in vying for new clinic space that was being generated. Assuming this administrative responsibility early in my career was a mixed blessing. It drew from my time directly devoted to my laboratory, but it provided me with a bigger picture as to how the NIH, and in particular, the NCI functioned. When Dr. Lutzner was given a second sabbatical year, Dr. Rabson asked me to be the Branch Chief in 1981, a position I held for 24 years, including three years as Acting. I was pleased to assume the responsibilities of Branch Chief, since in contrast to being a department chair in an academic health center, there were not many administrative meetings that I was required to attend. In addition, during those many years, I had the great fortune of working closely with Dr. Rabson, who was inspirational in always focusing his decisions on scientific excellence and scientific opportunity, both clinical and basic.

Mentoring Before It Became a Fashionable Term

One of the most satisfying aspects of my work at the NIH has been the opportunity to work with many very bright, energetic, and enthusiastic research fellows who have come to my laboratory and to the Dermatology Branch of the NCI (Fig. 11.8).

I have always had certain requirements for working in my laboratory. These include having some training in dermatology, having some research experience (although for some US-based fellows I have overlooked this requirement), having a laboratory to return to if coming from another country and having the ability to speak and understand English. Most of the fellows have come from the USA, though many have come from Europe (Austria, Germany, France, Italy, England, and Belgium) and Asia (Japan and Korea). I have always run the lab by giving each fellow his or her own project. In recent years these projects have often intersected. I feel that it is critical to create a collegial atmosphere as opposed to a competitive one. Over the years, I have employed many college students and even some high school students, many of whom are now either physicians or medical students. Since the inception of programs for medical students at the NIH about 20 years ago, I have had just two medical students working in my laboratory. Medical students

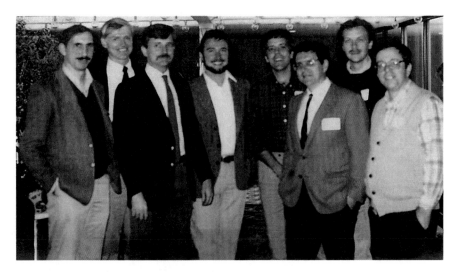

Fig. 11.8 Me with US-trained fellows at Immunodermatology Board Exam in the mid-1980s. Drs. Jo-David Fine, Tom Lawley, Russell Hall, Kevin Cooper, Wright Caughman, me, Kim Yancey, and John Stanley (*left to right*)

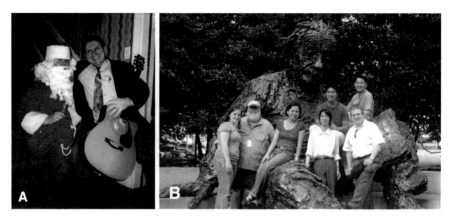

Fig. 11.9 Me with Jay Linton and others (*left to right*): Emily Nelson, Jay, Tinky Nograles, Fumi Miyagawa, Brian Kim, and Young-Hun Cho

require considerable supervision, and I have only had students in the lab when I felt that I could provide adequate time for my direct supervision.

A very important element in having a successful laboratory program is infrastructure, including both personnel and resources. The intramural research program has provided both over these many years. One of my best decisions was one I made about 30 years ago when I hired Jay Linton, who had been an animal caretaker at the time. Jay has taught and mentored all of my fellows and many others in the Branch over these past 30 years (Fig. 11.9).

Science Administration: Yet Another Challenge

Throughout my career I have actively participated in the professional organizations that I felt provided important support for dermatologists and immunologists. Being a member of scientific program committees, nominating committees, and editorial boards has provided me with important perspectives as to how the infrastructure of science functions. In addition, I learned a lot from participating in NIH study sections as well as peer review groups of professional and lay organizations that had grant programs.

Because of my scientific and clinical activities as well as my interactions with professional and lay organizations, I was offered many opportunities to become a dermatology department chairman at various medical schools in the USA. However, at an early stage in my career, I decided that I did not want to do this for several reasons. First, I wanted to continue to focus on my research. I also very much enjoyed what I was doing as Dermatology Branch Chief (for many years we were the major source of academic dermatologists). Finally, I did not want to spend my time recruiting dermatopathologists and dermatological surgeons, who are critical to the financial viability of dermatology departments.

For many years, I felt that I would be very happy continuing as Branch Chief for the remainder of my career. Although salaries were limited, I had sufficient income to care for my family, particularly because the Montgomery County School System was excellent and my three children attended public school. Also, in the mid-1980s, with President Reagan's encouragement of public-private interactions, scientists at the NIH were allowed to legally consult for private industry. This opportunity not only enhanced my income, but also enabled me to learn about a whole new dimension of the health science industry. With NIH permission, I was able to consult for major pharmaceutical and skin-focused companies. These experiences also enabled me to mentor several of my fellows more knowledgably about potential careers as scientists or managers in industry.

In the early 1990s, I was approached by NIH search committees who were seeking physician-scientists to lead various NIH centers and, in one case, an institute, and asked if I was interested in becoming a candidate. I listened and asked about the scope of responsibilities but did not pursue this further because the mission of these centers and institute were beyond my interest and expertise. In 1995, when asked to consider the position of Director of the National Institute of Arthritis and Musculoskeletal and Skin Diseases (NIAMS), I was intrigued because I felt that I could contribute in at least a few of these subject areas, skin and immune-related rheumatic diseases, and could learn about the others. When I learned more about this position, I realized that no one could be an expert in all of these areas, and I could use the expertise I had scientifically, clinically, and administratively to positively impact the work of the NIAMS. After going through the rigorous search process, I was asked by Harold Varmus, then the Director of the NIH, to become Director of the NIAMS in August, 1995, a position that I have held and have enjoyed immensely for the past 14 years.

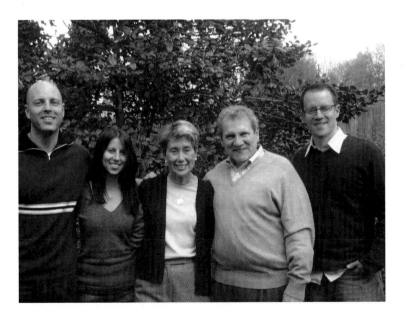

Fig. 11.10 My family: Ken, Karen, Linda, me, and Mark (*from left*)

Summing Up

So, to what do I attribute my becoming a physician-scientist? My father, who would not permit me to join the Coast Guard after high school; my brother, who has been a constant role model and inspiration; my teachers, whose enthusiasm for dispelling dogma and for approaching clinical medicine with constant curiosity; and my wife and children, who were always pleased with the lifestyle that we were able to enjoy while I was employed by the NIH. Indeed, my sons, Mark and Ken have pursued similar paths in public health and epidemiology, one as an internist and the other as a dermatologist (Fig. 11.10).

And, to what do I attribute my success? My choice of the NIH as a place to launch my career (little did I know that I would still be here 35 years later!); my colleagues at NIH, who have been more collegial than one could ever imagine; my fellows, who have consistently brought fresh ideas and excellent questions to the table; my core value of the importance of work/play/life balance; and my own commitment to experience the many dimensions of clinical and laboratory science, as well as my enthusiasm to learn about the administrative underpinnings of the complex, wonderful organization we know as the NIH.

Twelve
Journeys from Bedside to Bench and Back

Jeffrey C. Murray

My career has been based on a series of fortunate events, hard work, and the ability to connect with terrific collaborators who have also been friends and colleagues. In addition, I embrace the Danish view of life of achieving happiness through low expectations, so that I almost always feel as if I am the luckiest person on earth.

I grew up outside of Buffalo, NY in Tonawanda as the oldest of five children in our family. We lived next door to one of my mother's nine siblings, who had eight of my first cousins, so I was always comfortable playing a supervisory role for children. Ours was a classic 1950s childhood, growing up on the border of the country with farms next door and spending most of our time outside in the woods and fields or at play. I skated on ponds, played baseball in yards without formal organizations, and delivered my paper route by bicycle in the summer and by sled in the winter. I can't remember a single time, whatever the weather, that my mom or dad would have even thought about giving me a ride in the car, no matter what the weather. Thus, over time, it might seem natural that I would have gravitated toward Pediatrics. Since I also had a brother with Down's syndrome who had been taken from my parents as a young infant and placed in an institution, I also had a direct connection to genetics and through that, pediatric as well as social issues. A few events stand out from my time as a child. When I was four, I likely had polio, as I developed meningitis during the polio epidemic in 1954. I still recall the terror of having a spinal tap and feeling as though the doctor was trying to kill me. When I was 6, I was hit in the eye with an arrow when we were playing "cowboys and Indians" with, amazingly enough, real arrows! I recall the blood streaming down my face, my mother's hysteria at seeing me, and weeks of wearing an eye patch. At about 10, I tripped and fell through a glass window, lacerating my thumb and hand deeply. I ran to the bathroom to stop the bleeding and recall telling my very upset mother that it was going to be OK but that she would have to take me to the hospital for stitches. I think even then, I had an odd ability to step outside of myself

J.C. Murray (✉)

Departments of Pediatrics, Epidemiology and Biological Sciences, University of Iowa Carver College of Medicine, Iowa, IA, USA
e-mail: jeff-murray@uiowa.edu

D.A. Schwartz (ed.), *Medicine Science and Dreams*,
DOI 10.1007/978-90-481-9538-1_12, © Springer Science+Business Media B.V. 2011

and see a situation as others might see it. I think this has helped me in my work as a pediatrician. I also recall my father's relating a story of him coming upon an elderly man who had been passed by several others and was unable to get across a street crossing in heavy snow. My dad had assisted him in getting across and then to his home. This impressed upon me that sometimes you have to be the one to take charge and do the right thing, even if it's "not your job." Finally, on our occasional visits to the institution in which my brother Gregory lived because of his Down's syndrome, I recall being overcome by the pathos of the living conditions, the fear of the scary adults I felt as a child, and the isolation that less advantaged individuals must feel.

My first formal exposure to biomedical sciences came in tenth grade, when my biology teacher Mr. Pine (who also served as my wrestling coach) instilled in us a fanatical interest in understanding the descriptive nature of biology. While I must admit that a large part of this was motivated by his desire to have his students score 100 on the New York State Regents Biology Exam, it nonetheless captured my imagination and led me to begin exploring the boundaries of what we learned for the first time. I remember being particularly excited by genetics, specifically by doing crosses where I could expand the number of genes and loci as much as I liked, and also by his enthusiasm and excitement over the fairly recent discovery that the number of human chromosomes was 46 and not 48. I distinctly remember Mr. Pine conveying to us what a critical finding this was, how it completely changed our understanding of what people thought they knew about science, and how important it was to remain open to new ideas and concepts, even in the face of what might be dogma that was decades old. I think this early lesson, that even what is known and thought to be true can be wrong, has enabled me to keep an open mind about scientific investigation and helped our lab group in being willing to look at old problems with new lenses. Throughout high school I enjoyed the sciences and mathematics. As I was thinking of college, these were the primary disciplines I wanted to study.

During the summers between high school and college and after my first year at college, I worked in a quality control laboratory at a large chemical manufacturing plant. This was a truly eye-opening experience for me at the level of the real world workplace and real world workers. My job was to test batches of chemicals made to bind sand into molds into which molten metal was poured to make car parts. The chemicals were highly toxic (formaldehyde and nitric acid) and we had no masks, no eye protection, no ventilation, and no mechanical safety protection from the large mixers and molding apparatus I worked with. I developed almost daily nosebleeds from chemical exposure. Once I had a 55-gallon drum of nitric acid explode and cover me with no eye wash or safety shower available. I could not see for two days afterwards from corneal burns and was docked my pay for those days for missing work. This experience inspired my lifelong support for unions for workers. I also received countless burns on my hands and arms from handling hot bricks of test molds without protection. My fellow workers in the manufacturing plant were terrific workers with an amazing mechanical and technical knowledge but were in many cases illiterate. For me, a smartypants high school kid headed to college, this was truly eye opening. And for them, I also fulfilled some stereo-types about college kids when, on my first day at work, I mistook a large, circular sink for the urinal and was using that sink accordingly when two of the plant floor workers came in. When their hilarious laughter stopped, they suggested that I might want to look in the next room for the real urinals. While I was known as "college boy" for the rest of that summer, by the end I felt they were my friends. I had in fact learned an enormous amount about motorcycle riding and repair from the very guy who conferred my nickname. You only need to be caught urinating in a sink once to be able to remain humble ever after about any skills you think you might have.

I went to college at MIT in Cambridge based on my interest in doing physics or math. I had been at the top of my classes in these subjects in my small high school in Rocky River, OH, but at MIT I quickly realized that I was now at the bottom. Over my first two years there, I went down the mathematical and technical hill of majors from Physics, to Chemistry, to Chemical Engineering and finally settled on Humanities (English) and Biology as a double major. I took five years to complete these at a time when many of us where extending college by a year as a legiti-mate way to avoid service in the military and an almost certain posting to Vietnam. I remain embarrassed by what I sometimes feel was my cowardice that I could mask by a nonetheless truly felt anti-war sentiment. At MIT, I was fortunate to have a series of undergraduate part-time jobs working in laboratories, the last of which was in the lab of Dr. Gobind Khorana, who had recently won the Nobel Prize for being one of the three major figures in breaking the genetic code. He was by nature an organic chemist. Although I did not work for or with him directly, I did work with one of his very gifted postdocs, Dr. Marv Caruthers and his fellow postdoc, Hans Van de Sande. I was given tremendous latitude in exploring the boundaries of how one could assemble short stretches of DNA that had been chemically syn-thesized using recently discovered bacterial enzymes that could join the short DNA pieces into longer ones until an entire gene was created. It was the first time that I was able to participate in a genuine scientific enterprise of discovery where new outcomes were occurring on an almost daily basis. It also grounded me in the real-ization that to understand biology, one would greatly benefit from also knowing chemistry and mathematics. The functions of cells and tissues are chemical at their heart, and knowing mathematics enabled one to have an appreciation for statistics and the critical role it has in determining whether an experimental result is correct or suffers from a lack of sufficient information to make a firm conclusion. Over and over again, I have used the calculus and statistics I learned in college to help me judge the impact of an experiment. I think I especially benefitted from living in the pre-calculator era when we used slide rules. Slide rules give you the exact numeric value of a calculation but without its "order of magnitude" or power of ten. Thus a value of "2.3" could be 0.0023 or 23 or 23,000,000. On the slide rule, you need to be able to understand and measure independently that power of ten. Time and again this has enabled me to see (and help others see) that it is the size of the result that is critical and less so its explicit numeric determination. Thus, what is important is whether it is 23 or 230 and much less so whether it is 23.916752 or 24.196752.

Calculators (and their offspring, computers) can measure things to many decimal places that confer what appears to be meaning, but in the absence of understanding. I have enjoyed the interface of chemistry, math, and biology ever since this early introduction. It was at this time that I also gained confidence in my technical skills and the enjoyment I had when I discovered a faster, more efficient, cheaper, or in general, a better way to do an experiment.

I was exposed to many aspects of biology, and although all of us of an older generation can look back on the inefficiencies and slowness of the experimental work completed decades ago, I remain convinced that the ability to do a good and careful experiment is critical no matter what the technology available might be. It was also at this time that I realized that you often don't truly understand a method until you participate in doing it. No amount of reading can make you an experimental scientist (or indeed a medical doctor either); it is only by doing that you gain a feel for the subtleties of the work and sense for what can work better in the future. I feel grateful for the opportunity given in Dr. Khorana's Lab which enabled me to explore how I could best function in a scientific environment. It was also at this time that another of Dr. Khorana's postdoctoral fellows, Peter Loewen, first suggested to me that an MD might be the most advantageous degree to have if one wanted to do experimental science. I am not sure that even today I would agree with him on this, as I feel the lack of formal PhD training has limited my scientific abilities, but he was prescient in recognizing a path that would turn out to work for me by existing at the interface of science and clinical medicine.

It was also during this time that during one of the few genuine one-on-one encounters I had with Dr. Khorana, he related to me the story of his graduate thesis work in organic chemistry on a compound that he had been working on for months to prepare and whose only sample was present in one small flask in a solution that was a powerful acid. This generated a crisis when, in placing that flask on a stone counter, it cracked, and the precious synthesis work began to leak out. He showed me the scar on the palm of his hand that he obtained when ferrying the cracked flask to another room where it could be transferred to an available container and the burns that he suffered as a result. Whether it was his love of science or the investment in time and work doesn't really matter. In essence, this conveyed to me that you should be willing to make substantial sacrifices, even physical ones, to pursue your dream. I certainly know that I must appear to have made some sacrifices over time to continue my own career development. It seems to me that most of those sacrifices have really been made by my family. For me, the work has always been enjoyable and exciting and has never really seemed like work at all.

I was amazingly fortunate to have as teachers at MIT a number of individuals who have gone on to become major figures in biology but were unrecognized as such by undergraduates like me, who only thought of them as the people who were lecturing to us. David Botstein was a new Assistant Professor, and other more established figures such as Salvador Luria, Boris Magasanik, Ethan Singer, Jerome Lettvin, Philip Morrison, David Baltimore, and the aforementioned Khorana all provided course opportunities and discussion time and, in many cases, were genuine models of how one could pursue basic research and teaching.

I was in college from 1967 to 1972, a time of some political turmoil both in Boston and in the US, in general. While I had a few political encounters at that time, including learning that you really do want to get away from tear gas as quickly as possible, I did it more as part of the social and student milieu rather than because of any deep passion to right the wrongs of the world. While that later changed (I hope) to some degree, it did allow me to see at least that politics are a part of our lives, whether we are scientists or physicians or teachers.

Throughout college, I had no interest in medicine or applications of science and saw myself in the role of a Mr. Pine as a high school biology teacher. When college ended, I had the opportunity to stay on in the Khorana lab, and because I enjoyed the work and also because of the flexibility that research gave me to pursue my outside interests, I continued working there. It was during this time that I met my now wife, Ann Marie McCarthy, who had just finished nursing school and who was embarking on her own career in the healthcare profession. It was her stories of the patients she cared for and doctors she worked with (some heroes, some a bit villainous, at least in their personal lives) that first began to get me to see the real possibility of tying medicine to a research career. On one occasion, she told me of a patient of hers with cystic fibrosis who loved the Red Sox. As a big fan myself, I volunteered to take him on an afternoon out of the hospital to a game. Not knowing then as I do now that kids with CF have major problems breathing and digesting fats, I got us seats at the very top of Fenway Park so he could see better and let him eat hot dogs to his heart's content. Looking back now I know that his increasingly bluish color and fast breathing was likely a byproduct of our 200-step climb, and Ann Marie's relating to me his bowel habits for the next two days was an indictment of my suboptimal clinical care. I do feel he had a blast that day, and this has helped me ever since to see the little boy or girl who is inside of every sick child. Thus, after attending graduate school for one year, I made the switch over to medical school, having never had any sort of formal patient contact whatsoever and indeed, being an extremely shy science nerd, someone who was unlikely to be a force for patient care as well. But my early days as the oldest child of many at least let me see Pediatrics as a possibility, and I loved Ann Marie's stories of how you could really make a difference.

My one year in graduate school at Tufts was extremely formative, in that it was the first time that I had the opportunity to be truly independent in laboratory experiences, and I will be forever grateful to Professor Mike Malamy and others (Elio Schaechter, Lincoln Sonenshein, Eddie Goldberg, and Jack Levy) who gave me the opportunity to do, in some small way, and even if only for a few months, some independent research. I again thrived on the technical challenges of working out new experimental methodologies, and I still recall my own excitement (and I think Dr. Malamy's) when I successfully created two dimensional protein gels in the laboratory. I really enjoyed these small triumphs, and since that time have always instilled in my students that they will often be the first one after God to see or know or do something novel, and that this is an incredible privilege that the scientist has.

After dropping out of graduate school, a painful experience, as I had really been committed to enrolling in medical school, I very quickly embraced patients and patient-related care. I was able to work as a nurse's aid in a normal newborn nursery during my second year and had the first of what I am certain were many lucky coincidences in that I was chosen by lottery to spend the summer between my first and second year of medical school working for Dr. Murray Feingold, a pediatric birth defects specialist. This was the first time that I really had the opportunity to see how patient care took place, and the time I spent on rounds with Dr. Feingold and Dr. Lou Bartoshefsky, his senior resident, were incredibly formative for me. In addition, I had the opportunity to carry out a clinical research project on "The Birth Defect Complications of Maternal Type I Diabetes." There was also the opportunity to attend pediatric rounds, during which I was exposed to not only pediatric care, but also to the social and ethical dilemmas in pediatrics involving children born with birth defects or with major neonatal complications. I recall a discussion of a child with Smith–Lemli–Opitz syndrome and how the family and the physicians were working to decide if they should let the child die without aggressive interventions. I recall being struck with a profound sense of how doctors could not cure all things, but that even when no cures are possible, they can still play a critical role in the care of a family. I found that I really enjoyed the discussions that went with patient care, not only relating to their pathophysiology, but also to the social and ethical aspects of their care. I began to read extensively on the ethical aspects in biomedical literature and completely embraced the pediatric literature. Indeed, I believe it was during medical school that I probably spent the most intense time of my life reading the primary literature in the fields in which I was eventually to settle, pediatrics and genetics. I loved reading about new infectious diseases or syndromes, about new approaches to care, and about the science behind the problems as well.

After finishing my summer rotation with Dr. Feingold, I was certain I would be going into pediatrics and spent the rest of medical school doing everything I could to be successful in pursuing that dream. I worked several times at Northshore Children's hospital, a primary care community hospital setting, in Salem, MA, and saw practitioners like Bill Rowley and Marcy Mian, who provided terrific primary care in a pediatric setting. I fell in love with providing for the care of newborn infants, which I continue to enjoy to this day. Something about babies has really captured my brain and my soul, and I am never really happier than when in the nursery seeing a newborn baby and thinking about its potential for the future and the sort of life it may have. The opportunity to pursue research that might in some way benefit these most promising members of our society is, in itself, its own reward. At the end of medical school, I had choices to make about residency, and although I had many thoughts about trying to move to one of the major pediatric medical centers, I chose to stay at Tufts for my residency, as I believed I would receive outstanding clinical training there, and my wife's family all lived in the Boston area.

I had been fortunate indeed to marry Ann Marie during my second year of medical school, and she has been the center of my life since (although she probably does not realize this). I have learned more from her about family and love and children than from any formal mentor, and we have raised three terrific kids together while she has been wife, mother, PhD student, Professor, and all the other life roles a woman often has while being my greatest confidant and supporter as well. Our first child, Ryan, born at the end of my internship, taught me that you can be a fine pediatrician without being a parent, but that being a parent does give special insight into what a family feels like when they have a child in crisis. Our second child, Chris, taught me that even if the mother is a pediatric nurse practitioner and the dad a pediatrician, there can still be no shortage of long nights and scary moments as part of child rearing, and it can continue long past the age of the child's physical maturity. Our third, Katie, is the final light in our family beacon and that lets me sleep happily at night knowing that there are good people in the world who will continue to strive to make it better. Despite my many enjoyable interactions with colleagues and friends, I also know that at the end of my days, it will be family that means the most and that one should never sacrifice them for career.

I did indeed get terrific clinical exposure that is much different from how residency training takes place today. At Tufts, even as a fourth year medical student, I found myself in charge of a major pediatric ward service when doing a sub-internship. The dedicated intern became ill with chicken pox, and I had to take the intern's position. Dr. Barry Dashefsky, the senior resident at the time, took me under his wing. I found myself as a fourth-year medical student making diagnoses about infections and deciding on treatments, doing IVs and spinal taps without supervision, talking to parents about their child's illness, and determining if a very sick child needed to go to an ICU or not, all backed up by Dr. Dashefsky but doing the work on my own. I formed close working relationships with nurses and social workers and came to see medicine as a team approach where I could be much more effective (just as was true back at the factory I worked in after high school) by listening to and using the skills of people independent of their position but based on their ability and knowledge. This was a very powerful experience that allowed me to develop the confidence to make decisions on my own and to also recognize when I was outside of my depth and needed to get help. One other experience as a medical student also stands out as affecting my future thinking and teaching. I was working in Providence at Brown University in the Neonatal Intensive Care Unit (NICU), as a fourth-year student exploring my interest in neonatolology. One night, we were called to the delivery room to help with a baby about to deliver and whose monitors were showing it to be in distress. The mother was Portuguese and did not speak English and there was no one in attendance who did. The father was away at sea, a commercial fishman. There were six new nursing students watching their first delivery at the bedside. I was to take the baby from the obstetrician, carry it to a warmer bed and initiate any resuscitation that might be needed with a senior resident to guide me. As the obstetrician handed the baby up to me, the nursing students and I also saw that the baby was a true cyclops—one eye in the center of its forehead. One student nurse fainted, another began screaming, and I was overcome with what to do next. We rushed the baby to the NICU where it died a few hours later and soon proved to have Trisomy 13, a fatal disorder caused by an extra chromosome. This impressed upon me that prenatal diagnosis can be critical, not only for those families that might choose to abort such a severely affected fetus, but also equally so for those families, quite possibly this one even, who might not abort but who could at least be prepared for the birth of such a devastated baby. If we had known about this ahead of time, the dad could have been there with the mom; those student nurses could have been in another room seeing a normal delivery, and we could have been prepared to move the mom and baby to a room where they could quietly mourn the death together rather than undergoing the panicked and unexplainable separation. I retell it often as a parable of how information can have many uses and that lack of information does not make things disappear.

After finishing medical school, I moved onto pediatric residency and loved almost every month of that, although I had many failures and made many mistakes along the way. I learned a huge amount about patient care and for the first time, how bonded we become to our patients, so that in a way, when we lose them, it affects us for the rest of our lives. I can vividly remember the death of the first neonate that I took care of while in my first month of internship. I was in the midst of a very busy night with a senior resident for backup who I knew even then was weak and unhelpful. At one point they even pulled me out of the nursery to start an intravenous line that they had been unable to accomplish on a patient in another unit, causing me to miss valuable time with my own patients. I was in effect solely in charge of a 12 bed NICU as a first-month intern (unthinkable today) and while balancing the need to do task after task, I failed to see how sick one of the babies was becoming. By the time I started antibiotics it was likely already too late. While crying over that child's loss and feeling the guilt of whether I had made a mistake in management, I was chastised by an older nurse for showing weakness. I knew even at that time she was wrong and that it was only human to feel this type of compassion, and indeed even love for our patients, but I also recognized that I needed to be able to show to others I could be a leader at such times as well. From the mother of another patient, I learned that you never ask a child if you could listen to their heart when you have to; rather you ask "where would you like to be sitting when I listen to you heart?" This child was on the oncology service and subsequently died, and I remember how important it was for the child to be able to have some control, as well as for the mother to have control too. I made plenty of mistakes too, and you often learn much more from those than from your successes. One day, while standing in the nursery after I was done for the day, I was waiting for a fellow intern to finish so we could go home together. We were at the bedside of one of his patients while he was signing out to the night call person, and I noticed that the nurse was rather casually doing things with the IV and various tubes in the baby while the baby looked very blue to me. I was surprised at her and my friend's failure to be responding to the baby's appearance. I said to him that I didn't think his baby looked very good, and he responded "Murray, that baby is dead." In fact, the baby had just died and the nurse was removing the IVs and so on prior to taking the baby to the morgue. I became renowned afterwards for my ability to recognize illness in a child! I am grateful for these and many other lessons that I learned during my residency, and my only regret is that I did not stay on to do a Chief Residency, as I feel this may have put the capstone on my clinical training and career.

When it was time to choose a fellowship, I was torn between neonatology and genetics. For personal reasons I ended up choosing genetics, and I was amazingly lucky, mostly through Dr. Feingold's intervention, to get a position at the University of Washington under the guidance of Dr. Arno Motulsky in the wonderful Division of Medical Genetics that he assembled from internists, pediatricians, and basic scientists beginning in the 1950s. This was my last opportunity for formal training, and I had many mentors while serving as a fellow there. Dr. Motulsky was first and foremost, and I was particularly struck by not only his incredible clinical and scientific insights but also his compassion and warmth as a human being. While I was a fellow working under his guidance, he went to Israel to serve on a trial in absentia of Josef Mengele, the infamous physician geneticist at Auschwitz who had carried out extensive and horrific twin experiments. Because Dr. Motulsky was Jewish and had fled Nazi Germany at age 16, and because of his interest in genetics, he was asked to serve on this review commission. What I remember on his return is him telling us that Mengele had in fact been an outstanding physician and investigative scientist. Early on in the war, his experiments on twins (although horrible) made some sense scientifically. But, it was clear by the end of the war that he had made a descent into madness. Dr. Motulsky impressed upon us that since the pre-war Mengele had been viewed in a positive light by so many of his colleagues and indeed by his staff, yet had transformed so completely to evil, there is a risk for any of us in making a similar descent. I have always felt that this capacity for evil is something we need to guard against, and perhaps one of the best defenses is to demonstrate that good can be a far better approach to curing the world's ills than consensus evil.

I moonlighted extensively during this time doing some of the first air transports of infants and sick children from around the Pacific Northwest, including Alaska. This again cemented my interest in neonatology as a practice, even though I was formally trained in clinical genetics. I was lucky to have Dr. Motulsky gently guide me away from some scientific projects that were probably destined to be unsuccessful and toward an exciting discovery process using the new tools in molecular biology to identify DNA sequence variation in humans. I made a trip to a Native American family with a very unique genetic finding. This was the first of many trips to homes to collect DNA samples and a chance to see firsthand how much research can mean, even if the promise of useful finding are years off, to a family with a rare disorder who may feel abandoned by a medical system focused only on common problems. We also used Dr. Motulsky's own family to verify an interesting finding we made about DNA variation, an interesting twist on ethics we might not do today. During this time we were able to identify several new DNA variants in humans, a remarkable discovery for the time. This gave me my first introduction into human recombination, linkage disequilibrium, gene mapping, DNA sequencing, and other arcane aspects of the human genetics world and set the stage for the rest of my scientific career.

It was during this time that, after giving a presentation at the American Society of Human Genetics, a graduate student, Ken Buetow, came up to me and, in the nicest way possible, told me I had some really interesting data but that I had analyzed it in an extremely unsophisticated way. Typical of my lack of insight, I ignored Ken for a bit, but when he called me again a month or two later, it set the stage for what has turned out to be a life-long collaboration from which I have benefitted far more than Ken. We were almost perfectly suited for collaboration in that he had terrific quantitative and analytic skills and a great insight into the biology of the problems, while I had clinical skills and laboratory technical skills. We collaborated first on studies of individual genes and the mechanisms of inheritance in humans, eventually building a genome center together after my move to the University of Iowa for my first faculty position. We both benefitted from the creation of the Center for the Study of Human Polymorphisms (CEPH) by the great French immunologist and humanitarian, Jean Dausset. Dr. Dausset created a resource of DNA samples and computer programs that he made freely available to the scientific community for studies of human inheritance. It was this ethic of open sharing and rapid communication that I believe set the later stage for the Human Genome Project's work to similarly ensure that DNA sequence generated from public funding should go immediately into open database repositories, thus greatly advancing the speed with which scientists could exploit new information to assist in disease discovery, a great advantage over the old model of waiting one or two years for formal publications to make the data available. I believe this ethic of open sharing and communication is one of the most important legacies of the genome project.

This was also the opportunity for Ken and me to begin to build a program investigating the genetic causes of a complex birth defect, cleft lip and palate, which has proven to be the centerpiece of my life's work. It is not possible to thank Ken enough for all that he did for me, especially early on, when we were both in career-building phases. One of the greatest joys I have had in science has been to see his own considerable success in the area of cancer. It is with these close collaborations where individuals compliment each other so well and where they evolve into genuine friendship that it makes science all the more worth doing. Perhaps the most exciting time of our collaboration came at a human gene mapping meeting in Finland in 1985. One night at 2 or 3 o'clock in the morning while listening to some Scandinavian headbangers in an adjacent dorm room, we came up with the idea of linkage disequilibrium walking. Although it is now commonly accepted that applications of the "HapMap, SNP, and CNV" technology enable one to find mutations through surrogate markers and linkage disequilibrium, at the time, Ken and I had a major insight into this question. We had already identified this to be a common phenomenon for human DNA variants, where in essence one could take a known variant to make predictions about a nearby variant that might be contributing to a disease risk. Ken's work in graduate school had been to study this in the hemoglobin system, and we soon went on to demonstrate this phenomenon in several other human genes. In trying to convince some of the leading lights of the genetics field that this was a possibility, we also were met with skepticism that was legitimate, I am sure, but also has resulted in my always feeling that I should listen carefully to what may seem like the naive musings of youth. We were unable to convince some geneticists, even with data in hand, that we were right, and we were prevented from publishing Ken's first findings on this because of the skepticism. Although I have written a number of papers over my career that I feel made important contributions, the one I am perhaps most proud of is a smaller, less-frequently referenced paper on mapping of the plasminogen gene in which Ken and I outlined the theory of linkage disequilibrium walking, which has led to the many successes of genome-wide association studies that we see today. Indeed we were able to apply this to both cystic fibrosis, in which our findings were at first rejected by some of the leaders in the field as being too unlikely, and later on to Huntington's disease, where we were able to use the information to assist the Huntington's community in switching the focus of their search for the gene from a location likely based on incorrect data to that where the gene eventually was found to lie. That work was carried out by my first graduate student, Rita Shiang, and is perhaps the single most important piece of work in which I was able to participate, although one where our role is largely invisible.

While in fellowship at the University of Washington, I was contacted by Jim Hanson, who had also done his fellowship at the University of Washington under the guidance of the father of dysmorphology (the study of unusual appearing children). Jim asked if I would be interested in taking a look at an available faculty position at the University of Iowa. I had visited Iowa City once while doing a residency search and had enjoyed the community, but my wife, who had been raised in Boston, was committed to our returning to New England and told me not to even bother looking. Nonetheless, I swayed her, and it was clear from my first visit that the position was perfectly suited to me in that it had a well-established clinical genetics program that a new assistant professor could fit into without having to carry out program-building work. There was also a strong commitment to bring human molecular biology onto a campus that already had outstanding programs in biochemical genetics, clinical genetics, and cytogenetics. After visiting, Ann Marie said that it would be fine for us to come to Iowa City for a couple of years before making our final move back to Boston, and so we journeyed to Iowa City with our two young children, Chris and Ryan.

That move proved to be the last of my academic career, except for two sabbaticals, and I am sure I have never made a choice that has turned out so very well. Most of my other choices, even including medical school, residency, and fellowship, I can second guess and say that I might have been better off going to one or two other places. But, for my academic start as a new assistant professor, Iowa proved to be perfect. Ann Marie quickly identified a teaching position that fostered her own nurse practitioner career and eventually led to her faculty position and PhD. Our children thrived and our third child, Kaitlin, was born here, thus enabling us to have a child in each of the three major cities where we have lived in the USA.

Dr. Hanson was the perfect mentor in that he gave me full reign to do the research that I wanted to do, and he protected me from excessive clinical burdens while providing the opportunity to continue to grow and learn clinically through the wonderful Regional Genetics Program that he had established in Iowa. I was able to work at the interface of neonatology through my work on the inpatient service nursery and to build a molecular biology laboratory that established me as scientifically independent. I was also very fortunate to work with basic geneticists such as Gary Gussin and Bob Malone, who had built a PhD genetics program and who welcomed a pediatrician into their basic science community, which greatly benefited my scientific growth as well. The incredible collegial environment in Iowa really enabled me to get my programs off the ground.

I was also very lucky in that after writing my first unsuccessful NIH grant, Dr. Sam Fomon in the pediatrics department sat down with me and went over the "pink sheets" or the grant review statement, which in that pre-internet/PDF time were indeed still pink. Although he did not understand the science of what I was doing, he could read between the lines of the reviews very effectively and enabled me to make a very strong and positive response so that I was able to be funded the next time around. This need to help junior faculty in grant writing is now often taken as a matter of course in academics, but at the time it was unusual and proved a great benefit to my application efforts. I also believe that spending so much time as an undergraduate reading and writing English literature provided me with sufficient writing skills to be able to tell a story in a way that could be understood by a scientist. Efforts at learning to write will never be wasted on a scientist. It was also at this time that I met Holly Ardinger, at that time a genetics fellow, and I began to develop my interest in cleft lip and palate. I had always been struck by the terrible disruption that clefts cause in the facial structure and also by the fact that they can be discordant even in monozygotic twins, yet retain a strong genetic component. Since I was becoming familiar with the new tools of molecular genetics as applied to humans, Holly, Ken Beutow, and I developed the idea of a project in which we would carry out gene mapping to try and identify the genetic components of this common complex birth defect. Through Dr. Hanson's intervention, we were welcomed into the embrace of the craniofacial clinic, at that time under the leadership of Drs. Hugh Morris and Janusz Bardach, that enabled us to ascertain and enroll our first patients into the study. Within a few years, we were able to publish our first papers identifying a gene association with cleft lip and palate, and very shortly thereafter, mapping the gene for a dominant form of clefting, the van der Woude syndrome. We had been turned on to the van der Woude syndrome by Rich Pauli, the genetics division head at the University of Wisconsin-Madison. Rich pointed out that this dominant condition resembled the common form of cleft lip and palate very closely. Rich proved to be extremely prescient in this assessment, and although it took us almost 20 more years to identify the specific DNA mutation that confers a major risk to cleft lip and palate, that mutation turned out to be in the gene in which more damaging mutations caused the van der Woude syndrome, proving Rich absolutely right.

It was an exciting time to be in genetics, going to the yearly American Society of Human Genetics meetings or the human gene mapping meetings, where there was always an opportunity to learn about some exciting new development or technical advance. We got to be up close and personal with many of the leading lights of genetics including Drs. Jim Neal, Victor McKusick, Walter Bodmer. Newton Morton, Janet Rowley, Pat Jacobs, and others. These people were inspiring and also more than willing to talk to you at your poster or presentation about your ideas, and Ken and I learned a huge amount from them. I had always been shy in my approach to others, but the genetics community made it easy for young scientists and physicians to join in and benefit from their wisdom and to (most times) listen to their ideas. By the same token, the craniofacial community also welcomed us in, and we were able to rapidly expand the size of our program.

The rest of my career was characterized by two major events. The first was our moving from mapping single genes to taking on the task of generating genome-wide linkage maps through the use of a microsatellite approach. We were contacted by Dr. Jim Watson at NIH's Human Genome Institute about whether we would be interested in applying for a Genome Center using new technologies developed by Geoff Duyk and Val Sheffield and building on the insightful work of Jim Weber in the use of microsatellites in human gene mapping. The five of us, including Ken and myself, put together an application for a Genome Center. I pulled the last double all-nighter of my career getting it finished, and we were successful in our application. The first couple of years of the Genome Center were exciting, as we identified literally hundreds of new markers and were able to participate in generating some of the very first genome-wide linkage maps for humans, which have served as the framework for gene mapping work that continues to today. It was also my first exposure to the political side of science and perhaps the only truly negative experience that I've had in the scientific community when tensions between colleagues began to make themselves apparent, and I realized for the first time that to be successful, one had not only to pursue the science, but also maintain the friendship side. Ken and I retained our strong and close collaboration throughout the genome phase of my career, but I ceased to be interested in working at the industrial scale that genome work now required.

It was during approximately the same time that I read a paper by Kaare Christensen, a physician-epidemiologist in Denmark who had taken up the work of Paul Fogh Andersen. Fogh-Andersen was a Danish cleft palate surgeon who had described the complex nature of the genetics of cleft lip and palate for really the first time in the mid-1940s (and who included paper on clefting by Josef Mengele in the reference list of his brilliant thesis). Kaare had written a very beautiful paper on using the Danish cleft database, and I wrote to him to see if he would be interested in collaborating. This was perhaps, after Ken, the second most successful and lucky connection of my career, in that Kaare and I have now been working together for almost 15 years, first on cleft lip and palate and more recently on preterm birth. Again, we seem to be very well suited and complementary to each other. He is a terrific clinician and epidemiologist who understands the nuances of databases and, indeed, has built many of them in Denmark. I continue to have my interests in the laboratory and technical sides and understand some of the clinical aspects of clefting, and this has enabled us to build very strong and powerful approaches to gene and environment identification as contributors to clefting. Besides this, much as it was true with Ken, Kaare has become a genuine friend, with both of us having a strong interest not only in our careers and scientific and medical interests, but also in each other's families and lives as well. I was very fortunate to be able to spend a sabbatical year in Denmark, and it was during this time that many of our changes in approach and scale to clefting took place. This parallels a similar time in 1990 when I was also fortunate to have my other sabbatical in the lab of Dr. Kay Davies in Oxford, where I learned the British approach to science of collegial interaction and discussion and also a wide range of technical skills under her tutelage. I'll be forever grateful to Kay and Kaare for taking a very unproven American under their wings and allowing him the opportunity to grow to learn, and for also providing a home away from home for our family, who enjoyed living in "foreign" lands as much as I enjoyed the science.

Throughout all of these scientific efforts, my work could not have proceeded at this pace if it weren't for the combination of the incredible support of my wife, Ann Marie McCarthy, as well as the joy and enthusiasm that has been brought into my life by our three children, Ryan, Chris, and Katie. Even on those days that didn't turn out so well, I was always eager to come home to the family and see the children growing and thriving in the Iowa City community. The tight-knit community and the friendly interactions there enabled us to make many friends outside of medicine and science, and living here has greatly enriched our own personal lives. Ann Marie sacrificed many years of her own career advancement, both to take care of our children and also to allow me to grow and to travel, and as a result of that I always feel that I've incurred a debt I can never pay. Nonetheless, Ann Marie's successes have exceeded mine in that she has not only done extremely well scientifically, but also she has developed substantial administrative skills as well. Unlike myself, who has never had any administrative skill, she has advanced up the ranks in the College of Nursing, and I believe is a highly thought of chair in the area of maternal and child health. She has also served as an inspiration for her ability to multitask, something that I've not always been so successful at myself.

Almost all academic success is dependent on having good students and postdoctoral fellows who can bring new insights and hard work to the lab and generate the data and advances so necessary to keeping science moving. I've been particularly blessed right from the beginning with my first student, Rita Shiang, who was a major force in both our linkage disequilibrium and clefting work. Andrew Lidral was a DDS/PhD student who brought new insights into statistical analysis into our lab and who has gone on to have his own world class program in cleft lip and palate, the very model for how one hopes one's students can exceed oneself. Andrew also helped bridge our new collaboration with Mary Marazita in Pittsburgh. Mary replaced Ken as my primary analytic collaborator when Ken's interest diverged more into the area of cancer, and this has also proven to be highly successful in that Mary is just as smart and just as selfless as Ken in giving credit and in carrying out work in a timely and efficient manner. It's hard to believe that I could have identified one collaborator in this area who could be so helpful, let alone two. With Mary, our work has been able to continue without missing a single beat. The lessons from Mary are that there are often good folks waiting in the wings, and you can build successful connections at many times during a career.

There is one final brick in the house of my career that has had perhaps the biggest single impact in how my work has progressed and how I hope to have an impact on the world. In my cleft work I had been incredibly lucky early on when John Phillips at Vanderbilt introduced me to the organization Operation Smile. My current interest in social justice and international health arose from my first trip to the Philippines in the late 1980s, which made me aware for the first time of the incredible discrepancies between healthcare and social and economic status in the USA and many parts of the rest of the world (Fig. 12.1). On my very first trip, I saw children living literally on the garbage piles in Manila and saw tiny children not in school but selling cigarettes on the street to survive and calling a lean-to made of plywood a home. When I contrasted this to the lives of my own children, I could not help but

Fig. 12.1 Me on a carabao. This looks like a fun ride in the Philippines but I was picking nits and chiggers out of my legs for weeks after

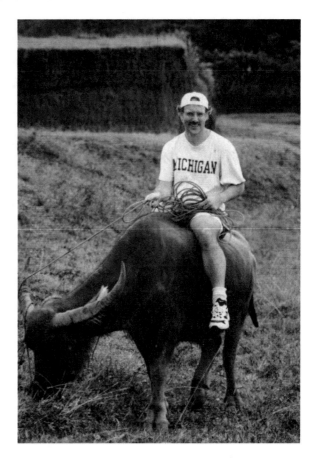

be overcome by emotion. I worked in public hospital wards where children were dying of tetanus, measles, and starvation, causes of death that were inconceivable in the USA. Operation Smile, under the direction of Bill and Kathy McGee, has done an amazing job of providing surgical and related services to tens of thousands of kids around the world with cleft lip and palate. The hundreds of volunteers that I've come in contact with over that time serve as a daily inspiration to me and to my laboratory members for how important it is to give beyond yourself to provide something back to the rest of the world that is so much less fortunate than we are (Fig. 12.2). It also never fails to reinforce to me how much all of us love our children equally and want the best for them, whether we come from the wealthiest family in American or the poorest family in South Asia or Africa. This work has occasionally led me to proselytize in my lectures for the role of the scientist or physician-scientist in addressing issues of social justice. While I know that this may sometimes be not well received in a scientific setting, I very strongly believe that this is a critical component of our work. Scientific research, and medical research in particular, has no real value if it can't be delivered in a timely and effective manner to the people

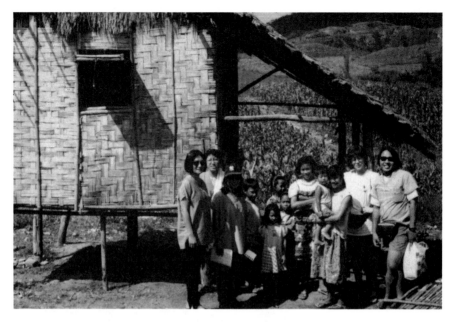

Fig. 12.2 Our nursing team with a family outside a traditional nipa hut in the Philippines during a trip to follow-up surgeries of children with cleft lip

who need it most, and even the most basic science-oriented student needs to understand and to embrace the ethic that at least a small portion of their time should be given to thinking about how they can do something directly to address the many mismatches in economy and law that exist in the world. Over this time I was also able to learn more about these through my contact with numerous physicians who not only felt similarly to the way that I did, but who also were far more effective than me in doing something about it. Physicians such as Dr. David Schwartz who did a sabbatical in my lab and later directed the National Institute of Environmental Health Sciences, Hatem El-Shanti who came from Jordan, Jorge di Paola who came from Argentina, and many others have instilled in me the understanding that we all need to work together toward the common goal of improving health. This needs to be not only through our research and our medical care, but also through addressing the social and legal ills of the systems as well. I hope that my students have not been overburdened by my preaching in this manner, but I've come to believe that it's one of the most important lessons that I can impart to the next generation and that our science lacks full meaning unless done in context. We should be challenged on a daily basis in our laboratories to consider why our experiments costing millions of dollars per lab should take precedence over providing those most basic health needs now (clean water, immunizations, and nutritious food) to the billions without access. I now oversee international programs in Brazil, the Philippines, India, and elsewhere, and in each of those places have parents ask me why we are doing research when it is so obvious that there are needs that could be met now with that

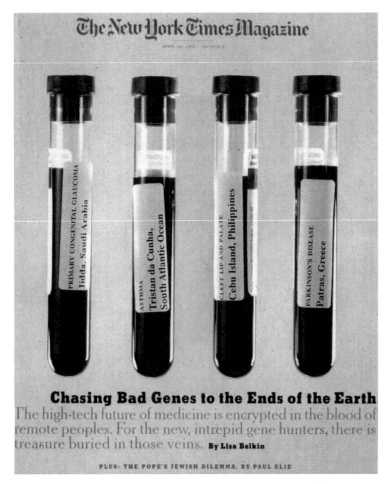

Fig. 12.3 A cover from the New York Times magazine with an article by Lisa Belkin raising the ethical issues of collecting DNA for genetic studies in less-developed countries. (The author acknowledges that in this instance he was unable to trace or contact the copyright holder for permission to reproduce this material. The author has included complete source references for all such material and takes full responsibility for these matters. If notified, the publisher will be pleased to rectify any errors or omissions at the earliest opportunity)

money (Fig. 12.3). When a single DNA chip costs more than the yearly income of many families and when we have sequenced the DNA of dozens of obscure organisms at costs of hundreds of millions of dollars, we need to ask daily if what we are doing is right. We should never fail to envision the mother of the child dying from preventable conditions such as tetanus or malaria or measles while we spend money on DNA sequencing the tenrec genome.

Thirteen
Life Comes to One

Erika von Mutius

My Family

I was brought up in a German family after World War II. My father's family had lived as small landlords with intense bonds to the land, its people, and the animals around them in former German Silesia, and were deracinated war refugees. My mother's family was made up of four generations of physicians. The most prominent family member was my maternal grandfather (Fig. 13.1), born in 1870, who became a physician as his father had been. He joined the first German expedition to the South Pole led by Dr. Drygalski, which voyaged on a sailboat from 1901 to 1903. After returning from his amazing adventure, he settled in Partenkirchen, Bavaria, in the south of Germany because he loved the mountains and was an excellent alpinist. He married a nurse, and both were highly respected for their immense dedication to their patients. I was 5 years of age when he died, so my personal memories of him are few, but my grandparents' house, the doctor's house, was the scene of many adventures for us children because of all the exotic things brought back from the expedition.

I was only a guest in that house during vacations and for festivities. My father had accepted a job at the International Labour Organisation in Geneva, Switzerland, as I turned 6 years old. I spent seven formative years around Geneva, where I started primary school in French. These years were free spirited—many children were bi- or trilingual, and it was normal to have several cultural backgrounds belonging to the maternal and paternal family and the place of residence, respectively. In my school class in Genthod, we had about 20 children from 11 different nations, and all sorts of European languages were spoken. French became my second language. These years taught me an open spirit and a love for the European cultural diversity, traits which would serve me well later when coordinating large PanEuropean collaborative projects.

My parents divorced and my mother went back to her family in Partenkirchen, where I completed my last school years. The bright spot in these rather difficult

E. von Mutius (✉)
Department of Asthma and Allergy, Munich University Children's Hospital, Munich, Germany
e-mail: erika.von.mutius@med.uni-muenchen.de

D.A. Schwartz (ed.), *Medicine Science and Dreams*,
DOI 10.1007/978-90-481-9538-1_13, © Springer Science+Business Media B.V. 2011

Fig. 13.1 Erika with her
maternal grandfather

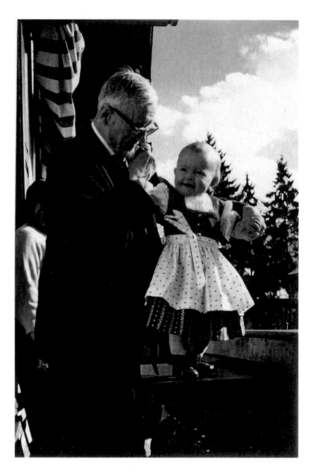

years for me was the formation of a very active and increasingly successful troupe of scholars playing theatre. I was not talented as an actress, but I loved the creative processes in building up a performance. I was responsible for costumes and loved to watch the metamorphoses of my friends once they stepped into an Elizabethan costume to play Shakespeare. This troupe became my life. I also met my first boyfriend, a student in medical school who was active in our troupe.

Medical School

After my final school examinations I was torn between two choices: I wanted to continue with literature and the arts, but I was also drawn to medicine by my boyfriend and family, which has generated physicians for five generations. Finally, I let life decide for me. I vowed that I would take a place at medical school nowhere else than in Munich. At that time—the 1970s in Germany—these positions were difficult to obtain. Otherwise, I would study German literature and the arts. I was offered a position in medical school in Munich, so I attended, but I still went to seminars in German literature studies and philosophy. Three times throughout my tenure in medical school, I came dangerously close to breaking up with medicine. I thought the learning was boring and that very little was logical or could be deduced by thinking. And medical school didn't touch the big questions of life, which poetry, literature, and art do so magnificently. At that time, medical school in Germany was very theoretical and allowed little contact with patients. The practical seminars were not inspiring; the teachers had neither time nor fun teaching styles, and some were rather arrogant. The final time I considered changing my life radically was after the last examinations. In Germany, a so-called unpaid "practical year" must be completed with three-month periods in internal medicine, surgery, and an elective subject. A friend who had worked on his doctoral thesis at the University Children's Hospital in Munich suggested that I pick paediatrics, and I fortunately gave it a try.

And I loved it! This was the first time in my prolonged struggle with medicine that I was captured by the challenge and the fun. These children were really sick but so full of energy once they were recovering. The work on the ward was hard and required long hours, but it was also very rewarding, interesting, and fun. I decided that I would apply for a job at that hospital. I was not the only one with such hopes, as Munich's Children's Hospital was one of the largest and most well-known paediatric hospitals in the country. Chances of being selected were small. I was interviewed and told, what I had expected, that there was no job for me. Five days later, I received a phone call in the morning telling me that there was a job available but that it would last for only three months with no prospect of prolongation. I took the job anyway, since it came with a salary. After all, I needed some money after all the years in medical school.

Paediatrics

Six weeks later I was told that I could stay at the Munich Children's Hospital if I would take on a project. At that time in Germany, there was a fierce political debate regarding the role of air pollution as a cause of croup. The Bavarian State Government had decided to fund a study on that matter and concluded that the money would go to the big university children's hospital in the capital of Bavaria, Munich. No proposal was needed; the political will was enacted. Here I was, a youngster in paediatrics, with no education and no experience in scientific work. My doctoral thesis had been a review of patients' charts and had been anything but demanding. It was decided that a colleague, Thomas Nicolai, would help me. So Thomas, who was not enthusiastic about his new assignment and his ignorant colleague, designed a study investigating children with croup admitted to our hospital. He planned to relate daily admissions to daily measures of various air pollutants. Thomas was of enormous help. I would not have survived this experience without him, especially given that I also worked on the wards in general paediatrics and later in neonatal intensive care. We designed a questionnaire, took throat swabs for viral cultures from the kids before discharge, and made every mistake in our research that one could possibly make. The study was a mess and was eventually published in a very low key German journal. I decided that I would never ever do this again.

The Chief of Paediatrics, Beat Hadorn, suggested that I should start another project since "money was abundant" at the Bavarian State Ministry for the Environment. I thought that if I designed a reasonable project, it would be so expensive that nobody would fund it. And I felt that asthma was much more important than croup. Meanwhile, I had also been assigned to look after children with asthma and allergies in outpatient clinics, a function that hadn't existed before at that hospital. At the end of the 1980s, epidemiological studies were scarce in Germany. The prevalence of asthma and atopy was unknown, and risk factors had not been investigated in German populations. Thus, Thomas and I designed a cross-sectional survey enrolling all children in primary schools in Munich and a rural area around Munich. Since the potential adverse effects of air pollution were still a major theme, we wanted to compare prevalences between urban and rural areas. We designed questionnaires according to our clinical history-taking approach and proposed to perform spirometry and cold air challenges as well as skin prick tests as objective markers of disease, much like in clinics. The budget for the whole package exceeded one million Deutsche Mark (about €500,000) and I felt rather secure that we wouldn't have to do the study, believing that surely they would not give so much money to a nobody like me.

Munich Asthma and Allergy Study

I was wrong. We got the funding, even without budget cuts, in the spring of 1989. Thomas and I drank a glass of sparkling wine to celebrate. Then Thomas disappeared for his two-year fellowship in Australia, and I was left alone with the conduct of the study and the regular work on the wards. Luckily, I had strong support from a very committed colleague from the local health authority, Edith von Löffelholz-Colberg. I hired a group of field workers and organized the study with the help of a statistical group at the Gesellschaft für Strahlenforschung (GSF) (Peter Reithmeier and Wolfgang Lehmacher). The biggest mistake we made in this study was that we randomly allocated field workers to different districts in Munich but had only one field worker for the rural area. He performed skin prick tests slightly differently than the rest of the group. Therefore, we could never reliably compare skin prick test results between Munich and the rural areas, one of our major outcomes.

German Re-unification

In November 1989, the Berlin wall fell. I remember these days like yesterday, sitting in front of the television and not believing my eyes. The imminent changes were perceptible in the demonstrations after the peace prayers in Leipzig every

Monday, which gradually became mass demonstrations despite the threats issued by the German Democratic Republic (GDR) government in late fall 1989. The people wanted freedom and their own rights, and these basic needs could no longer be ignored. The pace of events was phenomenal, and one night the unimaginable became reality: people were standing on the wall, celebrating, in tears, and hugging each other in a place where once death and perfidy had reigned for so long. It is a great privilege that I could live such a rare moment in history: a peaceful revolution of the people.

Thomas and I had always argued that West Germany was just not polluted enough to show effects on asthma, but that studies on pollution levels such as those encountered in the GDR would prove that there is indeed an effect. Such studies had been politically impossible until this time. With the sudden opening of the German border, I thought there was an opportunity. But how would we find colleagues in East Germany? The iron curtain had been impermeable. Friends of mine working for television spent weeks in East Germany during the months after the fall of the wall. I asked one friend if she could look out for some physicians interested in air pollution. Through her various contacts, she finally found such a person in Halle, Hans-Heinrich Thielemann. She also helped with arrangements in Leipzig, which had been, on paper, a partner University of Munich, and helped identify Christian Fritzsch. I invited them and their teams to come to Munich in June 1990. I will never forget the immense obstacles we had to overcome to contact them. To make a phone call to East Germany (and vice versa), one had to dial for about three hours to finally get connected. I will also never forget their amazement when they finally arrived in Munich; all hotel rooms had a bathroom with bathtubs and running hot water, all meals on the restaurant menu were really available, and the lights in the shop windows were lit at night. It was a humbling experience. They were wonderful people, full of excitement and optimism for a better future.

We did not have any funding, but the spirits were high. We decided to start a study in Leipzig right away. We copied questionnaires in Munich, collected all our lung function equipment from the Munich survey, and my brother helped to transport it all to Leipzig in my mother's VW van. Helgo Magnussen sponsored a cold air challenge device, and we instructed the colleagues in Leipzig to perform exactly the same study as in Munich, with the exception of skin prick testing which we could not afford. The statistical team at GSF entered the data and performed the statistical analyses. We were all incredulous when we saw the results, which indicated less asthma and hay fever in polluted Leipzig as compared to Munich. We discussed whether the data needed to be re-entered. We thought this result could not be right, but in the end it was right.

Stephan Weiland

Meanwhile, Stephan Weiland (Fig. 13.2) had appeared. Stephan was a physician who trained in epidemiology at McGill and upon his return had a dream. Like the big cardiovascular MONICA study, he wanted to establish a large survey for

Fig. 13.2 Stephan Weiland

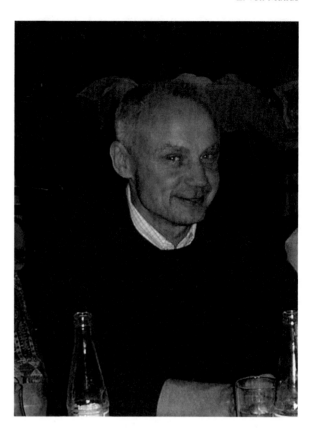

asthma. Ulrich Keil, his boss, had contacts with David Strachan and Ross Anderson in London and Neil Pearce in Wellington, New Zealand. Stephan invited them to Bochum for a meeting—the first meeting of what would become ISAAC, the International Study of Asthma and Allergies in Childhood. This meeting on a grey December day in 1990 at the University of Bochum was decisive for me. Stephan and I started our close collaboration, which turned into a long-lasting friendship until his tragic premature death in 2007. I also met for the first time Fernando Martinez, who had come as a substitute for Ben Burrows, from Tucson, AZ. My English was very poor. I understood all discussions but could not express myself. So I kept quiet, but I liked Fernando's approach based on his solid clinical background.

A few weeks or months later I showed Stephan our first East/West German findings. He immediately understood the impact and offered to help write the paper, as he was fluent in English after his fellowship. I travelled on several weekends to Bochum, where Stephan and I wrote the first paper on the East/West German findings. Stephan also strongly recommended that I should leave for a fellowship to the USA or Canada. Given that Fernando was the only American I knew and that he had impressed me at the first ISAAC meeting, I asked him if I could come for a fellowship to work with him. At the second ISAAC meeting one year later, he confirmed that I would become his first fellow. Meanwhile, the political land-scape in Germany was strongly in favour of collaborative studies between East and West Germany. I applied for a second survey in Halle and Leipzig, East Germany, to include skin prick testing to corroborate the questionnaire data. We received the funding, and after collecting this new data set and obtaining funding for a fellow-ship, I left for Tucson, AZ in the summer of 1992, having passed my paediatric specialty exams.

Fernando Martinez

My fellowship in 1992 and 1993 was fantastic and drastically changed my life. Fernando was a dedicated, inspiring, immensely supportive, and enthusiastic men-tor. I was in Tucson before he became the director of the Arizona Respiratory Centre, and every day he came into my office, and we discussed and worked together on the East/West German data set. Under Fernando's mentorship, my two souls finally found each other: the clinical soul and the intellectual soul with its desire to better understand. Fernando was the perfect teacher. He uncovered skills in me that I had not known before. He was the first who recognized my potential and talents, fig-ured out what was good for me, not for him or anybody else, and encouraged me to engage in creative scientific reasoning. This is when I really became hooked. It was a productive year with five papers written together in these 12 months.

The most important of these papers, which had a strong impact on all future work, related to our discussions in search of an explanation for the marked East/West differences. Fernando knew of a paper published four years earlier which had not received much attention until then. In this paper, David Strachan had proposed what would later be called the "hygiene hypothesis," which proposes that a hygienic envi-ronment predisposes children to the development of allergies and asthma. That is, conditions of extreme cleanliness during childhood fail to stimulate the immune system properly, leading to more allergies later in development. He described and interpreted his observation that children with increasing numbers of older siblings had less hay fever than children without siblings. Fernando and I replicated this observation in the German data. I presented the brand new findings in spring 1993 at a US–German meeting at Harvard. I believe this was the day on which the "hygiene hypothesis" took off. My German colleagues took the idea over to Europe, and soon many more studies corroborated these observations.

After one year of intellectual inspiration and excitement, I went back to Germany, my funding having expired. I was full of dreams, ideas, and concepts for further research but was put back full-time into clinical work. I was able to escape neonatal intensive care but was required to work full-time in outpatient clinics. I became more and more desperate to return to research, having finally found my true destination of being a physician-scientist. Sonia Buist was important in these days comforting and morally supporting me. Fortunately, Stephan and I had written a grant together which was awarded six months after my return. I threatened to give the money back if the chief of paediatrics would not agree that 50% of my time would go to research.

In reality, my time free of clinical work was only 20%, but this was still a big step forward. Stephan and I did the ISAAC Phase II Study in Germany, with much better funding than ever before. I could afford a half-time secretary, which was incredibly helpful.

I also decided that I wanted formal training in epidemiology, not just the hands-on experience. I had spent three weeks in the summer of 1991 at Tufts University in Boston taking courses in epidemiology and statistics, which were taught among others by Ken Rothman and David Hosmer. They were very inspiring teachers, and I understood for the first time the potential of epidemiology—which can be much more than counting peas. In 1997–1999, I spent three summers in the "Clinical Effectiveness" program at the Harvard School of Public Health. These were wonderful experiences; an excellent faculty, highly interesting and clever students from many different countries, and a concentrated learning atmosphere made me a highly motivated student. I graduated from Harvard with a Master of Science in epidemiology in 2000.

Charlotte Braun-Fahrländer

After my return from Tucson, I renewed ties with a colleague and good friend of mine, Charlotte Braun-Fahrländer (Fig. 13.3), an epidemiologist in Basel. Charlotte had a strong interest in air pollution when I first met her while we were finishing the croup study. We designed and exchanged many questionnaires and discussed study designs and findings from the literature. Stephan Weiland and she are the loyal and true companions of my career. She has always been enormously supportive. Charlotte had performed a large survey across Switzerland, the SCARPOL survey, where she also looked into urban/rural differences and indoor sources of air pollution. In our first study in Munich and its surroundings, we had observed that children exposed to coal and wood heating indoors were at significantly lower risk of asthma, airway hyperresponsiveness, hay fever, and atopy. In fact, I remember clearly that Peter Reithmeier, the statistician in our first working group in Munich, had pointed to these low odds ratios, telling us that this was the only relevant signal in the data that would be worthwhile exploring further. He was right, but at that stage we could not make any sense out of these data and did not publish the findings. At the end of my fellowship in Tucson, Fernando and I interpreted these data in light of the East/West comparison, proposing that a traditional lifestyle in West Germany was associated with protection from asthma and allergies as we had observed in East Germany, where indoor coal heating had been prevalent.

Charlotte had incorporated the identical question into the SCARPOL survey. She called me one day and told me that she saw the same strong protective effect of indoor wood and coal heating. In autumn of 1993, she called me again and told me that in her data, this effect was explained by the fact that most people who still heated with coal and wood indoors in Switzerland were farmers. She had included on her team Markus Gassner, a physician living in a small village in Grabs, Switzerland. He had performed yearly school examinations in his village and had observed that

Fig. 13.3 Charlotte
Braun-Fahrländer

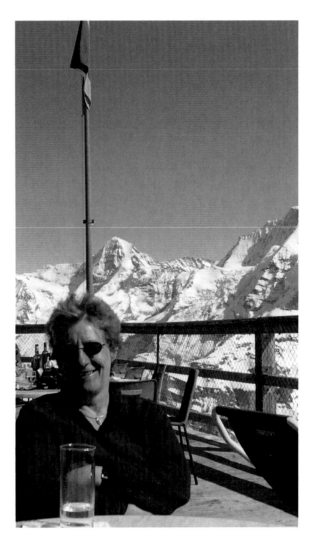

children from the farms there did not present with hay fever. Charlotte had listened to Markus Gassner and had incorporated one question about farming into her
SCARPOL questionnaire. At first sight of the protective farm effect, Charlotte did
not trust her data, having enrolled relatively low numbers of subjects. She repeated
the survey a few years later and confirmed her original observation. Meanwhile, I
got the opportunity to participate in a questionnaire-based study of children entering
primary schools across Bavaria. I also saw a strong inverse association between farm
upbringing and asthma and allergies. Inspired by our ideas, Josef Riedler who had
returned from his fellowship in Australia, had also started a cross-sectional study in
rural areas around Salzburg.

It took me a while to realize that our farm observations needed to be seen in the context of the "hygiene hypothesis." I had been invited to a workshop on the role of fungal exposures in the USA, where I met Jeroen Douwes. We talked about farm studies during the coffee break, and Jeroen told me about endotoxin, a substance in the cell wall of Gram negative bacteria, which was abundant in farm environments and was discussed as a risk factor for farmer's lung disease in adults. I suddenly realized that microbial exposures might be an important clue for understanding the asthma and allergy protective "farm effect." When I came back to Munich I called Charlotte and told her my new ideas. Meanwhile, she had been skiing in the Swiss Alps, in Mürren, where her neighbours were farmers. She went to see them and they told her about their observation that any small wound in the skin would rapidly suppurate when working in the stables. This observation and my newly acquired notion about endotoxin convinced Charlotte and me that microbial exposures were critical for the protective "farm effect." We had also seen in the first Bavarian farm study that among farm children, the frequency of stable visits was inversely associated with asthma and allergic outcomes, further corroborating this idea.

On a memorable day in 1998, Charlotte came to Munich to discuss our findings. We called Josef to ask whether he could come over from Salzburg in the afternoon to tell us about his observations as well. Luckily, Salzburg is just one and a half hours driving distance away from Munich, and Josef was available. Additionally, Dennis Nowak had just started his new position as Head of Occupational and Environmental Medicine in Munich. He had also performed farm studies in adults in Lower Saxony in the North of Germany. Charlotte, Josef, and I presented our questionnaire data and Charlotte showed her radioallergosorbent allergy test results. Josef called his co-workers in Salzburg and told us that strong differences were observed in skin test reactivity between farm and nonfarm children. Dennis also turned to his co-workers and confirmed strong differences in atopy between farm and nonfarm populations. We were all very excited and felt that we had an important observation in our hands. We were also thrilled by the idea that we could have discovered new land which would finally help us understand how to protect people from disease. Dennis knew how to measure endotoxin in dust samples. That day, we decided to join forces and begin a collaborative farm study including measures of endotoxin. The ALEX study had been born, which later received funding in our three respective countries.

We could indeed show that environmental exposures to endotoxin were strongly inversely related to asthma and allergies. We later also demonstrated similar protective effects for exposure to substances of Gram positive bacteria and fungi in the ALEX study and a subsequent larger farm study, the PARSIFAL study. We are currently in the process of refining the exposure assessment in a large collaborative farm study in Germany, Switzerland, Austria, and Poland, the GABRIEL Advanced Studies, and we hope to eventually identify the asthma and allergy-protective substances. The dream is to eventually apply this knowledge towards developing novel prevention strategies against asthma and atopy.

In the 16 years since my return from Tucson, I have been able to gradually increase my research time through a number of grants. I am currently spending about 25% of my time in clinical work, mostly related to childhood asthma and allergies. It has been a constant struggle between the two poles of clinical work and research, and this split has often been difficult. However, I strongly believe that both sides are indispensable and learn from each other. I am much more convinced of epidemiological concepts when I can see them applied in clinical work. In turn, patients and their mothers have often given me new ideas. Much of my work is now related to interdisciplinary approaches which involve collaborating with many colleagues from basic science. As each field has its own language, the dialogue must be learned, and the process of interdisciplinary work is challenging but very rewarding, because I am regularly confronted with many novel and exciting ideas. The asthmatic and allergic child is, however, still the focus and at the centre of all my studies.

My path to research was accidental and loaded with hurdles. My reluctance at the beginning had many roots, but first and foremost was my ignorance of my own talents and intellectual desire. My expectation for the future was having a family and raising kids, a traditional German female role where research and science are unheard of. Life has guided me towards what I love: medicine and science and most of all, the inextricable intersection of the two. I have been very lucky over the years. I have had and still have wonderfully supportive friends and colleagues, I had the best mentor in the world, and we had the luck to come across some very interesting observations. Fernando would say "life comes to one." For me that has been absolutely true.

Fourteen
What Is a Guy Like You Doing in a Place Like This? A Physician-Scientist in the Private Sector

Gilad S. Gordon

Unlike many contributors to this collection of biographies, I have spent most of my research career working as a physician-scientist in the private sector. In my career, the focus of my research has been on two different areas: health services research and clinical trials for new biotechnology products. The path I took in selecting the choice of both my research interests and the research location was interesting, full of challenges, spanned a variety of locations, and put me in touch with some extraordinary teachers and mentors. Below I have tried to provide a glimpse of the path and some of the key events that lead me to where I am today.

I was born in 1957 in Israel to an academic family where achievement was not only desired, but also was expected. My great-grandfather had written an interpretation of the Bible and was the first person to translate Shakespeare into Hebrew. His son, my grandfather, ran a prestigious publishing house in Jerusalem and was constantly surrounded by books and by friends who were authors. My father was born in Poland, but lived most of his life in Israel and was one of the young commanders who saved Jerusalem from falling to the Arabs during the Israeli War of Independence in 1948. After that war, he went to the University of California at Berkeley, studied engineering, met my mother, married, and moved back to Israel.

My mother was born in Philadelphia to immigrant parents of Russian descent. Her father owned and ran a pharmacy in Philadelphia and had enormous academic aspirations for his children. My mother, who is probably one of the smartest people I have ever met, went to the University of Pennsylvania and to graduate school at the University of California at Berkeley, where she studied biochemistry and botany. Interestingly, she was encouraged to go to medical school but chose not to do so because she felt that medicine as a career would not be compatible with having children and raising a family.

My interest in science certainly had its origins with my mother. Her curiosity and interest in the world around her captivated my childhood. She was fascinated by plants and insects. Walks in the park with her were always slow because we frequently had to stop to look and to try to name the living object that was the subject

G.S. Gordon (✉)
Department of Medicine, University of Colorado Health Sciences Center, Denver, CO, USA
e-mail: ggordon@orragroup.com

D.A. Schwartz (ed.), *Medicine Science and Dreams*,
DOI 10.1007/978-90-481-9538-1_14, © Springer Science+Business Media B.V. 2011

of her attention. She tried to get my brother and me to start a butterfly collection, but that was short-lived. I think it is still a source of disappointment for her that we did not complete the collection, as she has kept it in our old closet waiting for it to be finished. I remain very close to my brother who, although also interested in science, ended up pursuing a career in law and business.

In the fall of 1966, we moved to the USA for my father to complete his studies. He chose to get his PhD in Hydrology and Water Resources at the University of Arizona in Tucson. Moving to the USA was an eye-opening experience to say the least. In Israel, in 1966, there were no televisions, all the news was received through radios, and science was, for the most part, observational in very limited ecosystems. The USA, in contrast, was remarkable. One had television, the ecosystems were remarkably diverse (as we saw during multiple summer camping trips), distances were great, and, most importantly for me, the space program was in full swing.

As a 10-year-old child interested in science, nothing could be greater than the space program. I was captivated. My walls were plastered with pictures of the various space vehicles, I knew every astronaut by name, and I was hooked on space. When the astronauts landed on the moon in the summer of 1969, I was sure that Walter Cronkite was speaking to me personally. I vividly remember begging to stay up late and to wake up early to watch as much as possible of the landing and the first walk on the moon. I had mapped out my career as an astronaut, but was devastated to find out that I would not be eligible to fly because I wore glasses. Regardless, astronomy and physics were certainly going to be in my future.

In the fall of 1970, we moved to Reston, Virginia, a small town about 20 miles west of Washington, DC. Needless to say, one of our first trips was to the Smithsonian Institution to see the moon rocks and the various space vehicles. The Smithsonian, especially the Air and Space Museum, became a source of constant interest and fascination.

I started Herndon High School in Herndon, VA in 1971. One of the science teachers at the school was an older woman named Vera Remsburg who was both feared and loved (Fig. 14.1). Needless to say, I thought she was terrific and she, more than any other teacher, was instrumental in pushing me to science and to scientific projects. She taught us biology, but was concerned that the biology of 1971 was boring and involved primarily taxonomy and memorization. She seemed to have a sense of where biology was heading and tried to make it interesting, analytic, and relevant. For her, the future of biology was in studying the effect that man-made changes in the environment were having on the ecosystem. She made us read Rachel Carson's *Silent Spring*. Under her leadership and encouragement, a group of us began a three-year project to study the effect of building development on a local watershed. Every Sunday morning, we dragged ourselves out of bed at 6 a.m., went down to a local stream, and took multiple measurements of the water quality of the stream along a 10-mile stretch where new developments were being constructed. That project was the winner of the State Science Fair in 1974. Although the data we collected were rudimentary by today's standards, it was the first science project in which I was involved in defining a problem, setting up a project, analyzing the data, and seeing the results. This was science at its best, and I was captivated.

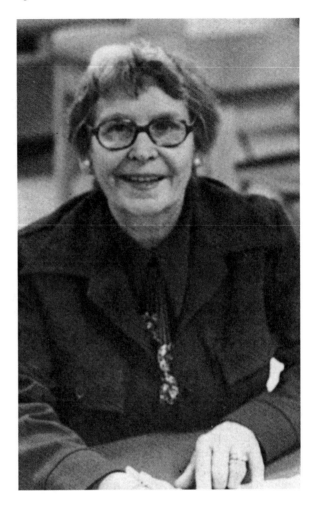

Fig. 14.1 Vera Remsburg (1976), an influential science teacher at Herndon High School in Herndon, VA

The results of this project helped define the problems of certain real estate developments in Northern Virginia. This project, combined with concerns about natural habitats, eventually led to a ban on development in certain parts of Fairfax County. As luck would have it, one of my interviewers for Dartmouth College was the developer whose work I helped stop. To this day, I consider it one of my greatest achievements that I was still waitlisted at Dartmouth, despite what was certainly one of the worst interviews imaginable!

However, despite the push into biology from Ms. Remsburg, I was still fascinated by astronomy and physics and tried to figure out a way to combine the two areas. I came across an article describing how a certain snail had approximately 365 rings in its shell today and its prehistoric ancestor had more than 400 rings in its fossilized shell. The question then arose as to whether the number of rings correlated with the number of days in a year, and thus whether the number of days in a year was decreasing over time. In other words, was the earth moving farther away from the sun? I combined a number of mathematical formulae and, using a dumb-terminal attached to a mainframe computer and using one-inch yellow tape, was able to show that this was indeed the case. I was ecstatic that I was able to, on my own, identify a problem, solve the problem, and relate it to a real-life observation. With Ms. Remsburg's encouragement, I submitted the work to various science competitions and was honored with various awards. In addition, she encouraged me to submit the work to the Virginia Junior Academy of Sciences, and it was selected for an oral presentation. This was the first time I had ever spoken in public about my research, and was I ever nervous? However, under her tutelage, I learned how to make a scientific presentation; I still carry that knowledge with me today. There was no question that I was going to go into science, but I still had the deep desire to go into physics rather than biology. That was soon going to change.

In the fall of 1975, I enrolled at Harvard and, true to my interests, immediately enrolled in an astronomy seminar taught by Alan Maxwell. When I mentioned to him my strong interest in astronomy, he took me over to the library and showed me the list of available positions for astronomers graduating in 1976. The list contained precisely one position, but it was a good one, in Maui. Needless to say, I was quite discouraged by the job prospects and, with the encouragement of my father (who was one of the most pragmatic men I have ever met) began to take a more pragmatic approach to my future. With that, the search began for other scientific areas to pursue.

Luckily, through a family friend, I was introduced to Dr. Dinkar Kasbekar, at Georgetown University Medical. I spent an entire summer in his lab pithing frogs and studying gastric acid secretion. This was my first introduction to the field of biochemistry, and it truly sparked my interest. Although it was not as glamorous as space travel, it was intriguing, and the questions were as interesting as any in astronomy.

In the fall of 1976, through sheer luck, I was introduced to Dr. William Haseltine, a man who had a most profound an effect on my career. At Harvard, we had to declare our major in the fall of our second year and, in the Department of Biochemistry, we were assigned tutors. These tutors were usually junior faculty who would meet with a group of five to eight students each month to discuss various topics and to serve as mentors to the students. I was lucky to be assigned to Bill, who had recently joined the Harvard faculty. Our group met with Bill at his house in Cambridge once per month. He was phenomenal and would continuously and enthusiastically introduce us to various aspects of the up-and-coming field of molecular biology. From him, I learned about the great discoveries in genomics and in recombinant DNA technology, and about the promise of this technology to improve the understanding of disease and to develop new medications to cure disease. His enthusiasm was contagious, and I wanted to follow in his footsteps. Sure enough, I was able to work in his lab and learned firsthand how to split genes, map genes, and sequence DNA. He introduced me to various leaders in the field, including Dr. Robert Gallo at National Institutes of Health (NIH).

During the summers after my second and third year in college, I worked in the lab of Dr. Gallo. These were heady times with the discovery of human T-cell leukemia virus-1 (HTLV-1) and the beginning work on the relationship of ribonucleic acid (RNA) viruses to leukemia. I was working on defining a certain part of the RNA virus called "Strong Stop RNA." We certainly did not know at the time that this work would lead, in the not-too-distant future, to some of the important discoveries regarding HIV.

Thus, in the fall of 1977, I was learning from the best and was as excited as could be about a research career in biochemistry. However, a number of events took place which pushed me away from a career in the laboratory and to a career in medicine. The first was a series of discussions which I had with Dr. Gallo, who was an MD, and with various other researchers who were PhDs. They all, without exception, recommended pursuing an MD as opposed to a PhD. Their rationale was two-fold. First, if I was to ever want to do research on human subjects, it is easier to do it with an MD than with a PhD. Second, given the geometric increase in research in biology, it was likely that this research would be quickly applied to humans and could be applied more easily if one had an MD. In addition, my father, to whom I was very close, was always concerned that I have a career where I could make a living, and this rubbed off on me. Thus, in the fall of my junior year, I officially entered the ranks of the pre-meds.

In the fall of 1977, a second event took place, which, in retrospect, had an important effect on my career. In response to the Asilomar Conference in 1975 which was a gathering to discuss what controls should be put in place to safely undertake recombinant DNA research, Harvard established a committee charged with overseeing the recombinant DNA work of its various faculty. This committee was composed of faculty, lay people from the city of Cambridge, and a student representative. Bill Haseltine had recommended me for this committee, and I served on this committee for a total of four years (two in college and two in medical school). As part of my role on this committee, I began what would ultimately be a lifelong passion of evaluating the role of science and medicine in society. I realized then that one cannot undertake research in a vacuum and that most research projects have a larger societal impact than the findings themselves.

In the fall of 1978, another event took place that, in retrospect, also profoundly affected my career. During this time, I was working in Bill Haseltine's lab and was applying to medical school. He called me into his office and, in a very nice way, told me that he would write me a great letter of recommendation to medical school and then went on to recommend that I not pursue a career in basic academic medicine, but rather look toward a career that was more multi-disciplinary in nature. He went on to explain that in the three years that he had known me, he saw that I was a good lab researcher, not great, and that my interests were too broad. In other words, he felt that for me to succeed in the lab, I would need to be super focused on one issue, and that my interests where much broader and would divert me from success in the lab. Needless to say, as an aspiring academic lab researcher, I was devastated. However, in retrospect, he was entirely correct, and I am quite grateful for his being so forthright with me. Because of his advice, I pursued a much broader and diverse career and have probably been much happier than if I had pursued a lab career.

As an interesting side note, during my 25th medical school reunion, I had a conversation with a former classmate, Dr. Alan D'Andrea, who worked with me in

Bill's lab in 1977 and who attended medical school with me. When I mentioned my conversation with Bill, he remarked that Bill had told him at roughly the same time that he, Alan, should go into academic medicine because he could focus on one issue. Sure enough, 30 years later, Alan is still working on the problem of DNA repair and is now one of the world's leading experts in the field. Bill certainly understood us well and provided each of us with the appropriate guidance to match our interests and personalities.

In the fall of 1979, I enrolled in Harvard Medical School in the Division of Health Science and Technology (HST). This Division was started by Dr. Irving London a few years earlier with the goal of training medical students in a very research-intensive environment. The group comprised 25 students, of whom roughly half went on to get a PhD in addition to their MD degree, and the vast majority of us now spend most of our time in research. This program was extraordinary. Every aspect of medicine was evaluated from the research perspective, and it provided me with a deep understanding of the human body, especially all that was unknown and yet to be discovered. As part of the program, we were required to spend one year doing a research project and that project would ultimately dictate my career path.

My entry into clinical research took place in Israel in 1982. I decided to spend three months working in the clinic of Dr. Zvi Laron. He is a pediatric endocrinologist at Beilinson Hospital near Tel Aviv. Dr. Laron is one of the most visionary physicians I have ever met. He has a very strong personality and created a well-respected clinic at the hospital. Because he was so well known, most children in Israel with endocrine problems were referred to Dr. Laron. He, in turn, was a very firm believer in the value of research and the value of population-based data. Therefore, every child that was referred to him, as well as their family members, regardless of diagnosis, underwent a full battery of medical tests. These tests were repeated periodically. On the basis of these findings, he was able to describe various new diseases which had been unknown before, such as Laron dwarfism. This syndrome is a rare autosomal recessive disease characterized by short stature despite normal- to high-growth hormone levels and is also associated with low somatomedin levels. More recently, as receptors were defined and evaluated, the disease was determined to be due to a variant of the growth hormone receptor. The original observation was based on only about 15 children and was drawn from the extensive data that he had prospectively gathered on all of the children who came to his clinic. This population-based data gathering was truly ahead of its time.

While studying there, I undertook a small study to evaluate the growth pattern in children newly diagnosed with diabetes, and because of these data, I was able to correlate the growth to various measures such as growth hormone levels and c-peptide levels. This was my first experience in clinical research, and I was fascinated.

When I returned from Israel in 1982, I began my fourth year research project as part of the HST program. Prior to starting this project, I spoke to numerous leading researchers to try to identify a project. Ultimately, I chose to work with Dr. Jeffrey Flier (the future Dean of Harvard Medical School) at the Beth Israel Hospital in Boston on a project aimed at determining whether insulin could be administered as an inhaled agent. We based our work on a couple of small studies from Japan that had shown some preliminary results. Insulin alone could not cross the nasal barrier, so various adjuvants were required to help facilitate the absorption. Early in the course of the study, I brought in one of my gastrointestinal professors, Dr. Martin Carey, who was an expert in bile salts, which, it turned out, where great adjuvants. Most of the work during that year evaluated various bile salts in combination with insulin with ongoing assays of blood glucose, and insulin levels. The project was a great success and clearly demonstrated that different bile salts lead to different levels of insulin absorption and different levels of nasal irritation. In addition, we showed that diabetics could control their blood sugar in the short term using this new technology. It was terrific to be able to use various disciplines to try to solve the research problem.

This work was quickly recognized as having commercial value and was ultimately licensed to California Biotechnology. About eight years later, when I was working at Eli Lilly and Company (which had in the meantime licensed the product from California Biotechnology), I was asked to do a careful evaluation of all the clinical data from multiple short- and long-term trials. To my chagrin, the chronic administration data revealed that the early drops in glucose in response to nasal insulin were not reproducible in the long run. Furthermore, there was hypervariability in that a given dose of nasal insulin could lead to a 20-fold difference in absorption. This was a level of variability certainly not compatible with a clinical product for diabetes. The project was ultimately stopped. I was there at the beginning and at the end.

In 1983, I started my residency at the University of Colorado Health Sciences Center in Denver where the head of the program was Dr. Robert Schrier. He had created a superb training program through his scientific work and his ability to attract and retain some of the brightest people in medicine. In addition, he was very personable and would, on a monthly basis, have gatherings for the residents at his house. I am still struck by the difference in attitude between Boston and Denver. I found medicine in Boston to be highly competitive, all consuming, and not enjoyable. In Denver, the quality of the people was similar, but there was a far greater attitude of camaraderie, a sense that life outside the hospital was important, and a strong belief in the value of the team in taking care of patients.

In Denver, I had the pleasure of interacting with one of the most remarkable men I have ever met, Dr. William Robinson. He is a Hematologist/Oncologist who was the ultimate triple threat—clinician, scientist, and teacher. Unlike many of the doctors in Denver, Bill had been born and raised in Colorado, but like so many others he had trained back east at Massachusetts General Hospital and had returned to Colorado. During my residency, I spent a considerable amount of time with him in multiple settings. As an attending physician, I never saw a more compassionate physician. He always took the time to talk to the patients and to the families about the grave prognosis and their various options. As a researcher, he ran both a basic lab and was involved in numerous clinical trials in which he insisted that we get involved. As a teacher, he not only made time for us on the wards, but also insisted that we interact outside the hospital. This often involved Thursday ski trips, when we spent lots of time talking and discussing medicine and various career options. It was through him that I began to appreciate that life as a physician-scientist could be balanced with outside interests. Although Bill tried to convince me to go into Oncology, I was anxious to get out of the hospital environment.

During my residency I had a very touching experience with a young patient named Webjorn Svendsen. He was 32 years old, from Oslo, Norway, and presented with widely metastatic melanoma. He came from a well-to-do family and traveled to Denver to try and get help from Bill Robinson. Unfortunately, by the time he arrived in Denver, his disease was wide-spread with numerous brain metastases and nothing could be done for him. He very much wanted to return to Oslo to be with his family, but was felt to be too unstable to fly alone. I was asked to accompany him and his girlfriend back to Oslo. This gave me a lot of time to talk to him about his life, his aspirations, and his dreams. He was a young man who was well-educated, full of life, and was struck down just as his life was beginning. He was quite philosophical and continuously reflected on the fact that cancer has no bounds and can strike a young man such as him in the prime of his life. He went on to ask why could we land a man on the moon, but not cure cancer. As I have gone on in my research, I continue to reflect on this wonderful young man and the need to assure that such men in the future can lead full lives.

The other key individual with whom I have shared numerous experiences is my close friend Jeff Berman. Jeff and I met during my first day in college and, thereafter, attended college together, attended medical school together, and completed the same residency in Colorado. Jeff is one of the brightest and most insightful individuals I have ever met and we spent many hours together, often on the ski slopes (Fig. 14.2), discussing medicine, research, and the role of medicine in society. He, more than any other friend, has been the one who always encouraged me to look beyond classic

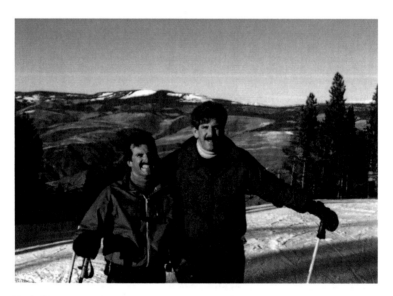

Fig. 14.2 Jeff Berman and the author skiing in Vail in 1986

academic medicine and to explore other options in medicine and research. Jeff is currently a cardiologist in Westport, Connecticut and has been heavily involved in developing electronic medical records for cardiologists.

I truly wanted to study the interaction of medicine in society from a different perspective than either the hospital or the scientific lab. I found that this interest could be developed through the Robert Wood Johnson Clinical Scholars Program, and I was fortunate to be accepted to the fellowship at the University of Washington School of Medicine. In the program, we were encouraged to pursue an additional degree. I was interested in the finances of medicine, and decided to get a Masters of Business Administration (MBA). Although the finance and accounting courses were interesting, I found that the human relations and management courses were much more valuable. I only wished that these courses had been required during the transition from internship to residency. As I reflected on that transition time, I realized that one went from being a front level MD to a manager of a team with no management experience. No wonder it was so difficult for all concerned.

During my training, I was once asked a very simple but telling question: "When you introduce yourself, which degree do you mention first, the MBA or the MD?" Initially I thought about the answer, since I was not treating patients on a daily basis. However, it soon became apparent that my life was medicine and that the MBA was merely an additional degree. Given the rapid increase in physicians getting additional graduate degrees, I often wonder how they would respond to this question.

During this fellowship, I concentrated on trying to understand the economics of health care. During the 1980s, questions began to be asked about the costs of care, the differential costs, the value of the care, and ways to contain the costs. The only difference between the discussions then and the discussions now, 20 years later, is that the costs of healthcare as a percentage of the Gross Domestic Product have gone up by a factor of two. I devoted considerable time trying to analyze the costs, the care, and the outcomes of patients treated in teaching versus non-teaching hospitals. Along the way, I had to learn statistics, research methodology, and how to evaluate quality of care and quality of life. Initially, I viewed this project as a mere statistical analysis of cost tables, but it soon became apparent that one would need to delve deeply into the types of disease, the severity of the disease in the patients, and the patients' socioeconomic backgrounds. Suddenly, bench research with well-controlled cohorts appeared to be much more manageable than health economic studies. However, I persevered, conducted the research, and was thrilled to be able to help show that teaching hospitals were not necessarily the more expensive dispensers of care.

In my life, I have traveled to many parts of the world and along the way have met some extraordinary people who have a very different view of the world and have made me think about my own world in very different ways. One person who comes to mind is an older Chinese physician named C.C. Chen, whom I met in 1988 in Chengdu, China. Dr. Chen had spent a considerable amount of time with Mao Zedong and was considered to be the father of primary care in China. He had been trained at Harvard in the 1920s, and after returning to China, focused his work on improving rural medical care. Reflecting on his own work with the Chinese health system, he asked me why in the USA we insist that every patient see a doctor rather than having a triage system where patients first see a nurse and then are referred on to a doctor who may manage multiple nurses at multiple sites. In other words, why not create a system similar to most other systems in business where a senior, more experienced, and more educated individual manages multiple less educated and less experienced individuals? The answer is obviously complex and is a result of the various aspects of American society. Nevertheless, it is these types of questions that frequently influence the type of research I ultimately undertake.

In 1988, I had to make what was perhaps the most difficult career choice of my life, that is, what to do with all of my wonderful training, multiple degrees, and multiple certifications? I interviewed with various academic programs, with various governmental agencies (including members of Senator Ted Kennedy's staff), with various private companies, and with several pharmaceutical companies. My initial thought was to go to academic medicine and to pursue my research interests in health economics. However, I was faced with the daunting problem that there was very little money to support this type of research and the most that I could be guaranteed was two years of support. As I evaluated the environment, I was struck that even though many people were talking about the problems of health care costs, few organizations were willing to support the research necessary to understand the problems before proposing solutions.

Along the way, I met Dr. Leigh Thompson, who was Vice-President of Eli Lilly and who, earlier in his career, had been the Chief Resident to my advisor at the University of Washington, Dr. Tom Inui. Leigh was a dynamo. He was probably the brightest physician I had ever met. He was a blur of ideas, most of which were extraordinary. He had been at Eli Lilly for a few years and was in the process of assembling a world-class research institute with a focus that went far beyond the traditional evaluation of the safety and efficacy of drugs. Leigh had a firm belief that one needed to study the role of drugs in society as a whole and had the obligation to report these findings in the medical literature. In order to accomplish this research, he assembled a group of physicians with backgrounds similar to mine to study the economic impact of individual drugs, to study the quality-of life-impact of drugs, to evaluate the large databases for safety issues with drugs, and to work with other companies to evaluate the economic impact of drugs as a whole. In addition, he insisted that I have an academic appointment at the University of Indiana School of Medicine. In essence, I was provided with a wonderful laboratory and a huge budget with which to conduct health-economic research. This opportunity was far superior to any other academic opportunity with which I was presented.

However, my main challenge was trying to convince my peers that research in the private sector was really valuable and not tainted. This was and continues to be an ongoing challenge. It was most dramatically illustrated at a Robert Wood Johnson Clinical Scholars Annual Meeting in 1988 when I presented my research work. One of the then clinical scholars rose up and asked me a very pointed question about how could I, in good faith, go into the private sector after receiving my training. He was clearly implying and stating that I had sold my soul to the devil. Before I could respond, Dr. Alvan Feinstein, a noted physician and epidemiologist from Yale, stood up and responded that, in his experience, the research from the pharmaceutical industry was usually less biased than that conducted by either the NIH or by NIH-sponsored physicians. He went on to say that the NIH-sponsored physicians needed to have positive results in order to continue their efforts and this, at times, unduly biased the interpretation of their results. Dr. Feinstein concluded by stating that all research is biased and that the challenge for all researchers is both to understand and to publicize their bias. I certainly agree and have always been very frank and open about who sponsors the research I am conducting.

I stayed at Eli Lilly for about three years and then moved to a biotechnology company in Boulder, CO. Over the last 20 years, I have conducted most of my research within the realm of biotechnology and pharmaceutical companies. In my first five to seven years, I concentrated on health economics and quality of life research. These were either standalone studies or were conducted as part of large multi-center, randomized clinical trials. It was interesting that the quantity of the data was huge and the quality was very high because of the nature of pharmaceutical clinical trial requirements. This permitted me to conduct careful evaluations and comparisons of different methods to collect economic data such as bill review, patient reported data, targeted data collection, and modeling. Such a database is so expensive to collect that it would be nearly impossible to do it in the context of a classic academic setting. Furthermore, most of the data were published, and through collaborations with international researchers, we were able to develop fairly sophisticated models for costs of care that can be applied in various health care systems.

Over the last 12 years or so, most of my work has been in setting up and conducting various clinical trials to evaluate the safety and efficacy of new biotechnology or pharmaceutical products. It is interesting that over the last 20 years, the amount of research dollars from the pharmaceutical companies has vastly eclipsed the amount of research money from the NIH. Furthermore, in 2007, the amount of research dollars from the biotechnology companies alone also surpassed the amount of research money from the NIH. The challenges of clinical trials today are enormous in that the diseases are often complex, the endpoints are not clear, and the variability in patients and in clinical settings is high. However, these studies have very clear value in that they lead both to an understanding of the role of the drug (good and bad) as well as to improved understanding of the disease. The vast majority of these trials is done in collaboration with major academic centers and are published in peer-reviewed journals. The key differences between drug studies and more traditional academic research is the subject matter of the studies, the location of the studies (often multi-center, international trials), and the source of funding. However, at the end of the day, both types of studies rely on well-controlled, well-designed studies that must follow sound research methodology. Anything less is unfair to the patients whose lives we are trying to improve and to society, which is ultimately funding all of these studies.

Mentors

I have often thought about mentors and the people who were the key influences on my life and the academic choices that I made. As I have noted above, I was fortunate to meet and closely interact with some extraordinary people who, in their own right, became well known and well respected for their work. Along the way, I also met and interacted with some wonderful people whose comments and thoughts have stayed with me for a long time.

The first significant mentor I had was Vera Remsburg, my high school biology teacher. She, more than anyone else, pushed me to undertake research projects at an early age. She was the one who saw the future of research as crossing various disciplines and encouraged me to look at the world through very wide eyes. She retired from teaching shortly after I left high school, but always kept in touch with me and always wanted to know how I was doing.

The second major influence in my life was Bill Haseltine, my tutor in biochemistry at Harvard. He instilled in me an enthusiasm for biochemistry, a love of research, and a wide view of the opportunity that recombinant technology afforded the world. In addition, Bill had an understanding of me and my interests that helped steer me into a research world which was far broader than the laboratory research I was doing with him.

The third influential mentor was Bill Robinson, the oncologist at the University of Colorado Health Sciences Center. Bill was the ultimate doctor and researcher. I have never met a more caring and compassionate physician, and whenever I face a difficult patient situation, I invariably ask myself, what would Bill say or do? In addition, Bill had a thriving research endeavor which spanned both the lab and the clinic. He was always enthusiastic about this work and loved to talk with great glee about this work. Bill was also the ultimate teacher. He always had the time and the energy to teach the residents and the students, never worrying that he was spending too much time explaining a complicated patient or a complex multi-faceted clinical problem. Bill somehow also managed to have time outside of the hospital to spend with me, to show me the sites of Colorado, to share his personal life, and to enjoy a good laugh. He showed me how he could balance the life of the academic physician with enormous skill, steadiness, and humor. Whenever I have had a problem, Bill has always been there to help.

Finally, the ultimate mentors were my parents. From my earliest memories, I remember them teaching me, encouraging me, and always being there for me. They had challenging lives growing up and had made certain decisions along the way that, given other circumstances, they would have changed. Rather than impose their views upon me, they always discussed my choices and provided sound advice that helped me enormously. Is that a mentor or the role of a parent? I do not know the answer, but am certainly grateful that they were always there for me.

In addition, I am blessed with a very supportive and mentoring family—my wife Cathy, my brother Liran, my children Oren, Roby, and Ari, my step-children Max and Liza and other family members who have been interested in what I was doing and who have helped in every way they could.

Conclusion

The path that I took as I became a physician-scientist was interesting, challenging, and full of fascinating encounters. Along the way, I met remarkable people, interacted with some of the best and brightest in our generation of physicians and scientists, and ultimately chose a path that was different from the one most of them had chosen. I chose this path of research because I felt that I could ultimately bring about change and improve health both by undertaking a different kind of research (health services research) as well as by having a different perspective on the research (that is, a pharmaceutical/biotechnology perspective) from that of the traditional physician-scientist in the academic setting.

I have been asked whether I would undertake this career path again. I often answer without any hesitation that I cannot imagine a more interesting and fulfilling life. The path to get here is long, the costs in time and money are high, the successes as measured by large milestones are relatively few, but the intellectual challenges and the ability to help people more than outweigh the costs. At the end of day, I gain great satisfaction from my work as a physician-scientist, as measured by the ability to improve the lives of people whom I have helped either directly as a physician or indirectly through my research.

Fifteen
The Jock and the Doc

Michael D. Iseman

1939: The Year of the Rabbit

Sitting in our neighborhood Chinese restaurant, between won ton soup and General Tao's chicken, I found myself perusing the Chinese 12-year zodiac. Born in 1939, the Year of the Rabbit, I was informed that those who entered the world under this sign were the "luckiest" of all. While I universally disregard my fortune cookies, I found myself thinking that the Chinese astrologers who came up with this system may have been onto something.

Looking back at my career in medicine, I have been the beneficiary of immense good fortune. This is not to present false humility or invoke mysticism. Rather, at many of the important decision nodes of my life, my choices were not reached by careful, rational analysis but guided by intuition and emotion. The homely expression for this is "following your heart." Mechanistically, this "visceral" process fostered a happiness which has substantially shaped my success, such as it is.

1953: My First Medical Hero

Dr. Carroll Nelson sat with a frightened eighth-grade football player on a Wednesday afternoon from 4:30 to 9:00 p.m. until his parents returned from an out-of-town trip. In a scrimmage, I had suffered a fracture-dislocation of my right elbow, shearing off the medial epicondyle and trapping the ulnar nerve in the joint space. The pain was beyond anything I could imagine, but due to my age, narcotics could not be given and surgery could not be performed without parental consent. Dr. Nelson, a general surgeon, was a soft-spoken man with a wry smile whose tender attention helped make the unbearable bearable.

After my parents arrived, I was taken to the operating room that night, where Dr. Nelson undertook the difficult task of restoring order to my elbow. Freeing the ulnar

M.D. Iseman (✉)
Division of Mycobacterial Diseases and Lung Infections, National Jewish Health, Denver, CO, USA
e-mail: isemanm@njhealth.org

D.A. Schwartz (ed.), *Medicine Science and Dreams*,
DOI 10.1007/978-90-481-9538-1_15, © Springer Science+Business Media B.V. 2011

nerve, placing a screw to anchor the medial epicondyle, and debriding the shattered joint, the wait began to see if my ulnar nerve would survive. Within weeks, it became apparent that the axon had been interrupted: classic loss of sensation of the fifth digit and the lateral half of the fourth, and, more frightening, the interosseous muscles—intrinsic to hand function—began to wither. By the end of the month, I looked down at a dwindling claw hand. Slowly, I learned to write my lessons left-handed. Even more frustrating was that I was relegated to the sidelines of basketball practice. There was, however, an unintended but positive consequence: learning to dribble and shoot left-handed!

Dr. Nelson gave me my first lesson in neurophysiology: although the ulnar axon had been interrupted, the sheath had been left intact. The nerve grew back, as Dr. Nelson explained, at roughly one inch per month. Thus, by the following fall, I was ready to put the pads on and resume my passionate affair with sports.

Years later, as Dr. Nelson lay near death in an Omaha hospital, I visited to pay my respects and thank him again for salvaging my arm. With his gentle laughter, "heh-heh," and a twinkle in his eye, he informed me that he'd never done such surgery before or after my case and, that indeed, he had done the procedure with a surgical textbook propped up on an easel in the OR! How could one fail to admire and wish to emulate Dr. Nelson?

1957: Go East Young Man?

As a high school senior in Fremont, Nebraska, I gave nominal attention to my studies. My world revolved around athletics, particularly football. Then, the dream of every boy who had donned cleats in Nebraska came true for me, when I received the offer of a scholarship at Lincoln. However, at my recruiting visit it became apparent that it would be difficult to reconcile the demands of big-time football and the pre-med studies I also wished to pursue. The coaches suggested that I take my science courses in the summer to avoid conflict with practice.

Zealous as I was about football, these competing priorities were a wake-up call. Consulting "The College Handbook," it seemed that my best chance to play football while preparing for a career in medicine would be the Ivy League. "Cowed" (pun intended) by the agrarian character of Fremont, I imagined that I would be happier in a smaller college rather than a great urban university. So, in a frigid January week of 1957, my father took me to see this new world. I returned home confident that I would like either Dartmouth or Princeton. Letters of acceptance still sitting on the kitchen table a week later, I received a call from Lucy Caldwell, wife of the Princeton coach. Interrogating me about my choice, Lucy finally asked, "Did anyone at Dartmouth agree to bake you chocolate chip cookies each month?" "No." "I will." "Well that's good enough for me."

Charlie Caldwell died of stomach cancer my freshman year, and I never had the privilege of playing a down of football for him (he is in the Collegiate Football Hall of Fame). But, true to her word, Lucy baked cookies monthly, hosted my girlfriend for her four annual visits to Princeton, and, in 1963 drove from New Jersey all the way to Nebraska for our wedding!

1959: Biology or History?

Autumn of 1957 was as close to "boot camp" as I had known. In addition to meeting classmates, trying to find my way around campus, and playing football, I ended up taking five courses, any one of which would have been a challenge for a homesick sod-buster: chemistry, biology, calculus, German, and Shakespeare. Attendance was mandatory and role was taken. I had six classes at 7:40 a.m. and a total of 44 hours in lectures and labs each week. To raise the survival ante, I came down with Asian flu in mid-October and spent five days in the infirmary. Stumbling around in a post-febrile daze the next week, I walked into a series of mid-term exams which had somehow escaped my attention. Princeton then graded on a 1–7 scale, 7 reflecting flagrant and offensive incompetency. My mid-term average was 5-minus! When I returned to Fremont for Christmas, my parents managed to stifle their reactions, but when I rang the doorbell at the Christensen's, my wife-to-be Joan couldn't hide her dismay. In place of the 205-pound lean-mean football machine, who had left in September (Fig. 15.1), now stood a 182-pound and thoroughly shaken young man.

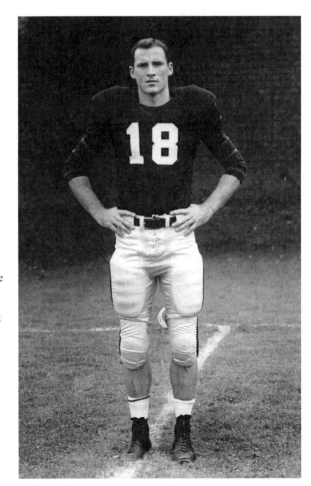

Fig. 15.1 *Young Warrior:* We played Yale for the Ivy League championship in the fall of 1960. Before 66,000 at the Yale Bowl and NCAA Regional TV, they prevailed 41-22 and went on to a 9-0 season, national ranking and the Lambert Trophy for Eastern football supremacy (ahead of Penn State and Pittsburgh). In those days we played both offense (wing-back) and defense (corner-back). Look at that hair!

The holiday went by in a blur and in the first week of January I was confronted with a harsh reality: I did not want to return to New Jersey and my final exams. Encouraged by family and compelled by the unacceptability of failure (coaches had imprinted on the adolescent mind, "quitters never win, winners never quit"), I returned to the cold, grey campus, buried myself in the library, and came out of my finals with a 3-minus average. The straight *As* from high school had never looked better!

The first two years at Princeton were an academic buffet: a little of this, a little of that. Toward the end of the sophomore year, we chose our major. With some trepidation I selected history. I thought it was my last liberal arts fling before delving into a career in biological sciences.

In retrospect, it was a great choice for me, as it provided a durable perspective on humanity. History, I came to believe, boils down to little more than an explication of the recurrent predictable phenotype of *Homo sapiens*.

The last great hurdle for Princeton students was the senior thesis. I had chosen Radical Agrarian Movements in the Midwest in the 1930s as my topic. My thesis advisor was a well-known modern American historian, Eric Goldman. I worked diligently and was rewarded with a 1-minus grade and encouraging comments from Professor Goldman. For the first time, I felt "scholarly." Graduating with honors in history and having been accepted to Columbia College of Physicians and Surgeons, I was ready to commence my life as an adult.

1961: P & S, Bootcamp II

During our freshman biochemistry course, I found myself second-guessing the decision to major in history at Princeton. "How did all my classmates already know what purines and pyrimidines were?" More candidly, my basic science aptitude was modest.

After a few visits with Dean Pereira about, "improving [my] performance," I persevered, until along came the physical diagnosis course in our second year. Perhaps it was proximity to clinicians and patients, but suddenly, medicine became what I had imagined it to be. My junior and senior years affirmed my choice.

Despite having the habitus of an orthopedist, my interests had gravitated toward the excitement of pathophysiology and differential diagnosis. The next question: where to commence my career in internal medicine?

1965: Bellevue, Not Just a "Loony-Bin"

Contemplating internship and residency options, I was attracted to Bellevue Hospital, and I was delighted to be selected for internship in the Columbia program.

The internship was an historical anomaly: six months of medicine, three months of surgery, and three months of "chest medicine." We were on call every-other-night for the year with two weeks of vacation. We had a small room in the hospital, which was ours for the year. Our annual salary was approximately $3,000, but we got *four* meals per day in the elegant "Café Bellevue."

The first day on call on the surgical ward was memorable. The temperature hovered near 100°, there was no air-conditioning, and the tasks of dawn rounds with seemingly infinite "scut-lists" were pressing down on me. I was urgently informed by the head nurse that "Mr. K"—four weeks post-pinning of a fractured hip—had been found unresponsive in his bed. In charge of the resuscitation efforts, I supervised the first-step of the protocol, which was to put this large patient on the floor so we could do chest compressions. I took his legs and the fourth-year student, Henry, and nurse each took an arm. Unfortunately, Mr. K was as wet and sleek as a seal fresh out of water. As we neared the floor, they lost control and his head snapped to the floor with a horrible "thud." Feeling like I was in a Kafkaesque dream, I came around for the head of the "beached" Mr. K to intubate him. Smartly snapping open the laryngoscope, there was no light—the batteries were dead. Meanwhile, the EKG machine arrived, but there was no paper in it. Unable to get routine intravenous access, Henry had commenced a "cut-down" on the ankle. Catching sight of Henry hard at work, I realized he had made the incision over the lateral malleolus, which was not the appropriate medial approach. At some point it dawned on me that Mr. K was as "blue as a squid" and "cold as a mackerel," in other words, he was dead. Almost certainly the victim of a massive pulmonary embolism, my patient's end-of-life dignity had been sorely violated by a medical novitiate. Soaked in sweat and humiliation, I feared it was going to be a long year.

Like most interns, the learning curve was steep for me—if it weren't, few could survive. In contrast to the nine months of fast and furious times during the surgery and medicine rotations, the pace and environment on the chest service were blessedly measured and excitingly instructive. The faculty was spectacular: John McClement, Julia Jones, Harry Fritts, Dudley Rochester, Ann Davis, Yale Enson, and Jane Walker, to name a few. Our major responsibility was managing patients in varying stages of respiratory failure and cor pulmonale. The primary diagnoses were Chronic Obstructive Pulmonary Disease (COPD) and kyphoscoliosis. For those retaining carbon dioxide and in heart failure, the remedy was the "iron lung" or Drinker Respirator. Developed to address respiratory failure due to polio, the Drinkers were roughly six-foot-long and three-foot-wide cylinders into which patients were rolled on a flat surface. The head and neck protruded from one end and were sealed by an adjustable collar. The other end was a bellows mechanism driven by an electric motor, which cyclically created negative then slightly positive pressure within the cylinder. The pressures and rhythms were fine-tuned by respiratory therapists or pulmonary fellows. There was one large ward in which as many as 10 to 12 ventilators may have been active. Lying on their backs, the patients looked up at an angled mirror on an inverted world. Assisted by this ventilatory support, oxygen saturations rose, carbon dioxide levels gradually fell, and acidosis was alleviated. True to the Bellevue-based Nobel Prize winning studies of Cournand and Richards, pulmonary artery pressure receded, diuresis occurred, and heart sizes magically shrank. I did not realize then that the hook had been set, but I was going to be a pulmonologist.

1967: Anchors Aweigh

Military service by physicians was compulsory in the mid-1960s. Under the Berry Plan there were three options: military service after completing internship and one year of residency, after completing one's entire residency or, jackpot, a stint at the National Institutes of Health or the US Public Health Service. The notice came that I was to be inducted into the US Navy in 1967. But, my orders were too good to be true! I was assigned to be an Assistant Epidemiologist at Preventive Medicine Unit 6 (PMU-6) in Pearl Harbor, Hawaii! Additional duties included technical officer at Project Shipboard Hazard and Decontamination (SHAD), also in Pearl Harbor (more to follow).

My responsibilities at PMU-6 primarily related to the struggle against penicillin-resistant gonorrhea, the bane of frisky sailors on leave in Asian ports. Fortunately, we inherited an inspired research program developed by my predecessor, King Holmes. King, who went on to a most distinguished career as a Professor of Infectious Diseases at the University of Washington, had initiated a brilliant research model in Olongapo City, Phillipines, which abuts the Subic Bay north of Manila. Subic was a deep-water port at which the largest navy vessels, including aircraft carriers, could dock. As a manifestation of local hospitality, there were approximately 220 bars in Olongapo. Prostitution was illegal, but over 5,000 "registered hostesses" were employed here.

Before King Holmes came on the scene, an average of 50% of the enlisted men who had taken shore leave developed "the drip." And with the evolution of penicillin resistance, therapy was problematic and morale was at risk. Dr. Holmes had established a system wherein 500 young women came in daily for cervical cultures. If positive for "GC," the women were to return to the center for treatment within 24 hours. A variety of regimens were administered, and the young women were compelled to stay in the dormitory for 12 hours, after which they were re-cultured to determine efficacy. By testing 2,500 patients per week, all of the workers were checked every two weeks. Over time, the incidence of gonorrhea following leave in Olongapo fell to approximately 5%. King Holmes should have received the Congressional Medal of Honor!

Project SHAD turned out to be an equally fascinating assignment. US Intelligence had determined that the Soviet Union had an ambitious program to weaponize anthrax. Our major mission was to determine whether ships at sea could be protected against aerosolized bacilli. Our "fleet" consisted of the mother-ship, a World War II (WWII) Liberty freighter, the USS Granville S. Hall (YAG-40), and five ocean-going tugs. Using non-pathogenic surrogate species including *Bacillus subtilis,* the tugs generated aerosols through which "the Granny Hall" bravely steamed portholes and hatches duct-taped down. Inside were high-volume air samplers to determine aerosol penetration within the ship.[1] Our research took us to

---

[1] At the time, I wondered if the threat of anthrax was real or the paranoid ideation of a "General Jack D. Ripper" (Stanley Kubrick's unforgettable character from "Dr. Strangelove"). But, in a

Eniwetok Atoll in the Marshall Islands, where the native population had been relocated due to post WWII atomic testing. Our project extended over nearly three months.

Most exciting, though, was the letter I received in Western Pacific: Joan was expecting our first child. Four months after our return to Hawaii, following a Saturday night visit to Shakey's Pizza, she awoke at midnight with "gas-pain." Following 8 hours of Lamaze, Tom came into the world. At 11 a.m. Sunday morning, mother and son doing well, I got into our car in the lot at Tripler Army Medical Center to drive across Oahu to our home on Kaneohe Bay. Driving up the Likelike Highway, I was simultaneously giddy and subdued, somber with the realization of my newfound parental responsibility and driving more cautiously than I could ever recall.

1969: Return from Paradise

The Columbia Medical Service at Bellevue was relocated to Harlem Hospital in 1968. Returning as a second-year medical resident in 1969, I felt as though I had been caught in a time warp. At Bellevue, we had observed the starched whites and neckties dress code. Under the intense cultural rebellion engendered by Vietnam, the interns in 1969 wore Levi's^{TM}, work shirts, and engineer boots. Unshaven and unkempt, they seemed the antithesis of our eager-to-please deportment just four years before! In my second month, one of the interns did not show up for a Saturday-Sunday call. Indeed, he reappeared on Tuesday looking thoroughly bedraggled. Howie's lost weekend had taken him to a rain-soaked farm in New York for a delirious rock 'n' roll and drug celebration. Woodstock marked a cultural shift to which I, as a very traditional Nebraskan, have never really accommodated.

1970: A Ramifying Career in Lung Disease

A number of the Bellevue Chest Service faculty had migrated north to Harlem. Prominently, Julia Jones was chief of the service and Dudley Rochester one of her lieutenants. Harlem had an old tuberculosis ward, which reawakened my interest in

---

truly improbable coincidence, I wound up 20 years later comparing war stories with my friend and colleague at National Jewish Health, Leonid Heifets. Holder of an MD, PhD and Doctor of Science in the old Soviet System, Heifets assured me that, indeed, the Soviets had a highly sophisticated program of weaponized anthrax. Then, 10 years later, Leonid and I were touring Russia to lecture on MDR-TB. We found ourselves in the city of Ykaterinberg, recently renamed from Sverdlovsk. Leonid, with a conspiratorial twinkle, told me in detail of the infamous Sverdlovsk anthrax disaster. In the laboratory where anthrax weapons were being produced, a chimney incinerator system failed and a massive plume of viable anthrax was released. An 80-mile diagonal swath of lethality drifted southeast of Sverdlovsk, killing thousands of cattle and unnumbered civilians. Turns out it wasn't paranoia.

this disease, and there was a very active Intensive Care Unit and ventilator program as well. It was an easy decision to accept the offer of a pulmonary fellowship for 1970–1972.

Serendipitously, an American College of Chest Physicians conference in Baltimore kindled my interest in a new instrument, the flexible-fiberoptic bronchoscope (FFBS). Pioneered in Japan by Ikeda, it opened the branching airways to direct visualization! Intriguingly, a young pulmonologist at the University of Kansas, impatient about waiting for operating room slots to allow placement of an endotracheal tube for introducing the FFBS, reported in Baltimore on a technique of transnasal introduction of the scope. Allegedly while sitting around the fellows' office, he had idly passed the scope through his own naris and, voila!

The Chief of Medicine at Harlem Hospital, Charles Reagan, had been head of the First Medical Service at Bellevue. Informed by Julia Jones of my interest in the FFBS, Charlie not only bought the instrument, but also paid for the week-long visit to Kansas to observe Joe Smiddy perform his magic.

Back in New York City, I was the fastest (only) gun in town. In addition to performing roughly 200 procedures during my fellowship, I took my fiberscope roadshow to numerous hospitals. A year later, when applying for a faculty position at the University of Colorado, I think the FFBS—not yet in use in Denver—opened the door for me.

However, my fascination with TB determined my senior-fellowship research project at Harlem. At a local conference, Julia Jones introduced me to the Grand Doyenne of the TB laboratory community, Gladys Hobby, PhD. Dr. Hobby ran the national lab for drug-susceptibility testing at the East Orange (NJ) Veterans Administration Hospital. Dr. Hobby had meticulously coiffed silver-blue hair, and she was always carefully and tastefully turned out, including an impeccable white lab coat. She had a ramrod posture and an authoritative way of issuing commands. Fresh from the Navy, I thought she would have made a helluva admiral.

She was interested in testing her hypothesis that careful, semi-quantitative acid-fast bacilli (AFB) microscopy could be used as an early surrogate marker of response versus non-response to therapy. I had several tasks in the study: identify new patients, obtain initial and follow-up sputa on them all, and transport the specimens in my car to Dr. Hobby's lab in New Jersey. There, working with two of the senior technicians, Tulita and Audrey, I prepared the sputum for semi-quantitative culture and microscopy.

A year later, Drs. Hobby and Jones gave me the opportunity to present the results at the Armed Forces-Veterans Administration TB Conference in Cincinnati, OH. Mouth dry and hands trembling, I got through the 15-minute talk. Barely had my words stopped echoing from the walls when one of the famous, old, hard-line TB docs leapt to his feet, challenging our analysis and asking a question (in reality, a mini-lecture) for which there was no answer. A few moments later, I returned to sit with Dr. Jones. Julia—a quiet Southern lady—leaned over to comfort me: "Don't mind him; he's always been an asshole."

1972: Denver General Hospital

While living in Dumont, NJ in 1971, Joan delivered our second son, Matt. Raising two sweet but energetic boys and looking after me (Joan has, for reasons that elude me, always referred to me as "high maintenance"), she began to yearn for a life more similar to that we had known growing up. Nebraskans always regarded Colorado as a glorious respite from the brutal summer heat as well as visual relief from the unrelenting plains. Thus, as I explored career options, Colorado ended up as our clear number one choice.

We had an ally already ensconced at the University of Colorado. Tom Neff, who grew up in Fremont and with whom I'd played high school football, was the new "chief" at Denver General Hospital (DGH). A one-man band, Tom was looking to hire an associate.

The visit to Denver was like a trip to Disneyland: DGH had all of the excitement and challenges of Bellevue or Harlem Hospitals, but was a modern, high functioning facility. Tom Neff, Tom Petty (then a rising star in pulmonary medicine), and Jack Durrance (Head of the Veterans Administration Hospital pulmonary program and a 24 K character) took me to lunch at a local dive, "The Riviera." Driving south at 60 mph on Colorado Boulevard in Jack's BMW, I thought that these guys really knew how to have fun.

Thus, in August 1972 I began a career on the faculty of the University of Colorado, which has surpassed any expectations I might have harbored. Introducing the FFBS to my colleagues in the Division, learning the Petty-model of respiratory intensive care from Tom Neff (one of the most gifted clinicians in the history of this storied program), and having the opportunity to teach internal medicine and pulmonary disease to med students, residents, and fellows was a joyous period.

In retrospect, I fit through a window in academic time when someone who was a hard worker, a good teacher, and a team player could forge an academic career. Never the recipient of a grant from the NIH, I was nonetheless of sufficient value to DGH and the medical school that I was retained and promoted. Having found the academics of medicine quite challenging made me, I believe, a better teacher. One of the adages of sports is that truly gifted performers make poor coaches. Due to their extraordinary natural abilities, they struggle to teach others to do what they do intuitively. That was not my case in medicine!

Ultimately, my pathway was shaped by a fascination with TB. I had been regaled in New York with tales of a wild guy in Denver who did odd things to motivate his TB patients to show up for therapy (bus tokens that could be transformed to wine, etc.); or, if they were recalcitrant, putting them in jail for non-compliance.

So, in my first week at DGH, I paid a visit to the notorious Denver TB Clinic. My first impression of John Sbarbaro was that he was the most enthusiastic physician I had ever met. In fact, the word "hypomanic" crossed my mind (37 years later, John—a dear friend and mentor—sustains the creativity, humor, and zeal that were manifest then, the Happy Unipolar Warrior).

Spending one afternoon per week in the TB Clinic with B.J. Catlin, a marvelous public health nurse who really made the Directly Observed Therapy program work, I collaborated with John and a medical resident named Rick Albert to write an article on the savings that accrued from supervised treatment. John also facilitated my involvement as the chairman of the American Thoracic Society (ATS) Committee, which produced a statement on TB contact investigation in 1977. Meanwhile, Tom Moulding, Director of the National Jewish TB Course, had given me the opportunity to give several lectures at the Course.

By the end of a decade, my favorite afternoon of the week was the TB Clinic, and the first articles that I read in journals were those related to tuberculosis. So, when Reuben Cherniack offered me a position as Head of the Mycobacterial Disease Division at National Jewish, it was an easy call.

1982–2009: A Field of Dreams

1983 was the modern nadir of TB in the USA. Tom Petty, who was a great supporter, quizzically inquired after my move why I had invested my academic future in a disappearing disease. I told him that I wasn't sure, but it felt like the right thing to do.

NJH (National Jewish Health) was in the process of evolving from a sleepy TB sanatorium to a model clinical and research facility. In addition to working on the TB program, I served as Reuben's Vice-Chairman of Medicine. Second-year residents from the University of Colorado rotated at NJH, and we had clinical fellows from the pulmonary and allergy-immunology programs. I took morning report six days per week for the entire year of 1982–1983. And, I was fortunate to be mentored in the nuances of TB and Nontuberculous Mycobacteria management by Marian Goble.

However, one of the things that became evident to others first and me belatedly was that I was a poor administrator and did not enjoy the process or, generously, I did not like administration and therefore did it poorly. So, Jim Cook, an MD doing research on viral oncogenesis at NJH, was named Head of Infectious Diseases and I was emancipated to "do my thing."

The primary mission of the NJH TB service from *circa* 1965 forward was the care of patients with drug-resistant TB. NJH had a philanthropic base, which allowed it to take on these complex cases for which remuneration was minimal or non-existent. Opening its doors in 1899 with the philosophy that, "None can pay who shall enter, none who enter shall pay," the TB program was a cottage industry, the de facto national referral center for advanced drug-resistant TB.

The NJH TB lab, headed by Leonid Heifets from 1981 to today, pioneered in drug-susceptibility testing for second-line and novel agents. From the menu compiled based on these lab results, we cobbled together regimens based on the NJH "Holy Trinity": three or more clean drugs (susceptible in vitro and not previously administered). Despite spending an average of eight months on our wards and being coaxed and compelled to accept nauseating, brutal medications like para-aminosalicylate sodium (PAS), ethionamide, or cycloserine and made deaf and/or ataxic from prolonged courses of kanamycin or capreomycin, treatment failed in nearly half of our patients.

Marian Goble embarked on a heroic page-by-page chart review of over 200 such patients treated between 1973 and 1983. The enterprise took nearly four years but resulted in compelling data, which appeared in a sentinel report in the 1993 *New England Journal of Medicine*: TB resistant to isoniazid and rifampin [dubbed by then "Multi-Drug Resistant Tuberculosis" or MDR-TB by the Centers for Disease Control and Prevention (CDC)] was associated with high failure and death rates.

Before the appearance of HIV/AIDS in the early 1980s, this information was of nominal and parochial importance. These old MDR-TB cases almost always reflected sequential treatment failures and were rarely associated with transmission to others. However, reports of epidemic spread of MDR-TB with high mortality rates among persons with AIDS appeared in the Morbidity and Mortality Weekly Reports of the CDC in 1989–1990. MDR-TB soon made its way to the New York Times and the network evening news.

Abruptly, our work at NJH grew to have national, then international implications. Ed Chan, my young colleague, took the lead on reviewing the post-Goble cohort of MDR-TB cases. In this timeframe, there were two important innovations: the fluoroquinolone (FQNs) antibiotics were found to be highly active against TB, and we had employed resectional surgery more extensively in the care of refractory disease.

Over the 15 years from 1984 to 1998, it was demonstrated that we had progressively employed the FQNs and, emboldened by observations of safety and the appearance of efficacy, had sent increasing proportions of patients to the operating room. Multi-variant analysis showed that surgery followed by FQN use were the most important interventions in our series of patients.

The use of surgery was substantially serendipitous. During my stint at Denver General Hospital, the Chief of Cardiothoracic Surgery was Marvin Pomerantz, who on his good days might have been described as "pugnacious." Eventually I came to think of Marv in Joe Namath terms: "it's hard to be humble when you're great." Marv had left DGH to go into private practice. But, I knew that during his training at Duke, he had done a lot of TB surgery. So in 1983, confronted with imminent treatment failure in a young woman from Pennsylvania, I asked Marv to come by to review the case. Before his retirement in 2005, "Carvin' Marvin" had performed resectional surgery on approximately 500 patients with MDR-TB or non-tuberculous mycobacterial lung disease.

Describing himself as a "dinosaur" in a New York Times interview, Pomerantz had virtually conserved a species that was nearing extinction, reinventing the discipline of surgery for lung infections.

TB Has Been Berry Good to Me

A character on a comedic television skit used to say with a thick Latin accent, "Baseball has been berry, berry good to me." Certainly, tuberculosis ended up providing singular fulfillment for this physician.

Among the opportunities that TB afforded me were stints as an Associate Editor of the *American Journal of Respiratory and Critical Care Medicine* and Editor-in-Chief of *The International Journal of Tuberculosis and Lung Diseases*, as well as consultancies with the CDC and World Health Organization.

The last quarter-century has witnessed critical events in the evolution of the tubercle bacilli, changes which brought focus on drug-resistance and, by implication, directly observed therapy. Both of these coincided with my career interests, making me a participant on the world's stage.

As an apostle of "Saint John (Sbarbaro), the Supervisor," I played a role in popularizing Directly Observed Therapy, a policy which has helped control TB transmission and substantially halted drug-resistance related to erratic treatment here in the USA. Using mainly the bully-pulpit of the NJH TB Course, we have strongly influenced America's TB control practices. Professionally, I believe this has been my major contribution.

"The Book": My Magnum Opus

How does one develop the audacity to attempt to write a book on a topic as broad as tuberculosis? In my case, it stemmed from organizing diverse lectures for the NJH TB Course. It is said that we learn far more by organizing a talk than hearing one. Amen!

Although we are teased in academics with the promise of every seventh year to spend in renewal, the Sabbath or sabbatical, few enjoy this privilege. My one retreat in 37 years came in 1992–1993.

Having found a publisher willing to take a flyer with me, I spent anticipatory months outlining chapters and organizing my files. We found a townhome for rent on the golf course at the Snowmass Country Club near Aspen, and moved in on November 1, 1992, amid an uncharacteristically early snow. Three feet of fresh powder fell in the Valley, with much more on the mountain. It became a contest between the writing muse and the long-suppressed ski bum impulse. Storm after storm came through, and the ski-lifts were running by the middle of November.

Dutifully, I set up 4' × 6' plywood on sawhorses and laid out my stack of references by chapter. However, the siren of Snowmass lured us up to the slopes regularly. Who knew how long the great conditions would last? Five months later, we were informed by the locals that, this was "the greatest winter in Aspen/Snowmass history."

Among the numerous miscalculations made in this endeavor, I had planned to learn to use the word-processor as I wrote (never mind the fact that I had been a dismal failure in high school typing, producing 20 words per minute with plenty of mistakes). Re-reading my early drafts, I recognized that my plodding manual dexterity was actually changing my written voice. After two marginally productive months, I surrendered my word-processing ambitions and bought the first of many packs of legal pads.

As the snow melted in April and May of 1993, I had compiled drafts of eight out of the 14 planned chapters. Taking advantage of Joan's skills, my penned pages were put into typed drafts. I returned to NJH in July of 1993, confident that I would finish the book by the end of the year.

Robbie Burns, the Scottish poet, wrote that, "the best laid plans of mice and men oft-times go awry." Well, my plans weren't that well laid, and they certainly went awry!

I had finished drafts of all the chapters by winter but then commenced an act worthy of "The Ed Sullivan Show." As I revised each chapter, I found additional references, old and new. By the time I had finished redoing the fourteenth chapter, the first chapter begged amendment. At an escalating, comedic pace, this went on for five more years.

My office was overflowing, and my piles metastasized to two large tables in the NJH library. At first it was nights, then weekends that found me literally cutting and pasting, lines crossed out, so many arrows that the pages faintly resembled Jackson Pollock's art. Not for a moment would I suggest it matched the pain of childbirth, but this gestation certainly involved years of intense labor. *A Clinician's Guide to Tuberculosis* (Lippincott, Williams & Wilkins) finally materialized in 2000, testament more than anything else to endurance. The book was well received and went through multiple printings.

Among the more positive comments about the book posted on Amazon's readers' website were some flowery words from "Tom Kazansky." TB is a small community, and I thought I knew most working in the field. The name was vaguely troublesome, and it rattled around my subconscious for several weeks. Then, the light bulb! My son Matt and I had regularly watched the Tom Cruise classic movie, "Top Gun" on DVD. Cruise's major competitor was a character played by Val Kilmer, Tom Kazansky. His code name in the movie was "Iceman," Matt's own nickname from college baseball. I was embarrassed but secretly pleased that Matt had given the old man a plug.

One last comment about "the book": at an ATS Annual Meeting after publication, Joan and I were at a reception. A colleague in the field, Richard Chaisson from Johns Hopkins, came by to offer some kind words. He said that the conversational style of my writing made it, "just like Iseman was in the room, talking with me." Without missing a beat, Joan replied, "and better yet, you can close the book and shut him up." Wives know, don't they?

Summary and Conclusion

After years of academic writing, this seems like an appropriate closure.

When David's invitation to contribute to this project came, it set in motion far-ranging and soul-searching reflections on my life and career. A few final thoughts:

- I still regard myself fundamentally as an athlete. My world view and relationships with others—patients, colleagues, and friends—have been shaped by a chivalrous code of competition and fair play.
- Among various sports in which I have participated, the last two sports to which I was introduced may have been the most influential.

- In the fall of 1963, my P&S classmate Jim Elting dragged me out to the initial practice of "The Old Blue Rugby Football Club." Guided by some skilled ruggers from England, Ireland, and South Africa, we rapidly became the dominant team in the East. A violent but subtle game, rugby called on the athlete to train hard on his own, to throw one's body about with reckless abandon (more hazardous than football due to the absence of pads and helmets) and—critically—to leave the pitch, bloody, and bruised, to drink beer and sing bawdy songs with the opponents, the same guys you were trying to decapitate an hour before. Sportsmanship!
- Fifteen years after we had hung up our cleats, Elting called me to ask if I'd be willing to learn how to row (Fig. 15.2). Jim had been a heavyweight oarsman at Yale and was trying to find a fourth to row with "The Yale Old Farts Rowing Association" (YOFRA), the ribald creation of my old friend. My mentor in Colorado was Jim's Yale classmate, John Cogswell, then an attorney in Denver. John and I bought a 2-man Vespoli shell, and he commenced boot-camp III, teaching me to row. On the water every morning at 5:30 a.m. on a local reservoir,

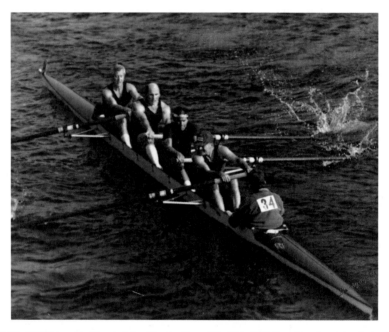

Fig. 15.2 *YOFRA at the Head of the Charles Race*: The Yale Old Farts Rowing Association four-man crew at the Head of the Charles Race in 1987. Our singlets were Yale blue with an orange stripe to acknowledge my Princeton origins. Passing under the Eliot Bridge toward the end of the race, the coxswain (#34 on his back) was telling us we had "only 70 more" strokes to the finish. In the first seat (with the Red Cap) was my med school classmate, Jim Elting. In seat #4 was John Cogswell. Coming off the oar of rower #3 (me) was a huge geyser. Rowing purists like to see nice, clean bladework. Critics commented that watching me row down a course was like a WWII movie with Allied destroyers dropping depth-charges over U-boats! My apologists said that although my technique was rough, I "generated a lot of power"

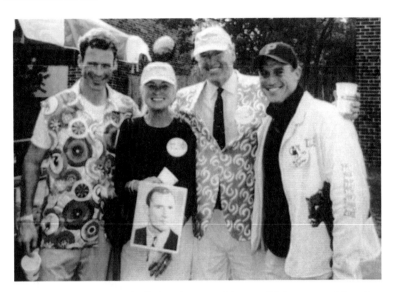

Fig. 15.3 *Going back to Nassau Hall*: Reunions are a big part of Princeton tradition. At my 40th in 2001, we were joined by Tom (on left), class of 1991, and Matt, class of 1993. Tom rowed his freshman year, played rugby the next three years and majored in history. After a year of ski-bumming at Jackson Hole, Wyoming, he got his Masters in Environmental Sciences at Michigan. After three years at the Department of the Interior in Washington, DC, he returned to Colorado to work with the Nature Conservancy. Matt pitched all 4 years including a complete game 2-1 victory over Dartmouth in 1991 for the Eastern Collegiate League Championship. He, too, majored in History and followed me to the College of Physicians and Surgeons where he, unlike the Old-Man, was Alpha Omega Alpha. Following a medical internship here at the University of Colorado, he had an epiphany—comedy. He moved to LA, joined a renowned improv group, "The Groundlings," and set out on his own. Currently he has regular roles on three weekly cable shows: "Sports Soup," "Clean House," and "Clean House Comes Clean"

John endured the indignity of being regularly capsized by a novice who "caught crabs" (buried the oar) with disheartening frequency. In the fall of 1985 we met in Ghent, Belgium for the World's Veteran Competition. In the four-man race, we lost by two feet to a German crew, but combining with another four man crew, we won a gold medal in the eights. Before retiring, we had won three golds and a bronze. Crew was the absolute essence of team sports. Technically, you must coordinate your efforts, and, physiologically, it demands you to completely commit your energy. Although a shell may look fairly calm to observers, inside the athletes are using every major muscle group. At the end of each YOFRA race over the five years we competed, I was near exhaustion. Endurance!

- At the end of the day my family means everything to me. It is easy to become self- or career-centered, especially in a field like medicine. Taking stock, though, I now realize that Joan made our home, which was the platform for everything that I have accomplished. She did the heavy-lifting in raising our sons, truly making possible all that Tom, Matt, and I had achieved (Fig. 15.3). Have I been lucky? Beyond any words!

Sixteen
The Making of a Medical Epidemiologist

Philip J. Landrigan

It was at the Communicable Disease Center, now the Centers for Disease Control and Prevention, that I made my transition in the early 1970s from physician to physician-scientist.

A decade earlier in 1963, I had entered Harvard Medical School firm in the belief that I would be a practicing physician, probably a surgeon. I had not made those choices through any very deliberate process, but mostly because I was deeply impressed by the kindness and clinical acumen of Dr. William Walsh, the family doctor in Boston who took care of me all through my childhood and adolescence, and by the surgical skill and profound humanity of Dr. Frederick Landrigan, my uncle and an ophthalmologist. Basically, I wanted to follow in the footsteps of those two splendid doctors. Surgery seemed like a good idea because I had always enjoyed making things with my hands, and besides it seemed very glamorous.

The first two years of medical school were mostly drudgery, a purgatory to be endured on my way to the promised land of the clinical wards. I made wonderful friends, many of whom remain dear colleagues to this day. And it was great to be in a class surrounded by extraordinarily bright and good people, many of whom have gone on to make major contributions to medicine and society, and some of whom became outstanding physician-scientists. But I still wanted very much to be a clinician.

Two very important experiences in my first two years of medical school were the summers I spent working in research laboratories, one on campus at Harvard Medical School and the other at Massachusetts General Hospital. Both were miserable. Teaching was minimal. Mentoring was close to non-existent. Interpersonal skills did not exist. I vowed never to work in a laboratory again. That is a promise I have kept.

Another important medical school experience was my three-month clerkship in surgery at Massachusetts General Hospital. The surgeons were great, many of them

P.J. Landrigan (✉)
Departments of Preventive Medicine and Pediatrics, Children's Environmental Health Center, Mount Sinai School of Medicine, New York, NY, USA
e-mail: phil.landrigan@mssm.edu

D.A. Schwartz (ed.), *Medicine Science and Dreams*,
DOI 10.1007/978-90-481-9538-1_16, © Springer Science+Business Media B.V. 2011

exceptional mentors. But to my surprise, I found that I just did not care for surgery. It seemed too impersonal, and the interactions with patients were too one-sided and transient. Cutting and sewing were fun, and I recognized the deep skill required to do surgery well, but by the end of the rotation I had come to realize that surgery was not for me. By contrast, I loved my time in medicine at Boston City Hospital and even more my rotation in pediatrics at Massachusetts General. I decided to follow one of those two specialties and eventually opted for pediatrics.

I did a combined medicine/pediatric internship at Cleveland Metropolitan General Hospital, and then I returned to Boston to do a two-year residency in pediatrics at Boston Children's Hospital. I received superb clinical training, and I developed a deep love for taking care of critically ill children. Among my mentors were outstanding physicians who were also superb scientists—Charles H. Rammelkamp, Jr., MD at Case Western, who as a military physician in World War II had done seminal work elucidating the links between streptococcal infection and rheumatic heart disease; Robert Schwartz, MD, also at Case Western, a renowned researcher in childhood diabetes; and Charles A. Janeway, Jr., MD at Boston Children's, a pioneer in the study of immune deficiency disorders in children. But despite the wonderful role models that those physician-scientists provided, I had not prior to my arrival at Centers for Disease Control and Prevention (CDC) given any serious thought to becoming a physician-scientist.

I made my decision to go to CDC in 1967 in the middle of my internship. I did not have any particular inclination toward public health or epidemiology, but the Vietnam War was on at the time, and there was a doctor draft that required every male physician to perform 2 years of national service. For most of my medical school classmates, that service was spent in the Army, Navy, or Air Force. But I had the good fortune to be guided by Dr. Rammelkamp, my chief of service at Case Western, who had worked with CDC scientists during his World War II years. He suggested that I perform my national service at CDC as a commissioned officer in the US Public Health Service (USPHS). I agreed and so Dr. Rammelkamp called his friend, Dr. Alexander Langmuir (Fig. 16.1), the founder and head of the CDC's Epidemic Intelligence Service. A few days later while I was in the on-call room at Cleveland Metropolitan General Hospital, I received a telephone call from Dr. Michael Gregg, one of Dr. Langmuir's close associates at CDC. Dr. Gregg asked if I was prepared to serve the nation. I said I was. He then asked me to stand and raise my right hand. He swore me in over the telephone and commissioned me as a Lieutenant Commander in the USPHS. He also gave me permission to finish my residency before reporting for duty in Atlanta.

I arrived at CDC in July 1970, five days after finishing my residency. Before I departed Boston for Atlanta, I reckoned that my time at CDC would be a sort of bump in the road, an interruption in my life's plan, an obligation to be fulfilled on my way to a clinical fellowship. Indeed, I had already pretty much decided to do a fellowship in pediatric neurology. I had chosen that specialty as I moved through residency because I was attracted to its academic foundations, its intellectual rigor, and the opportunity it provided to care for the very sickest children in the hospital. I started looking at training programs in pediatric neurology even before I went to

Fig. 16.1 Alexander
Langmuir, MD

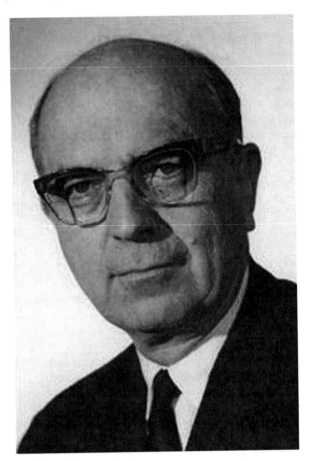

CDC, and midway through my first year in Atlanta I was accepted into the superb fellowship in pediatric neurology directed at Johns Hopkins University School of Medicine by Dr. Guy McKhann. My plan was to start training there at the end of my time at CDC.

At CDC I was inducted into the Epidemic Intelligence Service (EIS), an elite corps of "disease detectives" that had been formed by Dr. Langmuir 19 years earlier in 1951. The EIS is a remarkable program that continues to this day. Its mission is to provide a first line of defense against epidemic disease and to protect the health of the USA against epidemics and also against chemical and biological warfare. EIS officers, most of whom are young physicians, veterinarians, nurses, and epidemiologists just a few years out of training, serve as the nation's medical first responders. They are dispatched on as little as one or two hours notice to locations across the USA and around the world to combat disease. Over the years EIS officers have dealt with problems as diverse as cholera, polio, smallpox, poliomyelitis, Legionnaire's Disease, Ebola virus, toxic shock syndrome, AIDS, lead poisoning, hantavirus, obesity, 9/11, Hurricane Katrina, and H1N1 influenza.

Dr. Alexander Langmuir, the founder of the EIS, was a truly remarkable man. Dr. Langmuir, or "Alex" as my EIS classmates and I came to know him, was the person who most strongly influenced my transition from physician to physician-scientist. It was also he who imbued in me and in so many of my colleagues the concept that good science, while essential for public health, is by itself not sufficient to protect the health of the public. He taught us that science must always be translated into evidence-based action, that this action must be precisely planned in concert with our partners in the state and city health departments, and that it must be rigorously evaluated at every step.

Alexander Langmuir was a piece of work. He was a tall, bald, bespectacled, and commanding man with a deep voice. He was bright, detail-oriented, deeply driven, unencumbered by doubt, often bombastic, and fully capable of forcing an EIS officer to redraft a manuscript 40 times. He was happy to remind us that his uncle, Irving Langmuir, a physicist and chemist, had won the Nobel Prize in Chemistry in 1932. At the same time, however, he was an extraordinarily supportive mentor, teacher, and role model. And while it took more than a little work to get beneath his gruff exterior, the work was worth the effort, because down beneath it all he was a kind and caring man who lived and breathed through the success of his young EIS officers.

Alex was a Harvard College graduate. He received his medical degree from Cornell. He interned at Boston City Hospital and then earned a public health degree from Johns Hopkins. He worked for a few years in the New York State Department of Health in Albany and for the Westchester County Department of Health as Deputy Commissioner. During World War II, he was a member of the Army's Commission on Acute Respiratory Diseases at Fort Bragg, NC. He came to CDC in 1949. He stayed there, always as Chief Epidemiologist and Director of the EIS, until his retirement in 1970, a few months after the induction of my EIS class. He subsequently taught at the Harvard School of Public Health and then at the London School of Hygiene and Tropical Medicine.

In the nearly 20 years that Alex Langmuir directed the EIS, he built a program that became the wonder of the world of public health. He taught and mentored nearly 700 EIS officers. Under his tutelage, the EIS program became a major incubator for public health leadership. It has produced scores of professors of public health, preventive medicine, and infectious disease, dozens of state and federal health officers, more than twenty deans of schools of public health, two Surgeons General of the USA, and leaders of the World Health Organization. The EIS program has been replicated in countries around the world.

Alex Langmuir had three core teachings. The first was that epidemiology is the mother science of public health. While he had a certain disdain for highfalutin' biostatistics—"not needed if the epidemiology is clear"—he required every EIS officer of any background to have a good working knowledge of epidemiology and to know enough statistics to be able to do epidemiology in the field.

Alex Langmuir's second teaching was that epidemiology and the protection of public health depend absolutely upon a well-organized program of disease surveillance. He believed that there should be trained persons in every city and state across the USA with responsibility for recording the occurrence of each case and each death caused by the major infectious diseases and for reporting that information weekly to CDC. Alex believed that CDC then had responsibility to collate and analyze this information and to aggressively seek trends and anomalies in the data that might signal the emergence of an epidemic. He also considered it essential that CDC report back promptly to every person who had reported cases to keep them informed of CDC's findings and to continually reinforce their engagement in the process. He likened this sequence to a neurologic reflex arc, in which case reporting was the afferent limb, CDC the central processing unit, and feedback to state and local health officials (plus the occasional more direct response) the efferent limb. Alex created CDC's weekly publication, the *Morbidity and Mortality Surveillance Report*, the *MMWR*, to support the surveillance program and to disseminate its findings. Health officials, epidemiologists, and disease control specialists read the *MMWR* regularly. Funeral directors are also among its most faithful subscribers.

In Alex's view, a fundamental responsibility of EIS officers was to monitor the weekly surveillance reports submitted by the cities and states. That was a necessary and important task, though more than a little dull. But our second, much more exciting responsibility was to respond to anomalies in these data as soon as they became evident and to answer calls from state and city health officers the moment those calls came in. The constant goal was early detection of emerging epidemics.

Alex Langmuir's third core teaching was that epidemiology must always be practiced in the field and never from behind a desk. He believed absolutely in the importance of sending EIS officers out to the site of an epidemic as soon as a blip in the data was noted. He termed this "shoe leather epidemiology," and the symbol of the EIS became the sole of a shoe with a hole worn through it. To make it easy for EIS officers to travel quickly and to avoid red tape, he issued each of us a book of government travel requisitions (GTRs), blue chits that could be redeemed at the airport on a moment's notice for a ticket to anywhere on the planet. Alex encouraged us to use our GTRs liberally and to replenish our books as often as needed. What joy!

EIS officers were directed by Alex to characterize each disease outbreak by the three cardinal criteria of "time, place, and person." We were trained in the fine art of tracking the time course of an outbreak by building an "epidemic curve," a graph displaying each case of illness by time of onset. We were trained to plot the geographic spread of disease by making pin maps that depicted the location of each case. To determine which groups in the population were at greatest risk, we learned to tabulate cases by age, sex, occupation, diet, smoking status, and any other variable that seemed remotely relevant. We were expected to call in almost daily to CDC headquarters in Atlanta to report progress and to receive direction from Alex and his lieutenants. But most remarkably, when we were in the field, Alex left us alone. Seldom did he send anyone out to look over our shoulders. His trust in us was enormous, and that trust built an extraordinary confidence in him.

Alex Langmuir was a devoted, diligent, and uncompromising mentor. He taught us to think, and he taught us to write. He expected EIS officers to use the data on time, place, and person that we had so painstakingly collected in the field to develop hypotheses as to the source and mode of spread of each outbreak. We were expected to test our hypotheses, sometimes by collecting more data and sometimes by arranging for analyses of specimens at CDC's laboratories in Atlanta. Lastly, Alex expected us to write up each outbreak in pellucid English with the anticipation that every report would end up in either *JAMA* or the *New England Journal of Medicine*. Alex had on his staff a professional editor, Frances Porcher, a retired librarian and English teacher from South Carolina, whose sole responsibility was to work with EIS officers to produce stellar manuscripts. Alex thought nothing of taking an officer through 20, 30, or even 40 drafts to be sure that every fact was checked, every nuance precisely described, and every comma perfectly placed.

Some of the best and the brightest of Alex Langmuir's trainees stayed on at CDC to help him run the EIS program. Several of these extraordinary physician-scientists were also among my mentors.

Dr. William Foege, the charismatic Director of CDC's Smallpox Eradication Program, who later became CDC Director and then an advisor to the Carter Center and to the Bill and Melinda Gates Foundation, was among these mentors. Bill Foege's work bore eloquent testimony to the wisdom of Alex Langmuir's teaching that an epidemiologist must always study the data collected in the field before taking action. Bill's data-driven epiphany occurred during his work in India to control smallpox. He observed that smallpox still raged in India in the early 1970s, despite the fact that essentially 100% of the population had been vaccinated. He noted further that disease transmission virtually ceased during the monsoon season, when people were forced by the rains to stay in their villages. During those months the disease festered in only a few highly localized "hotspots" and spread no further. On the basis of these observations, Bill proposed a fundamental reconfiguration of the attack on smallpox. He proposed to drop the previous emphasis on mass vaccination and to focus instead on containing the "hotspots" by ring vaccination. Through vigorous disease surveillance at the village level, hotspots were identified on a daily or weekly basis especially during the monsoon months. Ring vaccination was then pursued aggressively. Within two years, this approach led to total eradication of smallpox in India. It was a brilliant and highly pragmatic application of the scientific method, and it saved the lives of millions.

Dr. Michael B. Gregg, the person who had sworn me in to the EIS over the telephone while I was still an intern, was another extraordinary mentor at CDC. Mike Gregg was the best scientific writer I have ever known. He served for many years as Editor-in-Chief of the *Morbidity and Mortality Weekly Report*. He was a quiet, dedicated, and extraordinarily patient man, the perfect foil to Alex's bombast. He was brilliant at discerning the core message of a manuscript and in helping EIS officers to shape their messages into publishable reports.

Dr. J. Lyle Conrad was Director of the Field Services Division at CDC. He was the man directly responsible for getting EIS officers out to epidemics in the most remote corners of the globe on a moment's notice. On one memorable occasion, Lyle requisitioned an Air Force two-seater jet fighter to carry an EIS officer with antiserum to an isolated airport in Idaho to fight an outbreak of botulism. Lyle had served in Africa as a Peace Corps physician before coming to CDC. He was deterred by no physical hardship or bureaucratic obstacle.

Dr. Clark W. Heath was a superb epidemiologist and the man who most guided my early thinking about the impacts of environmental hazards on human health. He had become well-known for his early investigations of leukemia clusters, and on that foundation he had helped to move CDC from an exclusive focus on infectious disease epidemiology to a broader emphasis that included chronic disease, disease caused by lifestyle, and diseases of environmental origin. Clark Heath taught me that there was more to epidemiology than outbreak investigation, and he opened my eyes to the fascinating worlds of planned epidemiologic studies and chronic disease epidemiology.

Dr. J. Donald Millar was a gifted leader who had begun his career in Africa with the Smallpox Eradication Program. He went on to become Director of the the swine flu program and then Director of the National Institute for Occupational Safety and Health. I served under him from 1980 until 1985. Don Millar was an expert at navigating difficult political waters. He taught me much about conducting public health in the face of political adversity.

The EIS class of 1970 of which I was a member consisted of 46 physicians, two veterinarians, and one statistician. Most of the physicians, I among them, had almost no concept of public health before we arrived at CDC and less still of epidemiology. I remember during my first week in Atlanta overhearing a discussion about denominators. I had not heard that term since high school algebra. Initially I could not recall whether the denominator was the top or the bottom half of a fraction.

Like every EIS officer, I began my CDC experience by passing through a basic four-week course in epidemiology and biostatistics—the "EIS course"—that is taught each summer to a new EIS class in the sweltering heat of July in airless basement CDC classrooms on Clifton Road in northeast Atlanta. Through this incredibly intense and highly compressed experience, we were taught the fundamentals of epidemic investigation, the techniques of disease surveillance, the principles of survey design, and the basics of evidence-based intervention against epidemics. The quality of the teaching and mentoring was extraordinary. While we did not fully appreciate it at the time, the EIS course was in fact a greenhouse for nurturing the early growth of an entire generation of physician-scientists. It was also a crucible for building *esprit de corps* and fostering life-long friendships.

By the end of the EIS course, all of us had at least a working knowledge of epidemiology and biostatistics. We were then each assigned to a duty station, about half of us to various programs at CDC headquarters in Atlanta and the rest to state and city health departments. We could not wait to get out into the field to conquer disease and subdue epidemics.

I was assigned to the Immunization Program in Atlanta and given responsibility for measles surveillance. My daily task was to review the weekly measles surveillance data. I was alert for clusters of cases that might signal failure of measles vaccine to provide durable immunity. This was very important at the time, because the live, attenuated measles vaccine had been introduced only a few years earlier, and the duration of immunity that it produced was still not known. Beyond that, measles surveillance took on an especially heightened intensity in 1970 because Alex Langmuir himself had publicly predicted the year before that measles would soon be eradicated from the USA.

In November 1970, I was dispatched by Lyle Conrad to my first measles epidemic. The location was Texarkana, a city in northeast Texas that straddles the Arkansas–Texas border with a population of about 50,000. As was common for EIS officers, I traveled alone. It was my first trip west of the Mississippi and my third ride on an airplane. I took Delta to Dallas and then Trans-Texas Airlines to Texarkana.

When I arrived in Texarkana, I found a raging epidemic. As is typical of measles outbreaks, there had been a few scattered cases, two to five per week, over the summer between June and August. But in September, as soon as children came together in large numbers with the opening of school, the epidemic exploded. At the time of my arrival, 40–60 new cases were occurring each week. By the time the epidemic ended, 633 measles cases had occurred in Texarkana.

I came very quickly to realize that there was a sharp disparity in measles incidence between the two sides of Texarkana. Altogether, 606 (95.7%) of the 633 cases occurred in Texarkana (Bowie County), Texas, while only 27 cases occurred in Texarkana (Miller County), Arkansas. A few hours of enquiry unearthed the reason for this disparity. It was not geographic isolation. There was a great deal of mixing between the two populations who readily crossed the border in both directions to work, shop, worship, and play. The explanation resided in a fundamental difference in public policy between the two states. The State of Arkansas, with a long history of Southern populism, believed in vigorous, publicly financed immunization programs, and more than 95% of the 6,016 children aged 1–9 years in Texarkana, Arkansas had immunity to measles. By contrast, the State of Texas believed then as now in private enterprise and did not operate public immunization programs. Texas required children to go to their private physicians and to pay for their shots. As a result, the level of prior measles immunity in the 11,185 children aged 1–9 years in Bowie County was only 57%.

I thought that I had fulfilled my responsibilities as an EIS officer as soon as I had plotted the epidemic curve and learned about this difference in public policy that I reckoned explained the epidemic. After four days, I returned to Atlanta where I gleefully presented my findings expecting a pat on the back and an opportunity to move on to the next problem.

Much to my surprise and chagrin, Alex Langmuir, Mike Gregg, and Lyle Conrad did not praise my rapid detective work. Instead they took me aside and chastised me sharply for having performed a sloppy and superficial job. They were very distressed that I had accepted the difference in public policy as the sole explanation for the outbreak and that I had not personally contacted every single case of measles to make absolutely certain that there was no evidence of vaccine failure. They instructed me to turn around and to go directly back to Texarkana.

While I was going through this painful moment, I was given some superb advice by Dr. Richard (aka Dick) Garibaldi (Fig. 16.2), my closest friend in EIS. Dick Garibaldi and I had known each other since we played Little League baseball

Fig. 16.2 Richard Garibaldi, MD

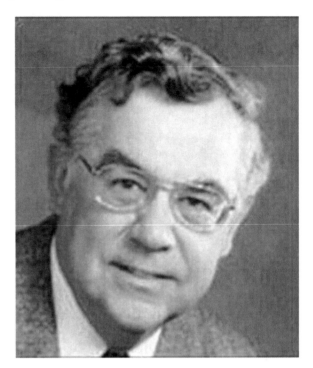

together in Boston, where he was a star pitcher and I was a second-string short-stop. We were high school and medical school classmates. He went on to become Chairman of Medicine at the University of Connecticut. Dick was a year ahead of me in EIS, and when I arrived there he already had a full year of experience at CDC. Drawing on that background, he offered me the wise counsel that "every epidemic is unique" and that the secret of extracting a great paper from an epidemic investigation was to find its unique point and to "push on it." Dick Garibaldi told me that the huge disparity in measles incidence between the two sides of Texarkana was absolutely unique (Fig. 16.3), and he urged me to get back to the field to characterize it as thoroughly as possible.

Back in Texarkana, I learned the hard way to do shoe leather epidemiology. Over a two-week period, I interviewed the family of virtually every measles case. I learned that 98% of the children with disease had never been vaccinated. I established with near certainty that the reason for the outbreak was indeed failure to vaccinate and not failure of the vaccine. I found that only 27 cases of measles had occurred in previously vaccinated children, and that six of these children had received vaccine with measles immune globulin prior to one year of age, a procedure now recognized as ineffective. I calculated that the efficacy of measles vaccine in protecting children in Texarkana against measles was a very acceptable 96%.

Another important lesson that became very obvious to me as I was doing my door-to-door interviews in Texarkana was that the disease was closely linked to

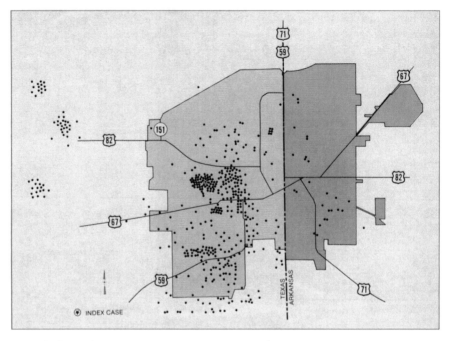

Fig. 16.3 Cases of measles, Texarkana, Tex-Ark, June 1970 to January 1971 (*JAMA* 1972; 221: 567–570) (Copyright©1972, American Medical Association. All rights reserved)

poverty and to minority racial status. The financial barriers to vaccination imposed by the State of Texas fell most heavily on poor minority families.

Once I had finished my investigation of the epidemic, I worked with Lyle Conrad and the two local health departments in Texarkana to organize an immunization program. Over 2,300 children were immunized, and the epidemic ended shortly thereafter. I returned to CDC and spent the next several months writing my report and taking it through innumerable drafts. The process seemed to take forever, but at the end and thanks to Alex and his team, I had produced a single-author paper that was accepted by the *Journal of the American Medical Association*. The thrill was extraordinary, and the lessons learned deeply engraved.

My second major epidemic investigation, the experience that sealed my transition from physician to physician-scientist, also took place in Texas. It was a study of lead exposure among children in El Paso. This investigation began with a telephone call that came in to CDC late one Friday afternoon from Dr. Bernard Rosenblum, the city health officer for El Paso, Texas. Dr. Rosenblum was a former USPHS officer, originally from New York City. He requested urgent assistance from CDC in investigating a possible epidemic of childhood lead poisoning.

Lyle Conrad asked me to go out on this investigation because he knew that I had seen children with lead poisoning during my pediatric residency in Boston. Because of the apparent large scale of the problem, he also dispatched my good friend, Dr. Stephen Gehlbach, another Boston-trained pediatrician, a fellow member of my EIS class who was assigned to the North Carolina State Health Department in Raleigh. Steve later became Dean of the School of Public Health at the University of Massachusetts. The two of us traveled together to El Paso in January, 1972. We expected to find children who had ingested lead-based paint, because that was the source of lead poisoning we had come to know in Boston. But instead we found something very different.

Steve and I learned when we arrived in El Paso that the focus of Dr. Rosenblum's concern was not lead paint, but rather the large quantity of lead that had been emitted into the air of El Paso by an ore smelter on the west side of the city. This enormous industrial plant had been in operation since 1887. It had capacity to extract lead, copper, and zinc from over 800,000 tons of ore concentrates annually. The smelter heated ore to high temperatures in enormous furnaces and then melted metals out of the mother rock. The waste rock that remained was discarded behind the smelter in great slag heaps. Dr. Rosenblum had learned a few weeks earlier that from 1969 to 1971, the smelter's stacks had emitted 1,012 metric tons of lead, 508 tons of zinc, 11 tons of cadmium, and one ton of arsenic into the air of El Paso.

The first question that Steve and I had to address was whether those emissions posed any threat to human health. The wisdom of the day, summarized in a National Academy of Sciences report, *Lead: Airborne Lead in Perspective*, was that there was no risk, only worry. But to test the validity of that received wisdom, Steve and I thought it would be a good idea to do some shoe leather epidemiology. We decided as a first step to conduct a pilot survey of blood lead levels among children in a nursery school located less than one mile from the smelter. Many of the children attending the school were the sons and daughters of professors at the University of Texas, El Paso (UTEP), which was located immediately adjacent to the smelter on land that had been donated by the smelting company. We found that 94% of the children attending this nursery had blood lead levels of 40 μg/dl or more, the level which at the time was CDC's official safe upper limit for lead in the blood in children. We realized we had a problem, and we returned to Atlanta.

After consulting with Alex and his leadership team, we decided to review environmental sampling data that the City of El Paso and the State of Texas were beginning to collect around the smelter. We started by looking at their data on lead in air. We learned that the average air lead level in 1971 at the downwind property boundary of the smelter was 92 μg/M3 (range 15—269 μg/M3). There was no federal air lead standard yet in place, but to put this number in perspective, an air lead standard was established a few years later under the newly enacted Clean Air Act, and it was set at 1.5 μg/M3. Air lead levels decreased rapidly with distance from the smelter and reached background levels at a distance of four to five miles. Levels of cadmium, zinc, and arsenic in the air were also highest at the plant boundary and decreased with distance.

Though it seemed improbable, the smelter managers raised the possibility that some source of emission other than the smelter might be responsible for these elevated air lead levels. They suggested two potential sources: a small lead battery recovery factory in downtown El Paso and lead emissions from the combustion of leaded gasoline by vehicles traveling across El Paso on Interstate Highway 10. We pursued both possibilities. We found that lead emissions from the battery plant were low and intermittent, and that they were minute in comparison to emissions from the smelter. We evaluated the possible contribution of automotive emissions by analyzing air samples from locations across El Paso for their content of lead and of bromine. The basis for this strategy was that lead was added in those years to gasoline in the form of tetraethyl lead bromide, and the ratio of lead to bromine in tetraethyl lead bromide as well as in automotive exhaust was known to be 2.6:1.0. Thus any airborne lead in excess of a ratio of 2.6:1.0 could be considered to derive from non-automotive sources. Air samples taken in February 1972 at a site 200 meters from the smelter showed a mean lead/bromine ratio of 62.8:1.0. This ratio declined with distance and did not reach a value of 2.6:1.0 until five to six miles out from the smelter. We had confirmed yet again that the smelter was the principal source of atmospheric lead contamination in El Paso.

To further define the geographic pattern of contamination, we examined the heavy metal content of surface soil samples collected at sites around El Paso. The highest lead levels were found immediately adjacent to the smelter (mean 3,457 ppm; range 560–11,450 ppm). Levels declined in all directions with increasing distance from the plant. Similar distributions, though less extensive, were seen for cadmium, zinc, and arsenic. The heavy metal content of household dust showed a similar pattern. Highest levels of lead in household dust were seen in Smeltertown, an adobe village on the banks of the Rio Grande immediately beside the smelter, inhabited mainly by poor Mexican families. The geometric mean household dust lead concentration in Smeltertown was 22,191 ppm.

Steve Gehlbach and I presented this information to the senior leadership at CDC. We realized that we were dealing with a medically serious and potentially politically explosive situation. To determine whether there existed a hazard to human health, we understood that it would be necessary to precisely document the pattern of blood lead levels in the children of El Paso and at the same time to carefully exclude the possibility that sources other than the smelter might be contributing to any lead exposure. We knew we would be under the microscope.

We went back to El Paso in July and August of 1972 with a team of 10 EIS officers and more than 20 support staff. Our plan was to do shoe leather epidemiology by undertaking a door-to-door survey of homes. At the same time, we planned to obtain multiple environmental samples. We divided the city into three roughly concentric circles along census tract boundaries with the smelter at the center. The outer margins of our circles were 1, 2.5, and 4 miles. The innermost circle included Smeltertown. In this circle, which was sparsely populated, we visited every home. In the two outer circles we used sampling survey techniques to select about 2% of houses.

In each home that we visited, we identified all children 1–19 years of age. We took a history of exposure to lead and of lead poisoning for each child. We collected venous blood samples and sent those samples to CDC for lead analysis. In each home, we collected samples of house dust and surface soil. We also took samples of paint from each home, and we measured the lead content of any pottery used for food storage or preparation. Our survey completion rate was 80%.

In Smeltertown, we found that 43% of 262 children had a blood lead level of 40–59 µg/dl. An additional 14% had levels of 60 µg/dl or more. Highest blood lead levels were seen in children 1–4 years old. In all age groups, blood lead levels were highest in the innermost circle and then declined progressively with distance. We found close correlations between children's blood lead levels and the levels of lead in dust and soil in their homes. We found lead-based paint in 25–30% of homes. Frequency of lead-based paint was nearly equal in all three areas, and there was no gradation by distance from the smelter. Use of pottery for food storage was uncommon in all three areas.

Our conclusion was that particulate lead emitted by the smelter was responsible for most of the lead absorbed by children in El Paso. After many drafts and much rewriting, we published our findings in *The New England Journal of Medicine*.

A striking finding in our data was that almost none of the children whom we examined in El Paso had any clinical signs or symptoms of lead poisoning, despite their often substantially elevated blood lead levels. This did not fit with the prevailing view of the time that lead poisoning was an all-or-none disease that either produced clinical symptoms or otherwise caused no harm. I discussed this unexpected observation with Dr. Herbert L. Needleman, a pediatrician and child psychiatrist at Harvard a few years older than me, whom I had recently come to know. Herb, who has become a life-long mentor and an iconic figure in lead poisoning research, was just embarking on his landmark studies of low-level lead toxicity. He encouraged me to look closely at the children in El Paso to ascertain whether they were suffering silent lead poisoning.

To investigate this possibility, I asked Dr. Rosenblum's permission to bring a CDC team back to El Paso in June 1973. Our goal was to see whether there was evidence of silent neurobehavioral dysfunction in children who were exposed to lead but had no obvious symptoms. Dr. Rosenblum extended us an invitation, and we arrived in El Paso. But once there we met a rude surprise. We were summoned before the Board of Health, Dr. Rosenblum's employers. The Board told us that Dr. Rosenblum had exceeded his authority in inviting us, that we were disinvited, and that we should return immediately to Atlanta. I was not pleased. I suspected intrigue, most likely instigated by the smelting company. I therefore instructed my team to stay quietly in El Paso for a few days while I used one of my ever present GTR's to travel to the state capitol in Austin to sort things out. In Austin, I met Mr. John Hill, the Attorney General of the State of Texas. I explained the situation to Mr. Hill. He told me that the Board of Health had acted improperly and that he would set things right. He instructed me to go back to El Paso and to get on with the study. I did so, and there was no further interference from the Board of Health.

In our study, we evaluated 46 symptom-free children aged 3–15 years with blood lead concentrations of 40–68 μg/dl (mean 48 μg/dl). We compared them with 78 ethnically and socioeconomically similar children from the same neighborhoods with blood lead levels <40 μg/dl (mean 27 μg/dl). To assess cognitive function, we tested each child using the Wechsler intelligence scale. Psychological examiners were blind to children's blood lead levels.

We found that age-adjusted performance IQ was significantly decreased in children with higher lead levels as compared to their less heavily exposed peers (mean IQ scores, 95 versus 103). Children in the high lead group also had significant slowing in a test of peripheral motor function, a finger-wrist tapping test. We concluded that lead emitted from the smelter had caused subclinical neurobehavioral dysfunction in the children of El Paso. We published our findings in *The Lancet*.

Our findings did not go unnoticed by the smelting company. They commissioned a rival study undertaken by a local pediatrician and a psychologist from the El Paso school district. Though their study was small, statistically underpowered, and methodologically flawed, it was portrayed by the lead industry as disproving our findings. The ensuing struggle took several years to play out and culminated in a most unpleasant public debate at the Society for Occupational and Environmental Medicine. Ultimately our findings on the subclinical neurotoxicity of lead were corroborated by Herb Needleman's work and further confirmed by numerous subsequent studies of children exposed to lead at low levels in North America, Europe, and Australia. Subclinical toxicity has now become a widely accepted concept in environmental toxicology, and it is a concept that applies to many toxic materials in addition to lead.

In the years following our studies, the smelter substantially reduced its emissions. Smeltertown was razed, and the families were relocated. Lead smelting was discontinued in 1985, and in 1999 the smelter closed completely, no longer able after years of legal wrangling to comply with environmental standards.

My work in El Paso marked a critical transition in my life. It was my first foray into chronic disease epidemiology. It was also my first contact with environmental medicine. What I found especially fascinating about the studies in El Paso was the opportunity they provided to trace a chain of causality from smelter emissions, to environmental contamination, to elevated blood lead levels in a large population, and finally to neurobehavioral dysfunction. The exercise was as elegant as anything I might have encountered in pediatric neurology. And beyond that intellectual stimulation, the work involved political intrigue, confrontation of truth to power, and an opportunity to use science to improve the lives of the poor and disenfranchised. The net result was that I became firmly hooked on research, specifically on research in public health. I made the decision to become a physician-scientist and to stay on at CDC to pursue a career in environmental epidemiology. After much soul searching, I finally called Dr. McKhann at Johns Hopkins and told him that I would not be pursuing a fellowship in pediatric neurology.

When I returned to Atlanta at the end of my work in El Paso, I was assigned to Dr. Clark Heath's chronic disease epidemiology program. With Clark's support and with the support also of Dr. David Sencer, CDC's far-sighted and dynamic Director who later became Commissioner of Health for the City of New York, I set up a new unit that we initially called the Environmental Hazards Activity. This little group, staffed initially by only three of us—Dr. Edward Baker, later Associate Dean of Public Health at the University of North Carolina, Dr. Malcolm Harrington, later Professor of Occupational Medicine at the University of Birmingham in the UK, and me—traveled across the USA investigating episodes of pesticide poisoning, toxic chemical spills, air pollution, and drinking water contamination. We undertook studies of heavy metal exposure around a number of smelters, most notably the Bunker Hill smelter in northern Idaho. Findings from these studies confirmed our data from El Paso. We were learning on the job, in classic CDC style, the new discipline of environmental epidemiology. Our unit prospered. Over the years it grew into CDC's National Center for Environmental Health.

After several years of this work, I came to recognize that if I were truly to become a physician-scientist, I must do more than pursue outbreaks. I saw that I needed more formal scientific training, especially in epidemiology as well as in

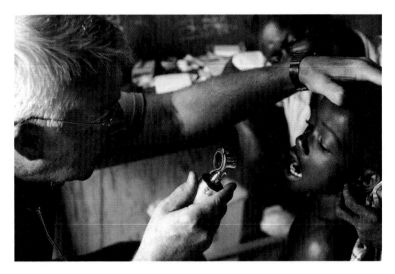

Fig. 16.4 Me with a patient

environmental science and toxicology. Until then, despite all the wonderful mentoring I had received from Alex Langmuir and his colleagues, I had no formal training in these disciplines beyond the four-week EIS course in July 1970. I therefore requested support for a year of graduate school, and I started looking for programs in environmental medicine. As it turned out, there were no training programs in environmental medicine in 1976. There were, however, strong programs in the related field of occupational medicine. Largely on the advice of my colleague, Malcolm Harrington, who had trained in England, I chose to do a course in occupational medicine and epidemiology at the London School of Hygiene and Tropical Medicine. CDC graciously sent me there for a one-year assignment beginning in July 1976.

By the time I had finished my course work in London, I had fully made the transition from physician to physician-scientist. I was poised to pursue a career that would combine a foundation in clinical medicine with a deep appreciation of the power of epidemiology to discover truth and to catalyze societal change. I was not what I had thought I would be when I entered medical school, but with the guidance of extraordinary mentors and the support of loving friends and family, I had found a wonderfully exciting and fulfilling pathway. I was prepared to play the part I would play in such grand endeavors in public health as the removal of lead from gasoline, the reduction of occupational exposure to benzene, and the control of exposure of children to toxic pesticides. I was ready for the work that I would later undertake with the US Environmental Protection Agency and the World Health Organization. I had acquired the tools I would need nearly 30 years later to help launch the National Children's Study.

My career as a physician-scientist has been a marvelous journey. I recommend it highly to any physician who feels the call (Fig. 16.4).

Seventeen
Curiosity, Hard Work, and Tenacity

Moira Chan-Yeung

The Early Years

I was born in Hong Kong, a British Colony in southern China, on the brink of the Second World War. I was the second of four children in a traditional Chinese family. On Christmas Day in 1941, when I was two years old, Japanese soldiers marched into the city, and our lives were forever changed. My father escaped to mainland China, intending to send for his wife and young children as soon as he found a steady job in free China. This plan never materialized, as he had a hard time finding a place to settle that was far enough from the advancing Japanese occupation. The rest of the family remained with our grandparents in Hong Kong. Life was hard, and we lived on the margin of starvation.

After the war, the hardship continued as the population of Hong Kong rose rapidly from 0.6 to 2.3 million in 1953, not only from returning families that had fled during Japanese occupation and a high birth rate, but also from the refugees who streamed into Hong Kong when the Communists defeated the Nationalists in China. This population explosion created enormous problems in housing, education, public health, and medical care. Post-war life in Hong Kong was difficult, and most people were forced to work long hours with meager pay and to live in overcrowded conditions. Tuberculosis reached over seven cases per 1,000 people in Hong Kong during this period.

Staying with our grandparents in Hong Kong turned out to be a blessing. Our grandfather taught us reading and writing in Chinese, so by the time of Hong Kong's liberation in 1945, we had not missed much schooling. Each of us was able to enter the primary school grade appropriate for our age, while many children in our classes were several years older. Later, we were admitted into two of the prestigious schools sponsored by the Anglican Church: my sister and I into the Diocesan Girls' School and my brothers, the Diocesan Boys' School. The school fees were high relative to the salary of most people. Supporting four children was a heavy burden for my

M. Chan-Yeung (✉)
Department of Medicine, University of British Columbia, Vancouver, BC, Canada; Department of Medicine, The University of Hong Kong, Hong Kong, China
e-mail: myeung@unixg.ubc.ca

D.A. Schwartz (ed.), *Medicine Science and Dreams*,
DOI 10.1007/978-90-481-9538-1_17, © Springer Science+Business Media B.V. 2011

father, who worked as a civil servant. To make ends meet, my mother worked as a teacher. We were often told that it was our duty to lighten the burden of the family by getting scholarships, so we not only had to be good, but also be one of the best in classes.

In the early 1950s, the government of Hong Kong coped with the rapid rise in school-aged children by pushing for massive primary school education. However, they made little provision for secondary school education, which created a pyramid system. Only 10% of young people of the appropriate age group were in secondary schools, while less than 1% were admitted into the local university—the University of Hong Kong (HKU). Competition for these places through public examination was fierce. Like most Chinese parents, my parents placed a great deal of emphasis on getting a good education and drummed into us the importance of these consequential examinations.

Medicine, Not My Choice!

My great grandfather was a notable mathematician and inventor, despite not having had any formal education. In fact, the government has erected a museum in his village to commemorate his achievement by displaying his inventions, including the machine for spinning silk, which led to the expansion of the silk industry and wealth in that province. My grandfather moved from mainland China to Hong Kong and was married at a young age according to custom. By the time he was 35, he already had 13 children. He ran an import-export business but lost it because he was too naïve and lacked acumen for the trade. My father obtained a degree in science in university, but he was unable to pursue his ambition in the medical career. The children in my generation were burdened with high expectations to achieve what the previous two generations had missed. At the time, a good profession that was always in demand, would ensure a good income, and would earn respectability was that of a physician. My brother, being a boy and the oldest in the family, bore the brunt of such expectations and most of the pressure. Being a girl, whose main duty was to be a housewife and to bear children, I was initially spared from this additional obligation.

While my parents saved assiduously for my brother's tertiary education, they could not afford or be expected to send a girl to university, even though I was the only child in the family to win a scholarship for my high school education. The only career choices available to me were through government subsidized training, either as a nurse or a teacher. After spending three years in a Catholic primary school, being an impressionable youngster, my secret ambition was to be a nun to serve humanity. To be trained as a teacher or a nurse was compatible with such an ambition.

Age 13, however, was a turning point. I came across a book in the library—the biography of Madame Curie written by her daughter, which broadened my outlook on life and opened my eyes to possibilities that I had not imagined. For the first time, I became aware that a woman could not only be a scientist, but also a Nobel Prize winner in not just one but two separate areas: physics and chemistry. I also learned the many difficulties and prejudices she had to overcome before her achievement was finally recognized. It was the contribution of her discoveries to medicine and to the well-being of humanity that led me to harbour a desire to become a scientist. This was a dream I did not share with anyone, lest I be ridiculed. At that time, my idea of a scientist was someone who studied physics and chemistry, subjects that were not even available in my school curriculum. With the keen competition, I might not even make it to the university. Nevertheless, the story of Marie Curie influenced my development during the teenage years, and inspired me to work hard and to persevere.

The first hurdle was overcome when the school arranged for me to take physics and chemistry in the boys' school and the remaining subjects in my own school. For the last three years of my high school education, I commuted between the two schools with another girl. My father saw, for the first time, the possibility that his dream of becoming a physician, which had ended abruptly by grandfather's failure in business as well as the Japanese invasion of China in the 1930s, could be realized not only in one but perhaps in two of his children. After my brother left for Canada to pursue higher education, my parents turned their attention on me. I was told that I had two important tasks: to enter medical school and to win a scholarship.

The overcrowded home environment in Hong Kong was far from ideal for a student who needed to study. For many years, our family occupied a small two-room apartment; the children slept in the living room. The few tables and chairs in the public library became favorite haunts for students like me. During holidays, we would arrive early before the opening hours to be the first in line to get a spot. By the later years in high school, having proven to my biology teacher how responsible I was in locking up and in looking after the place, I earned the permission to spend after school hours and weekends in the school laboratory, where I spent countless hours poring over intriguing problems in mathematics and physics. I loved the mental challenge of mathematics and the aesthetics in geometry. In my exploration of the sciences, I was having as much fun as other young people who were enjoying hiking, dancing, swimming, and other sports.

Because of the relatively high cost of university education, the education department decided that the first year of university should be taught as an extra year in high school. At that time there were very few qualified teachers in high schools who could teach subjects at the university level. I found that while the school provided us with opportunities to be exposed to science subjects, much of the learning and problem solving were self-taught, a practice that proved to be useful for the rest of my life.

My diligence paid off. At the end of the matriculation examinations, I was awarded one of the two King Edward VII Scholarships, given to the students with the highest marks for the year. At that time, there were around 40 places each year in the medical faculty in Hong Kong University (HKU) for a population of almost three million, with 10 more reserved for students from Malaysia and Singapore. A place in the medical school was coveted by many. The medical faculty, established even earlier than HKU as the Hong Kong College of Medicine in 1887, enjoyed an unusually high standard of teaching among Asian medical schools. Dr. Sun Yat-sen, the father of the Republic of China, was one of its first two medical graduates in 1892. The medical faculty in HKU was, therefore, better developed than the science faculty. Even so, I went into medicine with some reluctance. Despite the prestige it signified, when I was accepted into medical school, it meant to me an end for my dream of becoming a scientist. As an obedient daughter, I could not dream of going against the wishes of my parents!

After five years of medical school, one year of internship, and another three years of training in internal medicine, I was ready to receive the final touch necessary for all Hong Kong graduates who aspired to teach in the medical school or to become consultants in major hospitals—to gain membership in one of the prestigious Royal Colleges in the United Kingdom. At that time, only about 10% of graduates passed the membership examination. Examinations were held by each of the Royal Colleges (London, Edinburgh, and Glasgow), and candidates from local institutions and from the Commonwealth countries had the opportunity of trying their luck three times each year in each of the colleges. Today, the examinations and the MRCP (Membership of the Royal Colleges of Physicians) titles have a different meaning, as there are now many more choices, such as getting the specialist degree from Australia, the USA, or locally in Hong Kong.

I thoroughly enjoyed my years of training in Hong Kong, especially the *esprit de corps* in the group that I was trained with. This is what drew me back in later years, hoping to experience such kinship again.

Jack Pepys: The "Father" of Occupational Asthma

Professor Jack Pepys (Fig. 17.1), who headed the Clinical Immunology Unit at the Cardiothoracic Institute in London, kindly took me in for further training after I passed the much dreaded membership examination. A man with a moustache and a twinkle in his eyes, Professor Pepys became well known for his work on farmer's lung by identifying the thermophilic organisms responsible for the disease. He then moved on to study asthma caused by workplace exposures, using specific challenge testing to pinpoint the causative agent as well as to make the diagnosis for management. Four decades have passed since he published the method, and we are still using his very practical way of making the diagnosis. He also alerted clinicians and investigators to the occurrence of the late asthmatic reaction, which could be readily missed if not looked for specifically. Little did I know at the time that what I had learned in the eight months with Professor Pepys would form the backbone of my research in later years.

At that time, occupational asthma was definitely not something that I expected to spend much time with in the future. I was to return to Hong Kong and follow the footsteps of my mentors, to engage in busy clinical practice in internal medicine at a teaching hospital. The story of Madame Curie and the desire to be a scientist had long been forgotten. However, life has its twists and turns. Coinciding with the Cultural Revolution in China, riots broke out in Hong Kong in 1967 after I left.

Fig. 17.1 Professor Jack Pepys (painting by Mrs. R. Pepys)

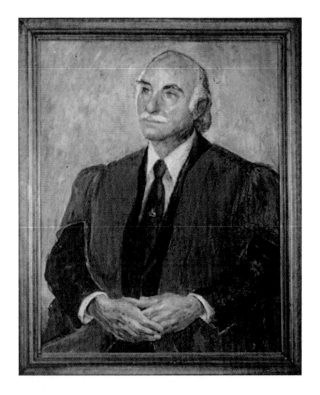

Looking back, with the red guards massing across the border, it was indeed a touch and go situation for Hong Kong. The stability of the Colony, under British law and order, suddenly became highly questionable. Many colleagues in Hong Kong left for Australia and Canada, among other countries. For my husband and me, who had just finished our studies in London, it seemed foolish to return to a smoldering hornets' nest of trouble. Our logical move was to apply for immigration to Canada, and to wait and see. We ended up in Vancouver, Canada after our British sojourn, for no better reason than the fact that several colleagues and my husband's sister had already moved there!

New World, New Life, New Challenges, and Clinical Investigations

Vancouver, once described by a famous conductor as a "cultural desert," was a marvelous place for outdoor life. One could swim in the sea or ski on the slopes, depending on the season. The medical school was still in its infancy, having been established in 1950. There were only a handful of full-time faculty in the Department of Medicine at the University of British Columbia (UBC), so having a faculty position (a position that I would have stepped into if I had returned to

HKU) was entirely out of the question. I was offered a job as a teaching fellow in the Department of Medicine working with Dr. Stefan Grzybowski, a specialist in tuberculosis. At that time, respiratory disease was not yet recognized as a specialty. The hard-earned title "MRCP" did not confer upon me any special privilege there. I had to sit with final year medical students for the qualifying examinations and take the specialty examinations.

While waiting to take these examinations, I came across several interesting clinical problems—exercise-induced asthma, allergic bronchopulmonary aspergillosis, and Western red cedar asthma. I studied each one of these problems, but it was Western red cedar asthma that caught my passion. Western red cedar (*Thuja plicata*), grown in the Pacific Northwest, is used extensively in local construction and in furniture making. It had been long known that asthma was common among these workers. Two clinicians had investigated this problem before me in Vancouver. They exposed workers with such complaints to Western red cedar wood dust in an attempt to reproduce the symptoms. However, the workers did not develop any asthma symptoms, and their lung function did not drop immediately after exposure to the wood dust as one might expect in asthma. The clinicians concluded that the workers were "allergic to work"!

Having observed the occurrence of late asthmatic reactions after challenge testing in Professor Jack Pepy's laboratory, I repeated the experiment but monitored the workers for eight hours after testing. While some workers developed an asthmatic attack immediately after exposure, more than half of them did not develop symptoms until four to six hours later. This observation was followed later by the discovery that plicatic acid, present uniquely in red cedar, was an agent responsible for asthma. At that time asthma was thought to be caused mostly by allergens. That a small molecule such as plicatic acid, with a molecular weight of only 440 Daltons, can cause asthma fascinated me, and I began to investigate every aspect of the disease. How does it cause asthma? Does it act as a hapten and combine with a body protein to become an allergen? Why is it that some patients develop only a late asthmatic reaction, others a biphasic reaction (an immediate followed by a late asthmatic reaction), and still others only an immediate reaction? Are these reactions mediated by different immunological mechanisms? What is the natural history of the disease? How frequent is the disease among those who are working with the wood dust? (Fig. 17.2) Why is it that only a portion of exposed workers develop asthma and others do not? Is there a dust level below which asthma would not develop in workers? Do people with Western red cedar asthma recover after they are removed from exposure? When I found that the majority of workers with Western red cedar asthma did not fully recover, as I thought they should when they no longer worked with the wood, I wanted to know whether this could be used as a model to study chronic asthma. For the next two decades, I pursued these questions one by one in earnest.

Life in the new world was far from easy. Even after I had completed the necessary qualifications to practice medicine as a specialist, had worked several years as a research fellow, and had conducted several studies, I did not have a faculty appointment at UBC. When the university finally appointed me as an Assistant Professor

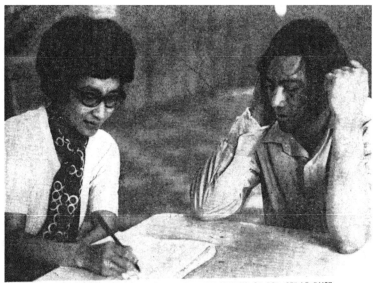

DR. MOIRA YEUNG CONDUCTS SURVEY ON EFFECTS OF RED CEDAR DUST

Fig. 17.2 Me interviewing a worker during a survey at a Western red cedar sawmill. This picture was copied from the Vancouver Sun newspaper published in 1974

in 1973, (the first female member in the Department of Medicine) my salary still came from research fellowships. I was not paid from the university budget until 1986; four years after I was promoted to full-time professor of medicine. During this period, UBC had expanded rapidly, and new recruits were not only given full-time salaried positions, but also laboratory space and operating budget for research. These privileges were not extended to me, even though I had arrived on the doorsteps of the university in the late 1960s. Yet I was happy with my work, which has proven to be fruitful. Moreover, my husband had already established his private practice, and remuneration was not a concern.

The Occupational Lung Disease Research Unit

Dr. Stefan Grzybowski was an opportunist who believed in not missing a chance to have fun in life. Stefan loved working, but he loved working more when mixed with fun. Trips to study tuberculosis in native people were often delayed until the hunting season so that moose meat could be enjoyed throughout the winter. Stefan believed in working for the underdog and that everyone should be equal. But, he also believed that certain groups, such as the upper class to which he belonged, should be "more equal" than others. Nevertheless, it was his "leftist" tendency that made him popular with the labour unions when the occupational lung diseases unit was established. This unit, his brain child, was created for my benefit before his retirement.

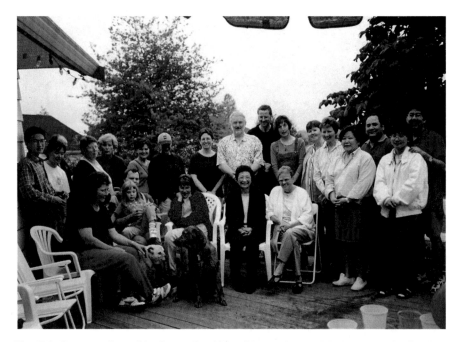

Fig. 17.3 Some members of the Occupational Lung Diseases Research Unit and their family taken in 1998

With the establishment of the unit, the team investigated most of the major industries in the province of British Columbia (BC), such as sawmills, grain elevators, pulp and paper mills, smelters, foundries, and bakeries. We insisted that all stakeholders should be involved in any health studies of workers. Thus, not only should the management be present, but representatives of the labour union as well as members of the regulatory agency should also be involved in all meetings. While these principles appeared to be a common sense approach, many health studies were carried out without such safeguards, and their results were often regarded as biased and discredited by either the labour union or the management. The results of our health studies led to much cleaner working environments for workers in BC. (Fig. 17.3)

David V. Bates: From Science to Public Policy

Dr. David Bates, (Fig. 17.4) the Dean of the UBC Faculty of Medicine, was responsible for my appointment. David was a leading researcher in respiratory diseases related to air pollution. While he was not directly involved in any of my research, he had shown a keen interest in my career over the years. When he attended my rounds, he always asked probing questions, which I was invariably unable to answer. His role in translating scientific findings into public policy had inspired me to engage in similar activities in the occupational arena. In my naivety, I did not anticipate

Fig. 17.4 Dr. David V Bates

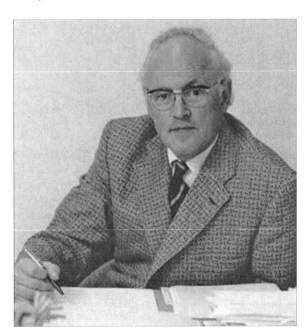

the amount of resistance that I would encounter, and my admiration for David's persistence increased with time.

In our epidemiological health studies, we included environmental monitoring and determined dose–response relationships between health effects and exposure. From the results of these and clinical studies, we came up with the threshold limit values for Western red cedar dust and for grain dust. The Workers' Compensation Board (WCB) of BC lowered the permissible concentration of Western red cedar dust from 10 to 5 mg and later to 1 mg/m^3 based on our findings. However, we had a great deal of difficulty in convincing Labour Canada, the agency responsible for the regulation of grain dust, to lower the threshold limit value, despite the fact that the American Conference of Industrial Hygienists had reduced it to 5 mg/m^3 based on our findings and those of other researchers.

The observation that the majority of workers with Western red cedar asthma failed to recover after the exposure was eliminated led to unanticipated ramifications. I had to address the issue of compensation for these workers. Although by then, the local WCB recognized Western red cedar asthma as a compensable disease, it was considered only as an acute illness. Despite many subsequent studies by other researchers showing the persistence of asthma after cessation of exposure to causative agents, long-term disability pension for these workers was not accepted by the WCB of BC for another decade.

I was also struck by the unfairness that patients with asthma were assessed only for respiratory impairment, which was based entirely on lung function tests as in patients with pneumoconiosis. Since normal lung function could be achieved with good treatment in patients with asthma, these patients were considered "not impaired." However, they could not return to the same job or to jobs that might expose them to irritant gases and fumes because of persistent nonspecific bronchial hyperresponsiveness (NSBH). I hardly considered these patients unimpaired. Therefore, in the late 1980s, I submitted a proposal to the WCB of BC outlining the management of patients with occupational asthma. For patients who did not recover, I proposed that the assessment of respiratory impairment be based not only on lung function, but also on the amount of medications necessary to control asthma and NSBH. A similar system was already in use in Quebec. My proposed plan was met with silence. I resubmitted the proposal in the early 1990s after the American Thoracic Society published our recommendations in a position statement. It was again met with silence. In the early 2000s, I had the satisfaction of knowing that the American Medical Association's recommendations for assessing respiratory impairment in patients with asthma included not only lung function, but also medication use and measurement of NSBH. Additionally, WorkSafe BC, previously the WCB of BC, finally published new recommendations for investigation and management of patients with occupational asthma, and they were not different from my proposal 15 years earlier.

Return to My Roots

I had left Hong Kong in 1966 with a Commonwealth Scholarship which stipulated that the recipient should return and serve his/her place of origin. This, and the fact that I had received years of free education in Hong Kong, weighed more heavily on my conscience as I grew older. By 1998, both our children were in university. With encouragement from my husband I went on a sabbatical leave to HKU, which turned out to be a permanent leave.

In my absence, Hong Kong had transformed into an international city with a population close to seven million. It now boasts eight universities and a number of colleges. My alma mater, a major university in the Far East, now emphasizes both teaching and research. It received the honour of being placed 18th in the World University Rankings in 2007 by the Times Higher Education Supplement and was named the best university by the Quacquarelli Symonds (QS) Asian University Rankings in 2009. Many colleagues in medicine are leading researchers in the world in their specialties.

I returned to work in the same teaching hospital where I was trained. The closeness and kinship among colleagues that I once enjoyed, having arisen from years of living under the same roof in the hospital whether we were on call or not, were no longer there. In the day of computers, cellular phones, and pagers, residents are allowed to live outside the hospital even when they are on call. Instead, I found comradeship within the respiratory community in Hong Kong, an honorable group of individuals. The respiratory physicians here placed themselves on the front line during the SARS epidemic without complaints, yet they did not receive the same kind of recognition and attention as some high profile "heroes" of this epidemic.

At the end of the epidemic, they provided invaluable recommendations on the use of nebulizers, lung function testing, intubation, and ventilation in patients suspected of having an infectious disease. I have had the honour of working with most of the chest physicians in the community on various projects during the past few years and have enjoyed their full cooperation. In turn, my contribution has been to point out the importance of the role of the chest societies in promoting public health policies, such as those related to environmental tobacco smoke and air pollution.

Reflections

I was very fortunate to be in the right place at the right time. My husband, in addition to providing financial security, has always been supportive of my endeavors as few men of similar social and cultural background would have. I am sure that if he had been less supportive, I would have followed an entirely different career path. My mentors were kind and generous and left me to develop my potential. I was trained in internal medicine, and while I learned how to investigate patients with occupational asthma from Professor Jack Pepys, I had no training in respiratory diseases, respiratory physiology, or epidemiology. Yet I carried out a number of clinical, immunological, and epidemiological studies using different methods. I learned techniques necessary for my studies from other centers with funds magically generated by Dr. Grzybowski, who also left his job to me when he retired, I became the head of the Respiratory division at UBC which the had held before his retirement. Whenever possible, I collaborated with others and relied on their expertise. There were times when I wish I had received a more solid basic training. When I mentioned this to Dr. Bates, he told me that it really did not matter all that much in my case. Such reassurance empowered me to move forward. My other mentor is Dr. Margaret Becklake. Margot, as everyone calls her, is loved not only by her juniors and students at McGill University, but also by her students worldwide. One of her great achievements has been the role she played as a model for many and especially female investigators. When I was still a very junior investigator, we met in a conference in 1970s and she invited me to dinner. The fact that she, at that time a renowned investigator, had given me, a research fellow who was not even working in her institution, personal attention had encouraged me greatly. My admiration for Margot increased with time as she is not only deeply committed to science, but also to teaching research methods to students in the third world. Our relationship ranged from teacher–student, co-investigators, colleagues, and friends over three decades. Her teaching and encouragement had been pillars on which I built my career.

Recently, I read about the enormous obstacles faced by women scientists in the early twentieth century as recounted by Sharon Bertsch McGrayne (*Nobel Prize Women in Science: Their Lives, Struggles, and Momentous Discoveries*). She wrote "... They were confined to basement laboratories and attic offices. They crawled behind furniture to attend science lectures. They worked in universities for decades without pay as volunteers—in the USA as late as the 1970s. Even today, 70% of American women physicists are married to scientists. As a result, the academic landscape was littered with husband-and-wife teams in which the man had the salary, job security, and prestige, and the woman assisted him at his pleasure." Compared to these women scientists, my career has been relatively easy, although I had to work very hard throughout my life, fulfilling multiple roles as a mother, wife, researcher, clinician, teacher, and administrator simultaneously at different times.

I have not designed my career to be a physician-scientist. The term physician-scientist came into existence after I had established my career. In my younger days, I wanted to be a scientist and do research in physics and chemistry to benefit mankind, but I entered medical school instead. My adoptive country, Canada, presented new challenges and new opportunities and allowed me to combine my training as a clinician and a scientist to conduct research. There were many frustrations and roadblocks along the way, but tenacity, hard work, and support from mentors solved most of them. In the end, although my accomplishments have been merely a fraction of those of Marie Curie, I have the satisfaction of knowing that my clinical and epidemiological research has also led to improvement of the health and well-being of those suffering from asthma.

Eighteen
Physician-Scientist: Linking Science, Medicine, and Public Policy

Gilbert S. Omenn

> *Do not ask what path to follow; go, instead, where there is no path, and leave a trail.*
>
> –Robert H. Williams, MD

Introduction

Forty years ago, soon after I came to Seattle in 1969 to be a Fellow in Medical Genetics with Dr. Arno Motulsky at the University of Washington, I went to meet the founding chair of Internal Medicine, Dr. Robert H. Williams. Dr. Williams was a world leader in endocrinology and especially diabetes. In the early 1950s, he famously recruited young physician-scientists from "back East," especially where he had been at Johns Hopkins and Harvard, by telephoning them and their spouses at home in the morning before they had a clue what the time was "out West" in Seattle! He was way ahead of his time in inviting spouses to participate early in the recruitment process. At a time when everyone seemed obsessed about identifying "role models," he had a plaque on the wall behind his desk, which read "Do not ask what path to follow; go, instead, where there is no path, and leave a trail"—as he had, from a start in rural Mississippi. I have found that statement very helpful for myself and for many young people and contemporaries I have counseled across a great variety of career paths. The explicit messages are, "Take risks, pursue your passion, override conventional wisdom, be creative, be bold." And don't look back on what might have been the obvious alternatives when pursuing what Robert Frost called "The Road Less Traveled."

A medical education opens numerous potential career paths. The "triple threat" combination of research, teaching, and clinical care, sometimes complemented

G.S. Omenn (✉)

Departments of Medicine, Human Genetics, and Public Health, Center for Computational Medicine and Bioinformatics, University of Michigan, Ann Arbor, MI, USA

e-mail: gomenn@umich.edu

D.A. Schwartz (ed.), *Medicine Science and Dreams,*
DOI 10.1007/978-90-481-9538-1_18, © Springer Science+Business Media B.V. 2011

with administrative or public policy responsibilities, is a foundation for a highly stimulating career with potentially important societal contributions and many personal satisfactions. I feel very fortunate to have experienced quite a range of those career opportunities.

Moreover, a successful combination of professional roles for groups of individuals leads to a successful model for academic healthcare institutions as well. Rather than lamenting the "tradeoffs" of research, education, and clinical care missions, those creating the strategic plan and reward systems of academic medical centers should seek to achieve synergies across these missions. After all, basic, clinical, and public health research advances bring excitement to the teaching venues and attract patients to the clinical services. At least this has been my experience.

Science can help all of us in framing and stimulating our thinking about the nature of the world and the nature of human interactions. Science and technology have long provided new means to address many of the grand challenges facing society, from economic vitality and national security to better health, more sustainable energy and environmental actions, better education, more effective global control of infectious diseases and population pressures, greater appreciation for diverse human cultures, and potentially even reduction in violence and irrational behaviors. Never have these opportunities been greater than today.

The Early Years

My parents, Leonard and Leah Omenn (Fig. 18.1), were second-generation Americans imbued with the notion that in America there are no limits on aspirations. At the same time, influenced by the deprivations of the Great Depression and the shocking oppression of Jews all over again in Europe, they felt it wise to develop skills and a profession "that society would always need," like medicine. They had gone to college during the 1930s. My mother completed a full pre-med program at Temple University and earned teaching credentials as well. She taught at Chester High School in her and my home town of Chester, PA (where William Penn had landed coming up the Delaware River in 1682) and got married before she could start medical school. My father grew up in Wilmington, Delaware, went to the University of Delaware and Temple Dental School, and set up a practice in nearby Chester, a bustling industrial city during World War II (WWII). They bought a home and set up a professional office so that my mother could assist and my dad could avoid commuting. He enjoyed playing with me and my younger brother whenever he had a convenient break in his schedule. He had a fine reputation as a specialist dental surgeon. Memorably, there were occasions when he would see patients who had been referred to him after some other dentist broke off a tooth. After carefully preparing the site, he would complete the extraction and state a (modest) fee. A few times patients demurred with "But it only took a few minutes," to which he would reply, "Would you rather I did it slowly?" Technical skills, good judgment, and good communication are all important.

Fig. 18.1 Leonard and Leah Omenn, parents of Gil Omenn, Chester, PA, and later Boynton Beach, FL

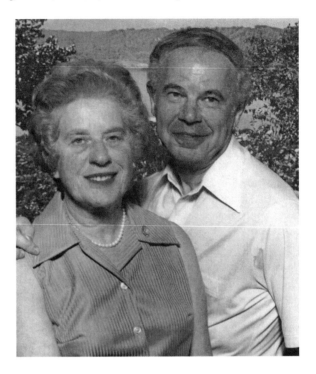

My parents were both good pianists. My father taught me piano; he was a taskmaster, who would assign a lesson, and then, if my playing fell short of high expectations, simply say, "Let me know when you are ready" and get up. Tough at age 8 or 9. My mother helped by reassuring me that further practice would be productive! However, my dad would proudly report that his patients appreciated hearing me play. He also liked to join me and my friends for various sports in the neighborhood and the vast city park beginning just a half block from our home, where I played some good tennis matches through high school. At school, I began clarinet for the band in grade four, alto saxophone in grade seven for the dance band, and oboe in grade nine for the orchestra. Our dance band won prizes three years in a row against the big Philadelphia high school bands. I played oboe for three years in the Philadelphia Youth Orchestra and clarinet in the Princeton Marching Band, which made the cover of *Sports Illustrated* in 1963. Music has remained a big part of my life. I have played piano informally in many homes, restaurants, and meeting sites around the world and served on symphony, chamber music, and musical society boards.

Our family had quite a disruptive but very interesting experience in 1953 and 1954. My father, who had been refused for service in WWII due to high blood pressure, was drafted by the Air Force when the military realized that they had a shortage of physicians and dentists during the late stages of the Korean War. He was offered rank of Major, commensurate with his specialty and years in practice.

We were sent to Wolters Air Force Base in Mineral Wells, Texas, 50 miles west of Fort Worth. I was in a group of eighth grade students who produced a local radio program and performed an operetta. I had to defeat the principal's son to win a table tennis tournament, with the final match held on the auditorium stage during school assembly. I had an advantage from playing against all comers at the Air Force Base Bachelor Officers' Quarters. I even tried out for the football team, but my dad showed up for an early practice at which I was the evidence of a shortage of equipment. I was relegated to full-time band!

Twelve months later, on an obligatory physical, my Dad was rediscovered to have quite high blood pressure, sent for an urgent diagnostic work-up by a Mayo Clinic-trained specialist at the larger base in Wichita Falls that yielded a diagnosis of "idiopathic malignant hypertension," and given a prognosis of three to five years survival and a medical discharge. This was quite sudden and disorienting to our family. It was also wrong, as my Dad survived to age 82, dying in 1997 of prostate cancer. In 1971, I persuaded him to go to the University of Pennsylvania to see highly regarded specialists, with the unfortunate results of a drug-fever from alpha-methyl-DOPA and a draining lesion from an unnecessary lymph node biopsy. Twenty-five years later, I assured him that he would almost surely die with, and not of, his prostate cancer. After a fine 18-month reprieve, he had a terrible final course. Neither he nor I was impressed with my advice or the reliability of medical decision-making. My mother managed to stay clear of doctors and hospitals into her nineties.

On to College at Princeton

I enjoyed math, science, and most other subjects in school. I had a junior high school principal who wanted me to go to Central High School in Philadelphia or apply to the Ford Foundation program for early college entry. My folks and I decided to stick with the standard course with all the enjoyable extra-curricular activities, especially since I was already a year younger due to having completed Grades five and six in one year. For college, I applied to Massachusetts Institute of Technology (MIT), Princeton, and the University of Pennsylvania, with an early inclination to consider physics at MIT and maybe patent law. Upon visiting the institutions, Princeton stood out, and it turned out to be a wonderful experience. However, it was a sobering experience when I realized how lacking my preparation had been. I was the only student in my calculus class who had not already taken some calculus in high school. Moreover, future math majors among freshmen were taking junior-level courses. Other classes were intellectually stimulating, especially biology, taught by Professor Colin Pittendrigh, an evolutionary biologist and co-author of the text *Life*, which espoused two memorable comprehensive themes: the capture, storage, and utilization of energy, as well as reproduction and the evolution of species. Nevertheless, after the end of my freshman year, my high school received a prize for my being ranked first and I was advanced to the junior year.

For my senior research thesis, I chose a project involving contractile proteins in the acellular slime mold, with electron microscopist and mathematical biologist Assistant Professor Lionel Rebhun as my mentor. Unfortunately, the strain I obtained from a friendly professor at Philadelphia failed to grow in my hands at Princeton despite many weeks of effort; it must have been the water! As time was running out, I approached my adviser about doing electron microscopy on this organism, which had not previously been done. The project yielded a worthy thesis as senior year was expiring and everyone else was relaxing. Three years later Dr. Rebhun wrote to me that, at a conference on this organism he had just hosted, a European scientist had reported unusual intracellular structures—these had in fact been very clearly photographed and described in my thesis, which was taken off the shelf for the visitor's approving review. This experience yielded two lifelong lessons: that students are more likely to benefit from projects in which the mentor has relevant experience, and that researchers must be adaptable about the feasibility of projects.

During those same closing weeks of undergraduate life, I was preparing a Latin Address as Salutatorian of my Class of 1961. Commencement was a beautiful day in front of Nassau Hall. The Address opened the program, of course, and confounded the assembled parents, families, and girlfriends as the graduates enthusiastically participated. Inserted in the graduates' programs was the printed Latin Address, embellished with footnotes such as "Hic plaudite," laugh, groan, etc. A key line referred to the decision of the Harvard Trustees that year to change diplomas from Latin to English, presumably reflecting the limited education of their modern graduates. So I toasted the Trustees of Princeton for maintaining the tradition. That remark became the "Quotation of the Week" in the Sunday *New York Times* News of the Week in Review!

The Value of Student Research Experiences

I was very fortunate to have a series of terrific summer research experiences. After junior year, I spent 1960 at the Woods Hole Oceanographic Institution in Massachusetts with Dr. Max Blumer characterizing previously unknown porphyrin compounds in Triassic sediment from Switzerland. Since these compounds were light-sensitive, I had to work at night with red light only. That left the daytimes available to attend lectures and discussions across the street at the Marine Biology Laboratory and to enjoy the beach. The project turned out quite well, with my first two publications, in *Nature* and in *Geochimica and Cosmochimica Acta*.

In 1961, I worked at Brookhaven National Laboratory, with Dr. Lewis K. Dahl as my mentor. He had grown up in rural Skagway, AK, where his father was a physician for the railway. He and his brother Bob (who became Chair of Political Science at Yale) would go hunting as teenagers only if they were confident that there were no other hunters for miles around. He graduated from the University of Washington and University of Pennsylvania Medical School and became Chief Resident at Massachusetts General Hospital, before moving to Rockefeller and then

Brookhaven National Laboratory for access to newly emerging radioisotopes for clinical research. He was particularly interested in the mechanisms of salt-sensitive high blood pressure and developed the Dahl strains of salt-sensitive and salt-resistant rats, which are still utilized today. He launched me on a side project about salt-sensitive hypercholesterolemia in these rats. I had a good lesson the first week. I suggested a modification of the blood pressure measurement technique, to which he replied, "Your idea is a good one, but I am more interested in the biological question, and the present technique is sufficient and reliable." This was a memorable pointer about keeping focus. When he and his wife went off on a long trip, I was turned over to a remarkable colleague, Dr. George Cotzias, who was in a still-early phase of devising the stunningly successful L-DOPA therapy for advanced Parkinson's disease, one of the most remarkable successes of translational and clinical research to this day.

On to Harvard Medical School and then Massachusetts General Hospital

My folks met me on Long Island and drove with me to Boston. The first student we met in Vanderbilt Hall was the president of the second-year class, who kindly offered the advice that, "You can't learn it all; you'll have to figure out what is really necessary." My dad's reaction, not surprisingly, was that, "It must be more effective and faster to learn the material than to try to figure out what is not necessary." Actually, I had a relevant experience at Princeton during junior year taking Political Science; a senior friend offered to study together for the final exam, stressing that, "I'm good on the 'cepts, and I'm sure you can help with the details." I've always thought it sad that some medical students complain about all the learning, since most lay people thirst for knowledge about medicine and human biology—as most newspaper and magazine editors would confirm. Anyhow, I found the material generally fascinating and enjoyed organizing its significance and challenging myself and our faculty, who seemed quite willing to respond. I developed a research interest in proteins and was referred to a junior faculty member, Dr. Thomas J. Gill, III, as a mentor. He, in turn, encouraged my desire to spend that first summer doing research in Israel.

I wrote to Professor Ephraim Katchalski at the Weizmann Institute. He replied that his brother Aharon Katchalsky, a Visiting Professor at Yale, would be willing to interview me there. That was a memorable afternoon, from which came an offer to join Ephraim's laboratory for the summer. I worked on poly-L-lysine and became friendly with young scientists who have been colleagues and friends ever since. Professor Katchalski (Fig. 18.2) took a lifelong interest in my career development and my scientific and science policy activities (I will mention him in a different context later. I also had an opportunity in November 2009 to speak at the memorial tribute to Professor Katzir at the Weizmann [1]). Returning to Boston, I worked three years with Tom Gill on synthetic polypeptides, employing fluorescence polarization to characterize certain properties.

Fig. 18.2 Ephraim
Katchalski/Katzir, former
head, Department of
Biophysics, Weizmann
Institute of Science, Rehovot,
Israel, and the fourth
President of the State of Israel
(1973–1978). Courtesy of the
Government Press Office of
Israel. Photograph by Moshe
Milner

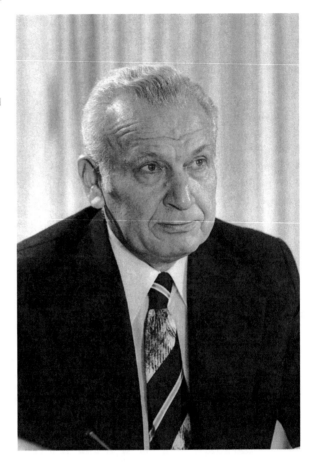

There were many other enjoyable aspects of medical school, including co-organizing a first-year spring symposium on "Mental Health and the Law" (inviting Judge David Bazelon and Professor William Curran), performing and playing the piano in the second-year show, serving as second-year class President, meeting the pioneering cardiologist Paul Dudley White (a household name after he had treated President Eisenhower) in an informal evening discussion with a few interested students, and many other events. Faculty mentors invited small groups of first-year students and attendings invited students on clinical clerkships to their homes, as my wife and I have in the decades since.

Another valuable lesson was finding something remarkable in the most ordinary of clinical case presentations. In August of my fourth year, a five-week-old boy was brought to the Boston Children's Hospital Emergency Ward with skin rash and diarrhea. The residents were unimpressed until the mother stated that she had had a previous child with the same symptoms who died before four months of age. The child was admitted for me to do the initial workup. During that

Sunday evening, I learned from the mother and aunt and from a phone call to Dr. Donald Merritt at Indiana University that this child was the twelth affected in a large Irish kindred with several first-cousin marriages. On rounds the next morning, the resident and I played a little game with our attending, Dr. Park Gerald, who always asked about the family history. I withheld the family history until asked, then unrolled a pedigree with the huge kindred over eight pages taped together! Over the next 5 months, I came back to see the child and family several times and talked with Dr. Alan Crocker and Dr. Sidney Farber about the many studies undertaken. Regrettably, this child died, too. I was given the privilege of writing up the case and the kindred as "Familial Reticuloendotheliosis with Eosinophilia" for the *New England Journal of Medicine*. The single-author paper received the Journal's annual student paper award, and this syndrome of combined immune deficiency became widely known as "Omenn syndrome." Over the decades I was asked occasionally to prepare review articles. The disorder was cured by French investigators with bone marrow transplantation in the late 1970s, and the cause of most cases was discovered in the late 1990s to be due to Recombination Activating Gene (RAG) mutations. The original article is on display in the Omenn Reading Room of the Jeffrey Modell Immunology Center in Building D of the Harvard Medical School, hopefully an inspiration to today's medical students and residents.

For Internal Medicine residency, I was part of a terrific cohort of 12 interns at Massachusetts General Hospital. I particularly enjoyed the Thursday Grand Rounds in the Ether Dome where Morton had first administered anesthesia in 1842. The 1965–1966 and 1966–1967 cohorts had a great variety of career successes, including practice in Bar Harbor, Research Director of Merck, Rockefeller Foundation program leader in Thailand, and three Nobel laureates (Joe Goldstein, Michael Brown, and Fred Murad). Of course, we worked 36 hours on and 12 hours off (actually Monday–Wednesday–Saturday–Sunday or Tuesday–Thursday–Friday overnights) for most months of those two years. I learned the necessity of working efficiently and getting off duty on time. When "my intern" arrived from Johns Hopkins in June 1966, I greeted him, oriented him, and told him I would stay that evening, but subsequently I would finish my notes and depart as soon after 5 or 6 p.m. as possible, and that I expected him to do the same on his nights off. Many years later when I was a visitor at Johns Hopkins, his nursing professor wife reminded me approvingly of that message!

Meanwhile, I suffered an occupational injury common to nurses and physicians from helping to lift heavy patients. I had had a maximal Thursday to Saturday stint in the Intensive Care Unit (ICU) with eight admissions. After noon on Saturday, I went to watch Sandy Koufax pitch in the World Series, stretched out on a sofa. At the end of the game, my back was a tight coil and I was unable to do anything but roll onto the floor and call the Emergency Room. I was advised to take four aspirin and repeat every three hours until my ears rang, which certainly did help. Monday morning was a late start due to Columbus Day, so I went to Orthopedics and was outfitted with a steel-ribbed corset, which enabled me to continue my regular schedule. Over the decades I had several recurrences, which were always managed with the aspirin regimen and the corset. I still prefer medical management of back pain unless very specific conditions are diagnosed.

I also pursued a research question during the two internship and residency years, the basis of hormone activities associated with certain cancers. The prevailing notion was chaotic synthesis of peptides in cancers; my alternative was production of exactly the normal amino acid sequence of peptide hormones produced in endocrine glands through de-repression in the non-endocrine tumors of the genes specifying those molecules. Surgery and pathology faculty were very supportive of my review of cases for the *Journal of Thoracic and Cardiovascular Surgery, Cancer*, and an invited commentary in the *Annals of Internal Medicine*.

Serving Our Country During the Vietnam War

In the 1960s, all young men were subject to the military draft. Medical Students were offered deferments under the Berry Plan to serve where assigned later as physicians. Many of us with academic medicine aspirations and early track records were assigned to clinical or research duty as officers in the US Public Health Service at the National Institutes of Health (NIH), while others served in the Indian Health Service, the Centers for Disease Control, or the military. One of my good friends among the surgical house staff was Dr. Bion Philipson, who became the first physician fatality in Vietnam. I have many times visited him through the black granite wall of the Vietnam War Memorial across Constitution Avenue from the National Academy of Sciences in Washington, DC.

I worked very productively on protein structure and function with Dr. Christian B. Anfinsen at NIH (Fig. 18.3), with a broad range of studies of the enzyme Staphylococcal nuclease. Anfinsen was a pioneer who deduced and experimentally demonstrated that the primary amino acid structure of proteins determines their three-dimensional active conformation, for which he shared the 1972 Nobel Prize in Chemistry. He loved to work in the lab himself. He enjoyed daily informal lunches in the conference room with the fellows and technicians. He had a splendid group of younger colleagues and visiting scientists, especially from the Weizmann Institute in Israel, where he eventually became a member of the Board of Governors. This period was a great time for the NIH Intramural Program, with many outstanding senior scientists before so many medical schools built up huge research faculties, and with the "yellow berets," young physician-scientists spared the risks of the "green berets" in Vietnam. We worked hard to try to make a difference through research in the lives of people everywhere. Several of Chris' trainees became prominent translational physician-scientists.

Two community activities bear mention from this period. Along with several others from the NIH, I helped form a chapter of the Medical Committee for Human Rights (MCHR). We worked with local leaders in DC to assist youth job training programs by providing much-needed medical exams. Later we provided "medical presence" at the 1969 Presidential Inauguration, which erupted in demonstrations and arrests. One of our volunteers, a community physician, resuscitated a National

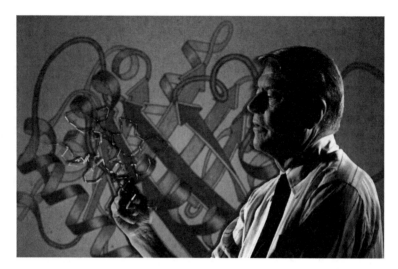

Fig. 18.3 Christian B. Anfinsen, Laboratory of Chemical Biology, National Institutes of Health, Bethesda

Guard soldier from Illinois on duty in the DC prison; Illinois Senator Everett McKinley Dirksen wrote a letter to MCHR thanking us profusely for our presence and service to all parties. This was a time when the House of Representatives Committee on Un-American Activities, a relic of the McCarthy era, subpoenaed our Chicago colleague, Dr. Quentin Young, to decry medical services to demonstrators (and a few police) in Chicago at the 1968 Democratic Convention. Meanwhile, in 1969, Sidney Wolfe and I persuaded Ralph Nader to address the national meeting of MCHR we were hosting in DC. After completing his work at NIH and residency in Cleveland, Sidney returned to became head of Ralph's Health Research Group, which has had tremendous influence on drug and device hazards for almost 40 years.

To Seattle for 28 Years

Everyone I consulted about pursuing a career in Medical Genetics encouraged me to go to the University of Washington in Seattle for fellowship training with Dr. Arno Motulsky and then consider applying to their institution for a first faculty appointment. I was interviewed in Bethesda by Arno's colleague, Dr. Stan Gartler, and was chosen for a position by Arno. When I received a US Public Health Service fellowship award, I learned from the fine print that the $9,000 annual stipend would be tax-free if I were pursuing a degree. I earned a PhD in Genetics while serving as a fellow in medical genetics. My fellowship proposal was focused on using affinity chromatography, newly developed by Pedro Cuatrecasas and Meir Wilchek in the Anfinsen Lab, to study inherited variation in thyroid-binding globulin.

By the time I arrived in Seattle, however, I wanted to do something more ambitious. I approached Dr. Motulsky about applying biochemical genetic techniques to the central nervous system and human behavior. He was delighted, saying he had hoped to find someone to do so for years. However, he warned me that it was high-risk, might not be successful, and would be viewed as "outside the mainstream of Internal Medicine." He gave me a stack of books and a list of articles to start reading. And he launched me on what would be a multi-faceted application of electrophoretic screening for polymorphisms of genes governing every step of glycolysis and as many other enzymes as we could find or devise specific stains; of pharmacologic agents for targeting certain enzymes, receptors, and reuptake mechanisms for pharmacogenetic variation; and of early techniques for assessing gene expression differences in different regions of the brain, using Cot curves for hybridization and isolation of single-copy DNA. I participated in the Winter Brain Research Conferences in Keystone, Colorado. Despite many fine publications, I cannot claim to have made a remarkable breakthrough on causes or therapies for specific diseases. I was fortunate to have funding from the National Genetics Foundation, a NIH Research Career Development Award, and the Howard Hughes Medical Institute (HHMI), and I have now enjoyed 40 years of stimulating interactions and joint publications with Arno Motulsky (Fig. 18.4).

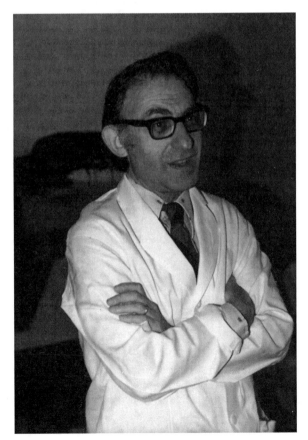

Fig. 18.4 Arno G. Motulsky, Division of Medical Genetics, University of Washington, Seattle, WA. Courtesy of Dr. Arno Motulsky and the University of Washington Division of Medical Genetics

Early in my time as a Fellow, Dr. Motulsky sent me in his place to an interesting conference on "Genetics, Environment, and Behavior." I presented our joint paper and became sufficiently involved in the conference that I was asked to serve as a co-editor for the resulting book. That experience led to many more as editor.

In 1970, I was on the speaker circuit for a hotly contested ballot initiative that liberalized indications for abortions in the State of Washington. Meanwhile, in our Genetic Counseling Clinic, we had patients in whom we were able to perform the first prenatal diagnoses with x-ray (thrombocytopenia with absent radii, TAR syndrome), with ultrasound (primary microcephaly), and with autosomal linkage (myotonic dystrophy).

An Interlude for One Year in Washington DC

While at NIH, I met Dr. Caro Luhrs, the first physician and third woman in the White House Fellows program launched by Lyndon Johnson and John Gardner in 1965, bringing about 15 young Americans to DC to work with members of the Cabinet or the White House staff and help them become more deeply engaged citizens for the rest of their diverse careers. Every year, she encouraged me to apply. Finally, in 1972, I did so. My Chief of Medicine, Dr. Robert Petersdorf, was skeptical that my activities as a Democrat would survive the Nixon administration's selection process, but I would be ineligible (more than 35 years old) if I waited four more years, and the program was supposed to be non-partisan. In May 1973, I was chosen for this program, and, after interesting interviews at several agencies, I was placed as Special Assistant to the Chairman of the US Atomic Energy Commission (AEC). My assignment was to staff an interagency work group on Project Independence, to reduce US dependence on imported oil. With a sense of urgency from the Arab Oil Embargo of 1973, we produced a fine report on time December 1. Dr. Dixy Lee Ray, the AEC Chairman and work group chair, surprised many by placing technologies to increase energy yield from fuels, enhanced oil and gas recovery, and cleaner coal production ahead of nuclear reactor improvements and long-term renewable energy sources. Thirty-six years later, as I said in my American Association for the Advancement of Science presidential address in 2006, that agenda is, unfortunately, still fresh.

Then I was secunded to the State Department and Undersecretary William Donaldson as part of a small group on cooperation with allies about energy R&D, oil sharing, and financing mechanisms. We went to Brussels twice, as I was involved in the R&D discussions. In May, when the Indians detonated a nuclear device in Rajasthan, near Pakistan, the French promptly offered to sell the nuclear fuel cycle to Pakistan. Ambassador to India Daniel Patrick Moynihan called for expert help. Seven weeks later, I was the person sent! First I went to Paris, meeting with the French minister who Dr. Ray and I had hosted at the AEC months earlier; he had noted her poodle and expressed the sentiment that he would be the most popular father in France if he could find a similar poodle for his 11-year-old daughter. Having made a mental note, Dr. Ray sent him the offspring of her poodle a few months later. I was welcomed warmly, as a participant in the whole saga. Soon after, the French quietly withdrew their offer of the nuclear fuel cycle to Pakistan. While in Paris, I arranged to have dinner with an American lawyer who had been a finalist in the White House Fellows competition. He brought to dinner an American friend, Martha Darling, who was moving to Seattle after four years consulting in Paris. She later became my wife, so in retrospect meeting her was the highlight of the trip.

I then made a stop in Israel, where I met in Jerusalem with Professor Katchalski, by then President of Israel and known as Ephraim Katzir. We had a warm personal discussion and then turned to diplomatic matters. President Nixon had just been to the Middle East, his final trip before his resignation, and surprised US experts and the world media by proposing to sell nuclear reactors to Egypt and Israel. President Katzir calmly informed me (and I cabled the State Department) that Israel would welcome an opportunity to help Egypt become less dependent upon Arab oil-producing countries and was confident that undergrounding and other security measures could make the reactors safe. Nixon resigned, and this idea evaporated. However, the exchange may have assisted in the journey to the Camp David Accord that President Jimmy Carter negotiated with Menachem Begin and Anwar Sadat. Remarkably, I was there in 1979 when President Carter brought Sadat and Begin to the White House lawn to sign the Accord. Meanwhile, in 1974, I had gone on to formal discussions in India, Nepal, Tokyo, and Hong Kong about nuclear matters.

Even after such heady experiences in the science policy world, there was no letdown upon returning home to Seattle, the University of Washington, and my young children from my first marriage. I was invited to speak about biochemical and genetic studies of the brain at a remarkable two-day program called, "The Majesty of Man," at Stanford in January 1975, along with a Stanford neurophysiologist. We were basically warm-ups for the conversations about the brain and the mind with Linus Pauling, Joshua Lederberg, and Artur Rubinstein, led by David Hamburg and Edward Rubenstein. Dr. Petersdorf, recognizing my policy interests, had proposed me as Program Director for the University of Washington Clinical Scholars Program, which was funded competitively by the Robert Wood Johnson Foundation. We had six Scholars per year, who have done remarkably well. Meanwhile, my renewed brain genetics research led to appointment as a Howard Hughes Investigator, and I resumed my inpatient attending responsibilities in Internal Medicine.

Back to Washington DC: The Virtues of a Physician-Scientist Background

In April 1977, Dr. Hamburg from Stanford, now President of the Institute of Medicine of the National Academy of Sciences, called to alert me that Dr. Frank Press would be calling me shortly. Yes, I was slightly aware from news in *Science* magazine that Dr. Press, a leading geophysicist, had been announced as President Carter's Science and Technology Advisor. Dr. Press did indeed call and informed me that he had a search on for a deputy in the life sciences and health domain. He was keen to meet me. I responded that I was coming at the end of the month for the annual Clinical Research meetings in DC and would be happy to meet with him. He told me that he had already ordered an airplane ticket for me and would appreciate my coming in three days! When I arrived, he had lined up the Director of NIH, the Commissioner of the Food and Drug Administration, the President of the National Academy of Sciences, and the President of the Institute of Medicine to interview me, to tell me I was needed in DC, and to promise to help me personally. It was a wrenching decision, requiring me to give up the HHMI position and put aside the research I had so recently worked hard to re-establish, as well as to leave my kids and now also Martha in Seattle. Moreover, I was committed to do my Internal Medicine attending for the month of June. I asked the White House operator to find Dr. Petersdorf, who was at an American College of Physicians meeting in Dallas. He took the call and said, "I know why you are calling; I've already been called twice." When I assured him I would not go until July, so I could meet my commitment (a very competitive assignment in our huge Department of Medicine), he cut me off, saying, "I will find someone to cover, or I'll do it for you myself." I started June 1.

I had a fascinating and productive two and a half years in the Office of Science and Technology Policy (OSTP); a report on OSTP during our time was published by Dr. Press in the January 9 and 16, 1981 issues of *Science* magazine (Fig. 18.5). Memorable projects and responsibilities included chairing a 22-agency task force on Human Nutrition Research, which the Senate Agriculture Committee had just assigned to the Department to Agriculture, rather than NIH; implementing

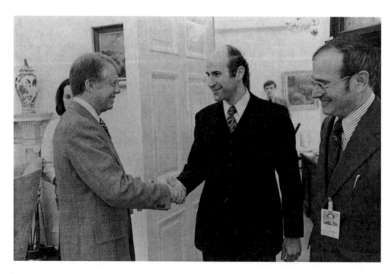

Fig. 18.5 With President Jimmy Carter and Dr. Frank Press, Science and Technology Adviser to the President, in The White House (1980). Courtesy of the Jimmy Carter Library

the President's theme of "basic research as an investment in the Nation's future" across all the Cabinet departments through close coordination with the Office of Management and Budget (OMB); trying to stimulate the biomedical community to appreciate and undertake "regulatory science," critical to rational, well-informed regulatory decision-making at FDA, Environmental Protection Agency (EPA), Occupational Safety and Health Administration (OSHA), and other agencies; and proposals deflected by NIH to fund cross-NIH initiatives from the Director's office and create potentially distinctive programs for the Intramural Program of NIH. A notable conflict occurred over a proposal from Health, Education & Welfare Secretary Califano for immunization against the "Russian flu," just two years after the much-criticized immunization of 40 million Americans against the "swine flu" of 1976. Califano wanted a program similarly large, so that a special budget line and appropriation would be needed, rather than a more focused effort which could be forced into the existing budgets. OMB relied on and cited my criticisms to pass back a zero for this request, which produced outrage from the Secretary. OMB held firm.

A particularly relevant experience for the theme of this book was a visit from a delegation of physicians from the American Medical Association (AMA). They were very skeptical about government and about the young physician they met in his stately office in the Old Executive Office Building. They pointedly described me as a "bureaucrat." When I pleasantly informed them that I was just back from my annual weeklong visit to Alaska, part of our Medical Genetics outreach from Seattle, during which I had seen 50 patients and their physicians with known or potential genetic disorders or birth defects, those MD-politicians were disarmed.

With a year to go in the President's term, there was a vacancy at a high level in the OMB. The OMB leaders analyzed their strengths and needs by program and department. They knew me very well from my regular participation in key sessions on agency budgets and appointed me Program Associate Director for a portfolio covering 53% of the whole federal budget (Health & Human Services; Education; Labor; Veterans Administration (VA); 60% of Agriculture; plus 24 other agencies). It was a difficult political year, after very high interest rates imposed by the Federal Reserve, the Iranian capture of American hostages and the failed rescue, the primary challenge from Senator Kennedy, and the draining re-election campaign against Reagan and Anderson. But the processes of government must go forward, so I had a lot of responsibility dealing with the departments' and agencies' budgets and working with others on such challenges as the Cuban and Haitian refugee crises.

In November 1980, Ronald Reagan was elected President. The incumbent still had to deliver a full budget proposal for what would be the 1982 Fiscal Year, just as President Ford had done in 1976. The day after the election, the Dean of the Woodrow Wilson School of Public and International Affairs at Princeton, Donald Stokes, on whose advisory committee I had been appealing for them to address science and technology issues in public policy, knowing I was on leave until July, called to offer me a visiting professor appointment and a chance to help them create such a new program emphasis. That turned out very well, with a flourishing program to this day. Then I was appointed the first Science, Engineering, and Public Policy Fellow at The Brookings Institution and wrote a book with economist Lester Lave on "Clearing the Air" about the Clean Air Act, as well as several joint articles about our "value of information" model for various schemes of testing for carcinogenicity of chemicals. My kids, Rachel and Jason, visited my very small office at Brookings and asked what happened to the desk and flags, big tables, and sofa of my OMB office! Finally, in spring 1982, Martha (who had served as a White House Fellow with Secretary of the Treasury Michael Blumenthal and then as Finance Committee legislative aide for Senator Bill Bradley) and I returned to Seattle.

Back to the University of Washington for Eco-genetics and then Public Health

The Dean of the School of Public Health & Community Medicine, Dr. Robert Day, focused on my well-developed scientific and policy interests in eco-genetics (the interaction of genetic and environmental factors in disease) to recruit me to be Chair of the Department of Environmental Health, while continuing my appointment in Internal Medicine. We turned a somewhat sleepy department into one of the national leaders. I gave up the lab reserved for me to recruit additional young faculty, all of whom progressed to be full professors and leaders in their disciplines. During 1982, I served on the National Research Council committee that produced the landmark "Red Book" on Risk Assessment in the Federal Government. A decade later, I was appointed by the Speaker of the House and elected by my fellow members to chair the Presidential/Congressional Commission on Risk Assessment and Risk Management; we held hearings each month around the country and published a two-volume report which has been utilized extensively in the USA and around the world as a framework for risk assessment. Risk assessment is a combination of science, medicine, and public policy.

Six months later, Day became President of the Fred Hutchinson Cancer Research Center and I was chosen to be the Dean of Public Health. Over the next 15 years, the Chairs and I led by example, with a high percentage of our time on competitive research grants (approximately 80% in my case) while fulfilling our administrative and teaching responsibilities. I moved my research to the Cancer Center, focusing on a long-term clinical chemoprevention trial of beta-carotene and vitamin A (CARET) to try to prevent lung cancers and heart disease endpoints and a series of analyses of the benefits of smoking cessation. I also co-founded the Consortium for Risk Evaluation with Stakeholder Evaluation (with Charles Powers, Bernard Goldstein, Arthur Upton, and Jack Moore) to deal with environmental contamination at the Hanford Nuclear Reservation in eastern Washington, established one of the first three Centers for Disease Control and Prevention Research Centers (focused on Keeping Older People Healthy and Independent), and led a Robert

Wood Johnson–W.K. Kellogg joint program called Turning Point to transform public health practice around the country. Every five years, I challenged myself and my colleagues to lay out a fresh strategic plan to justify continuing in the deanship.

A Big Move from Seattle to Ann Arbor, Michigan: Back to Medicine

After 15 years in public health, I had an opportunity to move back into the medical mainstream as the first Executive Vice-President for Medical Affairs (EVPMA) at the University of Michigan (UM). The immediate challenge was to overcome a reimbursement squeeze by Medicare, Medicaid, and the Blues that caused a (modest) deficit for the first time in memory at Michigan. The larger challenge was to bridge the common gulf between the academic approach of a medical school dean and the business approach of the hospital chief executive. We created the UM Health System, embracing the medical school, the hospitals and clinics, the M-CARE HMO, and life sciences technology transfer. We built a strategic plan on synergies across the missions of education, research, and clinical services (as mentioned in the Introduction to this essay). We turned around the financial picture and enhanced the surplus annually. We launched a Biological Sciences Scholars Program to compete for some of the very best new faculty candidates in the country; that group now numbers more than 50 junior faculty (several of them now full professors). Mid-career faculty took note and brushed off inquiries or offers due to the excitement of these developments in Ann Arbor. We invested in infrastructure for clinical research and clinical research training and in supporting technology development projects in the "valley of death" between discovery and validation. We had several splendid capital projects, including the Biomedical Sciences Research Building, featuring an inspirational "Flame of Wisdom" sculpture by Mexican artist Leonardo Nierman, and a magnificent five-story Omenn Atrium.

After five years as EVPMA, I was still able to compete for funding for a Michigan Proteomics Alliance for Cancer Research program project grant and help win one of the seven NIH Roadmap National Centers for Biomedical Computing while heading the University-wide Center for Computational Medicine and Bioinformatics and serving as an associate director for our Clinical and Translational Science Award (CTSA) grant and the Michigan Institute for Clinical and Health Research. Just as in the OSTP and OMB, the decades of experience as physician and as scientist provided a foundation for leadership responsibilities and for in-depth research and the testing of new ideas. I've been Chair of the International Human Proteome Organization Human Plasma Project Porteome since 2002. In our Proteomics Alliance, seven junior faculty have been awarded their first NIH R01 grants, allowing them to launch their independent research careers. This is quite gratifying. The associated publications have included proteomics applications to induced neurodifferentiation of human embryonic stem cells, discovery of sarcosine as a mediator and biomarker of metastasis in prostate cancers, characterization of alternative splice variants as a new class of protein biomarker candidates in cancers, and a comprehensive discovery engine for fusion genes in cancers.

Reflecting on a Career as Physician-Scientist

In 2004, the White House Fellows Association presented me the John W. Gardner Legacy of Leadership Award. Martha and I had the pleasure of knowing John and his wife Aida personally. His was a creative, fertile mind. He excelled both in the academic and public policy spheres. He prided himself on an action-oriented life, as he wrote in his book *On Leadership* [2]. His legacy includes the White House Fellows program, Common Cause, The Independent Sector, and the National Civic League. John wrote that leaders have the following characteristics:

1. They think longer-term—beyond the day's crises, beyond the quarterly report, beyond the horizon.
2. They look beyond the unit they are heading and grasp its relationship to larger realities—the larger organization of which they are a part, conditions external to the organization, global trends.
3. They reach and influence constituents beyond their jurisdictions, beyond bureaucratic boundaries. They may bind together the fragmented constituencies that must work together to solve a problem.
4. They put heavy emphasis on the intangibles of vision, values, and motivation, and understand intuitively the non-rational and unconscious elements in the leader-constituent interaction.
5. They have the political skill to cope with the conflicting requirements of multiple constituencies.
6. They think in terms of renewal. They seek revisions of processes and structures when required by ever-changing reality.

John Gardner championed leadership opportunities for people at every stage of life and at every level in the multiple communities in which we live. I have quoted him in my relationships with the members of my research groups and with the 15,000 people for whom I was responsible as CEO of the University of Michigan Health System. I share his conviction that every individual can develop leadership qualities. In addition, I thank my parents for instilling that sense of unlimited opportunity, a perspective we treasure in this great country, as well as a sense of responsibility to make a difference for others. In this context, we are proud of our son David, who at age 25 is now in his fifth year with Teach for America.

One of the most remarkable human attributes is curiosity. Inspired by Walt Whitman, I asked my 1965 medical school graduating class and their assembled families to think how curious and open to discovery nearly every child appears to be. Then I asked them to ponder what we do that suppresses that curiosity as children grow up, when questions are too complex or too embarrassing, at home and in our schools and workplaces. We could do much more to nurture curiosity at all ages.

Another important attribute is what W.H. Auden called "the capacity to suspend one's beliefs" or prior views and knowledge. The aim is to be open to learning—learning from fellow students, colleagues, workers, and visitors from other cultures and with other experiences; learning from the study of history and philosophy and science; and learning from observation and experimentation, from problem-solving as well as misadventures, in building a better future for our immediate communities and for the larger world.

This leads to a third crucial attribute of scientific thinking—the organized search for evidence and the skeptical probing of the available evidence. This applies to all kinds of decision-making. My own combined background in science and medicine has proved very helpful in policy and leadership positions. When I worked in the OSTP 32 years ago, the combination of science and medicine provided me with essential skills for this senior position. Upon reflection, I realized that science leads one to seek detailed knowledge and high predictive capability, dotting the "i"s and crossing the "t"s, while gaining a basis for generalization. By contrast, as physicians, we know that we must respond to the patient, decide on a therapy or test, and explain our advice or plan to the patient and family with whatever information is at hand or readily obtained. We must respond on someone else's timetable. This is exactly what happens in making policy judgments or administrative decisions, which generally depend on someone else's timetable.

I have found science tremendously energizing—from research at Princeton and Harvard Medical School to NIH, then Seattle, and now Michigan. From basic biochemical genetics, I became fascinated with the clinical and public health potential of genetics and the intersections of scientific discoveries, public policies, and law and ethics. Organizing a first-year Harvard Medical School symposium on Psychiatry and the Law connected me with Judge David Bazelon, who took me under his wing 12 years later when I came to DC in 1973 as a White House Fellow.

I took the "road less traveled" several times, applying genetic methods to the brain and human behaviors long before it was popular, focusing on differences in susceptibility among people exposed when the risk assessments for environmentally mediated disorders were only about the hazardous chemicals, developing major studies on prevention of cancers at a time when nearly all the research funding was going to treatment of patients already afflicted, moving from medicine to public health in 1981 and then back to medicine as CEO of a large academic health system in 1997, and returning to lab science and entering the newly emerging fields of systems biology and computational medicine since 2002.

We can all help our protégés and the diverse people John Gardner chose to call constituents to exceed our own accomplishments, to draw satisfaction from learning and doing what can benefit others, and to leave trails where no paths previously were recognized.

References

1. Omenn GS (2010) Ephriam Katchalski Katzir. Physics Today, pp. 57–58
2. Gardner JW (1990) *On Leadership*. Free Press, New York

Nineteen
Pursuit of a Patient-Oriented Research Career as a Physician-Scientist

Robert W. Schrier

In the 1850s, my mother's grandparents emigrated from Ireland at the time of the potato famine in that country. Bridget Kelly and John Moynahan married and settled in Lexington, Kentucky. Their son, James Moynahan, then married Ann Armstrong, and their third child was Helen Mae Moynahan, my mother. At 23 years of age she moved to Indianapolis, IN and entered the Indianapolis City Hospital School of Nursing. My grandparents on my father's side, George Schrier and Sophie Achopol, both emigrated from the House of Hannover, which is the present area of northern Germany and the eastern part of the Netherlands. This was probably why some relatives told me that they were of German descent and others that they were Dutch. My paternal grandparents married and moved to Seymour, IN where they became farmers. Their son, Arthur, my father, moved to Indianapolis where he obtained a job as a printer. He and my mother met and married in Indianapolis. My older brother, Dick, was then born, followed 18 months later by my birth, February 19, 1936.

In 1939, at age 29, our father developed extremely high blood pressure (malignant hypertension) with failure of the heart, kidney, and brain. At that time, there were no medications available to treat high blood pressure. He was hospitalized in Indianapolis at the Eli Lilly Clinic, which was associated with the Marion County General Hospital, where I ultimately had my rotating internship. Experts in high blood pressure were there, but no effective medicines to treat high blood pressure were available. Thus, the only treatment my father received was a barbiturate, phenobarbital. Similarly, in 1945, President Franklin Delano Roosevelt had an extremely high blood pressure of 230/130 mmHg (normal is less than 140/90 mmHg) at the World War II Yalta Conference with no treatment available. FDR died of a stroke a couple of months after Yalta. My father's fate was similar, and his premature death was devastating for my mother. I don't believe that she ever completely recovered emotionally from the loss of someone whom she loved very much. She always wondered whether his death had to do with his job as a printer. I also have wondered whether malignant high blood pressure in a young man of

R.W. Schrier (✉)
University of Colorado Denver, Aurora, CO, USA
e-mail: robert.schrier@ucdenver.edu

D.A. Schwartz (ed.), *Medicine Science and Dreams*,
DOI 10.1007/978-90-481-9538-1_19, © Springer Science+Business Media B.V. 2011

European descent might have been due to lead poisoning related to his profession as a printer. In the fifteenth century, lead was already important in the development of the printing press. At the time of my father's death, in addition to printing type, paint, gasoline, pipes, and many other items contained lead, even though lead was already known to have toxic effects. In fact, there was evidence of lead poisoning in ancient Rome. Moreover, lead is now known to damage blood vessels and cause high blood pressure.

My mother later married James DeVore, and they welcomed my half-sister, Geraldine Ann, into the family. James entered the Army during World War II and spent four years in North Africa, so my mother was in essence a single parent for several years. While our mother was a private duty and school nurse, Dick and I had substantial free time after school. Fortunately, my brother and I developed a passion for sports. In some ways, athletics took the place of a father for my brother and me. I did not remember my father since I was 3 years old when he died. Dick, however, had some memories and said that our father had a great love of baseball and took us to some games at Victory Field, the home of the minor league team, the Indianapolis Indians. At Thomas Carr Howe High School we both played baseball, basketball, and football. Dick was all-city in football and I was all-city in basket-ball. Sports contributed substantially to our opportunity to attend college—the first in our family to do so. Dick obtained a scholarship in football at Indiana Central College which is now Indianapolis University. He was the starting quarterback for four years, was all-conference three years, and established a four-year record with a total of 36 touchdown passes. He was also all-conference for three years in baseball.

During my senior year at Howe High School, Al Feasle, the Brooklyn Dodger scout who had signed Gil Hodges and Carl Erskine from the same summer base-ball team, P.R. Mallory, that Dick and I played for, called and asked me to attend the Brooklyn Dodger spring training camp in Florida. I was very excited but had already accepted a Rector Scholarship at DePauw University. I had been invited, and visited Indiana University and met with the head basketball coach, Branch McCracken, and visited Michigan State and met the head coach, Pete Newell—both were well-known basketball coaches. DePauw, however, had offered me a four-year academic scholar-ship which was more secure than an athletic scholarship. Moreover, my mother and the DePauw Director of Admissions, John Wittich (still a wonderful friend) empha-sized the importance of scholarship over athletics. I also thought that I could start as a freshman on the varsity basketball team at DePauw. That summer I broke my ankle sliding in a baseball game, so I was glad to have accepted an academic schol-arship. With respect to the Brooklyn Dodger invitation, I learned that at that time if one participated in any professional sport, he was ineligible to participate in any college sport. Although I certainly wanted a college education and liked baseball, my main desire as a Hoosier was to play college basketball (Figs. 19.1 and 19.2).

When asked to indicate my major at DePauw University, I was a bit perplexed. However, my mother was a nurse and she suggested a pre-med major. So a pre-med major it was. Nine of ten pre-med DePauw students switch from their pre-med major after their first year, most because of the chemistry and physics classes. I had never taken either class in high school, so I also was very intimidated by these topics.

Fig. 19.1 Three-time-All-Conference in Basketball and Baseball at DePauw University

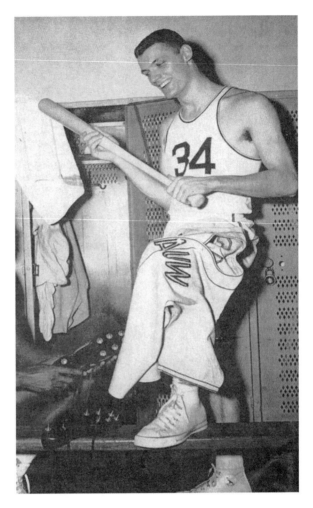

Somehow, however, I barely survived these classes and a very busy freshman year. In addition to my pre-med classes, I waited tables at a sorority house for my meals, started on the varsity basketball and baseball team, and was a Sigma Nu pledge. I was fortunate to break the single season basketball scoring record for DePauw during my freshman year.

My minor at DePauw University was philosophy-religion. In fact, as I look back, these courses may have had more impact on my life as a physician-scientist than the science courses. The desire not just to treat ill patients, but also to discover new means to understand, prevent, and treat illnesses perhaps began to percolate in my mind with these courses. Later, I also recognized that moral and ethical issues are frequently encountered in the practice of medicine.

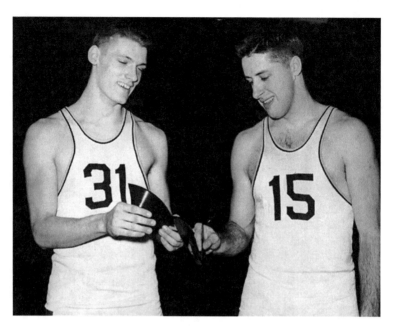

Fig. 19.2 "Breaking the Single Season Depauw Record" in basketball in the season which just closed were Bob Schrier, with 321 points, and Gene Loercher (*right*) with 309. Schrier is a freshman, Loercher a senior

After graduation, rather than heading straight to medical school, I applied for a one-year Fulbright scholarship to study anthropology at Johannes Gutenberg University in Mainz, Germany. It was a great year. The love of my life, Barbara Lindley, also a DePauw student, was taking a year abroad in Stockholm at the same time. We ended up traveling with an international student group to Leningrad and Moscow over the Christmas holiday. Barbara then transferred for her second semester to Gutenberg University to study German. I am not sure that was the reason, but nevertheless, we have been married for 50 years as of June 14, 2009 (Fig. 19.3).

After returning from Europe, I entered Indiana University School of Medicine and Barbara finished her last year at DePauw University. Shortly after her graduation, we married. Since we were both broke, we postponed our honeymoon but have made up for it over the years. Barbara began teaching English in high school and I continued with my medical career studies. During medical school and internship at Marion County General Hospital we had our two oldest children, David and Debbie. Since I had been told that my father died of Bright's diseases, a general term for kidney disease, I decided to review his autopsy. The autopsy revealed that he did not have primary kidney disease, but rather had necrotizing arteriolar kidney disease, which was typical for malignant hypertension as was his heart failure and encephalopathy. Nevertheless, it is indeed ironic that I ended up being a physician-scientist in the area of kidney disease and hypertension. It is now clear that hypertension can be either a cause or a result of kidney disease. Currently there

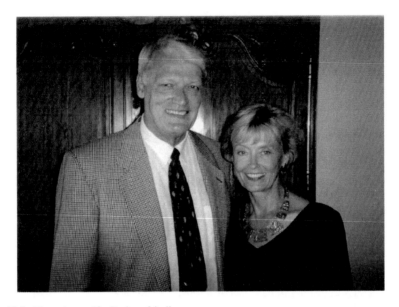

Fig. 19.3 Me and my wife, Barbara Lindley

are over 100 different medications to lower blood pressure in hypertensive patients, thereby protecting the heart, kidney, and brain.

During my rotating internship, I decided to pursue the specialty of internal medicine and was accepted into an excellent program at the University of Washington in Seattle. The time in Seattle was when I really became interested in patient-oriented studies. In spite of being on call every third night and having our third child, Douglas, I was able to publish several papers about patient-related problems in excellent clinical journals. These clinical problems included steroid-induced pancreatitis, fat necrosis mimicking erythema nodosa, kidney diseases related to penicillin homologues, and spinal fluid acidosis in pulmonary-related brain dysfunction. With support from the professor of medicine, Robert W. Williams, MD, a renowned endocrinologist, I next went to the Peter Bent Brigham Hospital at Harvard University where I launched my interest in clinical disorders of sodium (salt) and water. In Boston, during the middle of my first research year, in which I was studying kidney factors which were independent of aldosterone, the hormone that causes the kidney to retain sodium, I received a draft notice from the Department of Defense. This was in 1965 when we were in the middle of the Vietnam War. With a commitment of three years rather than the normal two years for drafted physicians, I was assigned to Walter Reed General Hospital (WRGH) and the Division of Metabolism at the Walter Reed Research Institute. This also was an outstanding experience, which enriched my interest in becoming a physician-scientist with a focus on patient-oriented clinical investigation.

On entering the US Army Medical Corp, basic training for physicians occurred at Fort Sam Houston in San Antonio, Texas. The temperature in San Antonio during the summer was in the 100s and the humidity was in the 90s. There had been a history of young military recruits developing heat stroke and dying during basic training. During my six weeks of training in San Antonio (summer of 1966), I certainly recognized how unacclimatized recruits who had been working in air-conditioned offices could develop heat stroke during basic training at Fort Sam Houston.

After San Antonio, I was pleased to be reunited with Barbara and the children at our new home in Silver Springs, Maryland, where we had our fourth child, Derek. The work at WRGH involved caring for injured soldiers transferred mostly from Vietnam. That summer we had our first soldier admitted for heat stroke and acute kidney failure. In recent years, there had been five such soldiers admitted to WRGH and all had died. We therefore were told by the career Army physicians that these recruits had multiorgan disease including the brain, liver, and kidney secondary to hyperthermia and thus heat stroke with kidney failure was a fatal disease. In reviewing the medical records of these five cases, however, an important observation emerged. Their acute kidney failure had been treated with continuous peritoneal dialysis, and yet their indices of impaired kidney function, blood urea nitrogen (BUN), and serum creatinine concentrations, continued to rise until their demise. These are the poisons normally eliminated by the intact kidney. This observation told us two things—the patients were breaking down their tissues, and releasing poisons into the blood stream. The peritoneal form of dialysis treatment was inadequate to remove these poisons. We also discovered that the major site of tissue breakdown was in the muscles. The initial clue was the finding of very high circulating levels of a muscle enzyme, namely creatine phosphokinase (CPK). Based on these observations, we proposed to use the much more efficient artificial kidney, i.e., hemodialysis, to remove the poisons from the blood in these young soldiers having acute kidney failure associated with heat stroke. That summer we had ten young recruits who had developed heat stroke and acute kidney failure during basic training in a hot humid environment. Aggressive treatment with the artificial kidney more effectively removed the poisons in the blood and allowed time for recovery of their muscle injury and acute kidney failure. As a result, eight of the ten soldiers survived their heat stroke, acute kidney failure, and damage to their other organs. We published these clinical results, which led to improved care of soldiers with heat stroke and kidney failure. These experiences lead to my life-long research career focused on the causes, diagnosis, and treatment of acute kidney injury.

During my military service, I was also allowed to continue a research interest in disorders of sodium and water homeostasis, which also had implications for military casualties. This involved several months of experimental research with Professor Hugh de Wardener in London. Our fifth child, Denise, was born in London. While this time in London prolonged my three-year commitment, the time with de Wardener was worth the extension. He had the unique capacity to ask clinically relevant questions which led to important hypotheses and patient-oriented research. "Prof" continues to be a friend and mentor for me.

After my time in the US Army Medical Corp, during in which I reached the rank of Major, I was convinced that I wanted to pursue a career in academic medicine with a focus on patient-oriented research. After visiting several university medical centers, I accepted a position at the University of California in San Francisco. In San Francisco, I became interested in the regulation of water excretion by the kidney. This is an important area because the body composition is two-thirds water. A hormone named antidiuretic hormone was known to normally regulate water excretion by the kidney and thereby to keep the amount of water in the normal body constant. However, abnormal water retention by the kidney was known to occur in diseases, including heart failure and cirrhosis. Moreover, the capacity of antidiuretic hormone to regulate the kidneys' capacity to maintain normal body water is drastically disturbed in patients with these diseases. In a series of five papers published in the *Journal of Clinical Investigation*, I and my research team demonstrated the mechanism whereby there is a constant release of antidiuretic hormone so that the kidney cannot excrete the water ingested. This important finding led to the hypothesis that this mechanism, termed non-osmotic antidiuretic secretion, accounts for the water retention in heart failure, cirrhosis, and other important diseases. We supported this hypothesis initially by measuring plasma antidiuretic hormone with a sensitive radioimmunoassay. More recently, with the use of drugs, which block the action of antidiuretic hormone, the abnormal water retention in patients with heart failure, cirrhosis, and other water-retaining diseases was reversed. These drugs are now clinically available to reverse the abnormal water retention by the kidney in heart failure, cirrhosis, and other diseases. From a clinical viewpoint, water retention which dilutes body sodium, causing so-called hyponatremia, has been shown to be a major risk factor for increased mortality in heart failure and liver disease and is associated with impaired mentation, gait disturbances, falls, and hip fractures. Thus, these new drugs that block antidiuretic hormone have important clinical indications.

Peter Agre received the Nobel Prize in Chemistry in 2003 for his discovery of the first water channel in the kidney. In our experimental studies in heart failure and liver disease, we had shown the clinical importance of these water channels, which are regulated by antidiuretic hormone. This was no doubt the reason that Peter Agre asked us to join him and his family for the Nobel celebration in Stockholm. This personal journey studying the non-osmotic regulation of antidiuretic hormone in important clinical diseases has been very rewarding and has been supported by funding from the National Institutes of Health (NIH) for over 35 years.

Next, we decided to focus our research on sodium retention by the kidney which is the cause of edema and pulmonary congestion in patients with cardiac failure and cirrhosis. There were many dilemmas and difficulties when studying sodium-retaining states in patients with normal kidneys, including heart failure, liver disease, and pregnancy. When the kidneys from patients with terminal liver disease are transplanted into patients with terminal kidney disease but with normal liver function, the kidney no longer retains sodium. Similarly, heart transplantation into patients with heart failure reverses the avid sodium retention by the kidney.

The enigmatic term "decreased effective blood volume" was suggested as the undefined signal for sodium retention by the kidney in patients with heart failure. This is because total blood volume is expanded in patients with heart failure and cirrhosis, yet the kidneys paradoxically continue to retain sodium. To make the body fluid volume regulation even more perplexing, the sodium-losing hormone, i.e., natriuretic peptide, is increased in renal sodium-retaining patients with heart failure or liver disease. Furthermore, the role of the sodium-retaining hormone, aldosterone, was dismissed because some of the sodium-retaining heart or liver failure patients did not have elevated plasma concentrations of aldosterone. Moreover, supraphysiological amounts of aldosterone in normal subjects did not cause edema because the kidney "escapes" from the sodium-retaining effect of aldosterone. Thus, taken together, there was little understanding for the mechanisms whereby normal kidneys retain sodium in patients with heart failure and liver disease and even pregnant women.

Based on this background, we proposed our hypothesis of body fluid volume regulation by focusing on the above apparent dilemmas. The hypothesis indicated that total blood volume did not provide the signal for normal sodium excretion by the kidney. However, estimates of circulating total blood volume indicated that approximately 85% is on the low pressure, venous side of the circulation and approximately only 15% is on the arterial side of the circulation which perfuses vital organs including the kidney. Based on our observations that the non-osmotic antidiuretic hormone regulation is accompanied by activation of the sympathetic nervous system and angiotensin, which constrict blood vessels, and aldosterone, we proposed that the integrity of the "arterial circulation," not total circulating blood volume, primarily provides the signal for sodium excretion by the kidney. Thus, arterial underfilling secondary to a decrease in cardiac output triggers the sodium retention by the kidney in low-output heart failure. Furthermore, we proposed that the stretch baroreceptors in the arterial circulation sense arterial underfilling not only by a primary decrease in heart function, but also by a relative underfilling which occurs with primary systemic arterial vasodilation. Specifically, with liver disease, dilation of arterial blood vessels in the intestinal circulation triggers arterial underfilling, which leads to sodium retention by the kidney. This Primary Arterial Vasodilation Mechanism of renal sodium retention and ascites formation in cirrhosis is now widely accepted by the hepatology community.

The next dilemma in addressing body fluid volume regulation in disorders, such as heart failure and liver disease, was the role of aldosterone and natriuretic peptides. Both of these hormones primarily act in the kidney at distal nephron sites of the collecting duct, where only 2–4% of filtered sodium remains to be reclaimed or excreted. Thus, the amount of sodium delivered to this distal nephron site modulates the sodium-retaining effect of aldosterone and the sodium excretion by the natriuretic peptides. In normal individuals, the aldosterone "escape" from the hormone's sodium-retaining action occurs secondary to increased sodium delivery to the hormone's distal site of action in the kidney. In contrast, in heart and liver failure patients sodium delivery to the distal nephron is diminished, secondary to effects on the kidney by the sympathetic nervous system and angiotensin. Thus, in heart failure patients there is a failure to "escape" from the sodium-retaining action of aldosterone. Perhaps most important, aldosterone antagonists act by competitively inhibiting the action of endogenous aldosterone on its receptors in the distal portion of the kidney. Thus, since heart failure and liver disease patients may have high plasma aldosterone concentrations, modest doses of aldosterone antagonists (e.g., 25–50 mg/dl) may be inadequate to block the sodium-retaining action of high plasma levels of aldosterone. Thus, in heart failure patients, modest doses of aldosterone blockers do not increase sodium excretion. In contrast, we demonstrated that the aldosterone antagonist spironolactone, at higher doses, reversed the renal sodium, retention in patients with advanced heart failure. High doses of spironolactone in this amount are currently accepted therapy in liver failure patients with excess fluid and sodium in their abdomen, lungs, and extremities. The failure of natriuretic hormones to increase urinary sodium excretion in heart and liver failure patients was also shown to be due to diminished sodium delivery to their distal site of action in the kidney. Thus, my career as a physician-scientist has involved patient-oriented research in acute kidney failure, as well as water and sodium disorders, such as those occuring in heart or liver failure.

Patient-related studies in the hereditary disease in which cysts in the kidney impair function, namely autosomal dominant polycystic kidney disease (ADPKD), and high blood pressure in diabetes mellitus are additional reasons why my 40-year career as a physician-scientist continues to be rewarding. ADPKD is the most common life-threatening hereditary disease (prevalence 1–400 to 1–1,000 US patients). It is more common than the combined prevalence of Huntington's disease, hemophilia, cystic fibrosis, Down's syndrome, sickle cell disease, and myotonic dystrophy. When I first arrived from San Francisco to the University of Colorado, there were many patients with polycystic kidney disease in the clinics. We therefore decided to study the disease in these patients. Over several decades, we developed the largest patient-oriented ADPKD research center in the world, with a database of over 3,000 patients. Scores of patient-oriented publications have emerged over the last three decades from our ADPKD Research Center. These studies resulted in defining the natural history of the disease, which was shown to begin in childhood. The discovery of early high blood pressure, heart enlargement, and activation of the angiotensin and aldosterone systems in ADPKD patients has led to early detection and treatment of high blood pressure. Moreover, in the era of end stage kidney disease treatment, cardiovascular complications are the major cause of mortality in ADPKD patients. Thus, the early and aggressive treatment of high blood pressure in ADPKD patients has been an important clinical advance in the care of these ADPKD patients. Currently, we have two ongoing NIH-supported clinical interventional trials in adults and children with ADPKD.

On arrival in Colorado, one of the first referrals I received was a patient with diabetes mellitus. This patient had diabetic kidney disease with a loss of 50% of her kidney function and large amounts of protein in her urine excretion. At that time, the medical literature indicated that this patient would need end-stage kidney treatment with either chronic dialysis or kidney transplantation within three to five years. I noted, however, that her blood pressure had not been well controlled. Thus, I instituted a more aggressive regime to control her blood pressure to less than 130/80 mmHg. I followed her for another 23 years before she needed and received a kidney transplantation. On this background, I hypothesized that more aggressive blood pressure control was needed in diabetic patients, independent of blood sugar control, to better protect their kidneys.

As principal investigator of the appropriate blood pressure control in diabetes (ABCD), we demonstrated the optimal level of blood pressure in diabetic patients necessary to decrease the progression of kidney and eye disease as well as to prevent heart disease and strokes. The obesity–diabetes epidemic is projected to be the worst world-wide health care problem in the future, both in developed and developing countries. A US health and nutrition survey estimated that only 17% of diabetic patients had their high blood pressure controlled. Once diabetic patients have increased urinary excretion of protein, 60–80% exhibit elevation of blood pressures. In our high blood pressure ABCD study, diabetic patients were randomized to a blood pressure of 135–140/85–90 mmHg versus less than 130/80 mmHg and followed for a mean of five years. The more aggressive blood pressure control significantly decreased all-cause mortality, which was primarily due to decreased cardiovascular complications. In the ABCD study of diabetic patients with the accepted normal blood pressure (<140/90 mmHg), patients were randomized for a mean of five years to no therapy versus lowering blood pressure to less than 130/80 mmHg. Those normotensive diabetic patients with more aggressive blood pressure control exhibited a significant decrease in progression of diabetic eye disease, decreased incidence of strokes, and stabilized kidney disease as assessed by urinary albumin excretion. Thus, early and aggressive control of blood pressure in diabetic patients, even before they become hypertensive, can decrease vascular complications, which is their main cause of morbidity and mortality.

In contemplating my career and passion as a physician-scientist, it is clear that I have not followed the sage advice of focusing on one area of research. I have, however, always sought to pursue areas of clinical research which addressed important areas of patient-related disease. There was an era in which academic advancement of a physician-scientist could only occur with a focus on basic science. This genre has, however, changed and a career in patient-oriented research is now being encouraged. As Chairman of the Department of Medicine, I launched a PhD program in Clinical Science based on the belief that rigorous training is just as essential for a career in patient-oriented clinical, as well as basic, biomedical science research. This PhD program is now one of the most popular post-graduate programs at the University of Colorado, Denver. Whether pursuing a career in clinical or basic research as a physician-scientist, an important ingredient for success is a passion for the work. I have been fortunate to have had passion over the past several decades for my patient-oriented research. One must also have patience in pursuing research, perhaps even more so in clinical than basic investigation. While the gratification in caring for an ill patient or teaching a medical student is relatively immediate, it may take a decade before realizing that one's patient-oriented research has actually enhanced the health of sick patients.

A challenging aspect of my personal career as a physician-scientist was my administrative responsibilities as Head of the Division of Renal Diseases and Hypertension for 20 years and Chairman of the Department of Medicine for 26 years at the University of Colorado (Fig. 19.4). For 16 years, I held both positions

Fig. 19.4 Me serving as Chairman of the Department of Medicine, University of Colorado, Denver, CO

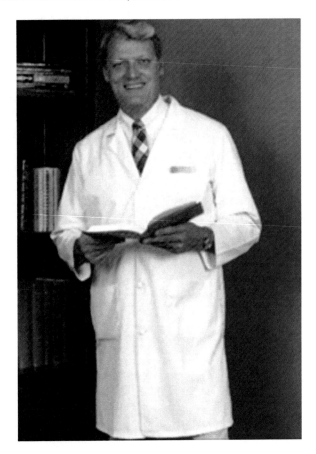

while trying to build other divisions in the department. While these administrative responsibilities limited my personal time for research, it gave me the opportunity to create an academic environment whereby careers of physician-scientists could be nurtured. Although as a faculty member in San Francisco I was offered opportunities to lead established and well-known kidney units at other institutions, I desired to make a contribution where there was little kidney presence, so I accepted the position at the University of Colorado. During my time as Head of the Division of Renal Diseases and Hypertension at Colorado, the faculty expanded from two to 20 full-time faculties, and the NIH research funding rose from none to approximately $10 million per year. A similar expansion occurred during my 26 years as Chair of the Department of Medicine in which the faculty expanded from 75 to 500 and the annual research funding expanded from $3 to $100 million. These administrative responsibilities were gratifying but required long hours to allow continuation of my research. With a family of five children, and now 13 grandchildren, my ability to stay involved in research was largely due to the tremendous support of my

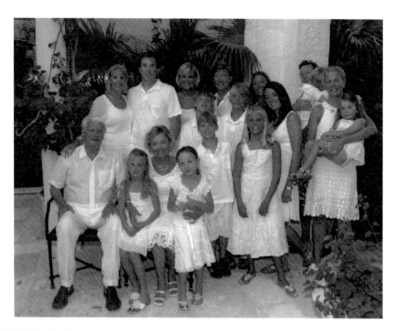

Fig. 19.5 My family

wife, Barbara, our children (Fig. 19.5), and the large number of renal research fellows who have worked with me over the years. Over 125 of these fellows now hold
leading academic positions around the world. As a physician-scientist, one of the
most gratifying aspects is to mentor the next generation of physicians committed to
advancing the biomedical knowledge in our profession. Moreover, when that knowledge has been shown to have a direct beneficial impact on the quality of patient
care, the feeling of gratification is remarkable.

While mentoring fellows in kidney disease from the USA and other developed
countries, it was quite obvious that there was an even greater need in the developing world. Therefore, for over 20 years as Treasurer, Vice-President, President, and
past President of the International Society of Nephrology (ISN), I focused on initi-
ating and developing programs to enhance the education and quality of physicians
caring for patients with kidney disease and high blood pressure in the emerging
world. This involved launching an ISN Fellowship training program for physicians from the developing world. As a result of this program, over 450 physicians
from third world countries in Africa, Latin America, and Asia have trained in outstanding kidney units in North America, Europe, Japan, and Australasia and then
returned to their home countries to care for patients with kidney disease, educate
fellow physicians about kidney disease, and perform patient-oriented research, particularly in the area of disease prevention and health maintenance. An ISN Sister
Renal Center Program was also developed whereby kidney and hypertension units
in developed and developing countries were paired. They share visiting professors
and fellows and join together in educational programs and patient-oriented research.

Frequently, equipment needs in developing countries, such as artificial kidneys, are also met. Lastly, the ISN Commission for the Global Advancement of Nephrology (COMGAN) holds an average of 50 educational programs each year in developing countries in Asia, Africa, and Latin America. Involvement in these international programs in developing countries has been an enormously gratifying aspect to my academic career.

At the present stage in my academic career as a clinician, educator, and scientist, I am frequently asked whether I would have made different decisions in my professional life over my 37 years at the University of Colorado. In general, I could not be more pleased with the professional path which I have chosen in academic medicine. I have thoroughly enjoyed the patient care, teaching, and research. I was offered, but did not accept, attractive Chairs of Medicine at more renowned medical schools including the University of Washington and Duke University. While I occasionally reflect on those opportunities, there have clearly been advantages to the stability and continuity in building a division and department at a single institution, while continuing a research career. Most important, however, was after moving seven times and having five children in 10 years during my early training, military service, and first academic position in San Francisco, the stability of raising our family with Barbara in the Rocky Mountain region has been extremely important for our family.

My department chair and mentor at the University of California San Francisco, Dr. Lloyd H. Smith, had recommended me for higher administrative positions above the department level. I only agreed to consider one such position, Dean at the University of California in San Diego. This experience made it clear to me that active involvement in patient care, teaching, and research is impossible in such a position. Yet these were the reasons that I had pursued a career in academic medicine. Perhaps the most important academic decision that I ever made was to reject that otherwise very attractive offer and to continue my career in academic medicine and translational research. Moreover, when I asked Dr. Smith why he never became a dean, he answered with his unique humor, "There is only one letter difference between Dean and Dead." Thus, for anyone who desires to pursue a career as a physician-scientist, great care must be taken when considering administrative positions.

As a young boy, I never dreamt of the possibility of becoming a doctor, even though my mother was a nurse. I did, however, dream of becoming a professional basketball or baseball player. Yet, I could never have imagined such a rewarding and gratifying professional life in medicine. While any honor that I have received has been appreciated and humbling, it has always seemed inappropriate to be recognized for something that I have enjoyed so much. I have to admit, however, that being elected recently to the Indiana Basketball Hall of Fame was very exciting. This is because, from a substantive point of view, much of any success which I may have had has been dependent, at least in part, on lessons that I learned growing up while participating in athletics. Among those lessons are the following:

- Hard work and persistence ultimately lead to success.
- Individual commitment to a team effort is critical.

- Ability to recover and move ahead from a setback or defeat is mandatory.
- Motivation is equally or more important than talent.
- Ability to enjoy the success of others and optimism are critical features of leadership.

These are just a few lessons that I have applied during my career in academic medicine as a physician-scientist.

Somewhat fortuitous, and perhaps subconsciously, given my father's demise from untreated high blood pressure (Fig. 19.6), my passion for patient-oriented research has focused on hypertension and kidney disease. Most importantly, if I had to summarize my passion for research as a physician-scientist, it has always been to answer questions which can improve the health of patients.

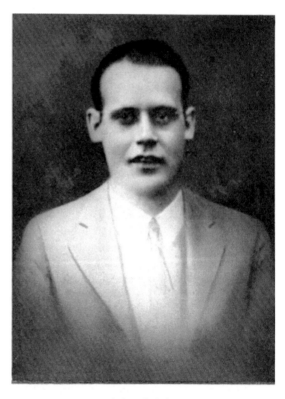

Fig. 19.6 My father, Arthur Schrier

Arthur Schrier

Twenty
What Went Right

Ralph I. Horwitz

My path to medicine was unremarkable. My parents loved me. My siblings irritated me. We lived in a working class neighborhood in Philadelphia where factory jobs and union membership were the common currency of everyday life. For immigrant parents with hopes of a better life for their children, there was only one path: success at school and a life in law or medicine. My brother chose law. I chose medicine.

My journey to medicine has always been much less opaque to me than my journey through it. I came from conventional circumstances and intended to pursue a conventional path. I admired physicians in practice and imagined that I would pursue a career like those of the physicians I had seen as a child. I would attend medical school and would hope to practice a sub-specialty in Philadelphia, where my parents' friends and family would see evidence of their success, if not mine. However, events in medicine altered that path and led me to a career that has emphasized clinical research and education. How did that happen?

After medical school at Hershey (Penn State University's medical school located in Hershey, PA), I made a fateful choice and headed north of the border to train in internal medicine at the Royal Victoria Hospital of McGill University. It was here at McGill that I started down the path that has shaped my subsequent career in medicine. It is this journey that I will describe in this essay.

Every new medical intern at McGill's Royal Victoria Hospital had a surprise awaiting them as they began residency training. Each of us was assigned a panel of patients to follow in the polyclinic where faculty and residents saw their outpatients. My panel was inherited from a previous resident who had finished general medicine training and was starting fellowship at another McGill Hospital. Fearful as I was to be the "real" doctor to these unsuspecting patients, I was grateful to have this former resident available to discuss my new patients.

I was surprised to learn how much I enjoyed caring for these patients and what a joy it was to develop a doctor–patient relationship outside the acute care setting. The older patients were often accompanied by their younger adult children, who

R.I. Horwitz (✉)
Department of Medicine, Stanford University School of Medicine, Stanford, CA, USA
e-mail: ralph.horwitz@stanford.edu

D.A. Schwartz (ed.), *Medicine Science and Dreams,*
DOI 10.1007/978-90-481-9538-1_20, © Springer Science+Business Media B.V. 2011

provided rides, listened to my assessments and recommendations, and offered support to their parents. Younger patients, especially women, frequently had their young children in tow and even brought them into the examination room if they were too active to be left alone in the waiting area. I was surprised to see how much I enjoyed these interactions.

One day I was examining a young woman who had annoyingly resistant hypertension when she surprised me with an appropriate yet challenging question. She had read a newspaper article the previous week about three research papers published back to back to back in the same issue of the prestigious British journal, *The Lancet*. All three papers had come to the same startling conclusion: a commonly prescribed anti-hypertensive drug (Reserpine) significantly increased the risk of breast cancer in women. My patient's blood pressure, which had proved quite resistant to treatment for a very long time, had finally been controlled with Reserpine after much difficulty by the resident who preceded me. The patient now wondered if she should stop the Reserpine to avoid the increased risk of breast cancer.

I had seen the three alarming papers myself the previous week and also wondered whether Reserpine should be avoided in women with hypertension. I had decided not to start my new female patients with elevated blood pressure on Reserpine, but I was uncertain what I should do with patients whose blood pressure was successfully (and in some instances, finally) controlled with the drug. For many of those patients, the alternative medications were unappealing options. Alpha-methyldopamine, Guanethidine, and Clonidine were available if a diuretic and Reserpine were insufficient, but these alternatives had disabling side effects in a substantial number of patients.

Even more frustrating, and a stronger reason for my indecision, was my lack of understanding of the published research. As a medical student, I had learned about cohort studies like those conducted in the Framingham Heart Study, and about randomized controlled trials that showed the benefit of hypertension control in patients like the woman who was now inquiring whether her treatment might cause more harm than good. However, the three papers indicating that Reserpine increased the risk of breast cancer had employed case-control studies, an unfamiliar study design to me. The investigators had studied subjects who already had breast cancer plus a control group of women without evidence of the disease. Somehow, by collecting data about prior use of Reserpine (and many other medications), the investigators concluded that the risk of breast cancer was twice as great in women who had used Reserpine as in women who had not. Then, in an act of statistical invention that was completely unfamiliar to me, they went further and concluded that prior use of Reserpine may have caused subsequent breast cancer in these women. It troubled me that the editors and reviewers of *The Lancet* apparently understood these studies and accepted them for publication. What did they know that I didn't? And even more troubling was that I didn't understand the statistical argument based on the odds ratio, which figured so prominently in the argument that Reserpine increased the risk of breast cancer in women. I should have admitted my ignorance to my patient and asked for time to learn more about the studies and their implications. But I was insecure. Besides, an author of one of the papers was Sir Richard Doll, who was famous for his pioneering research that had linked cigarette smoking to lung cancer. Surely someone so authoritative could not be wrong. Surely *The Lancet* would not publish research with erroneous results. I blurted out confidently that we should stop the Reserpine to protect her from developing breast cancer and assured her that we could switch easily to a different medication. I didn't know what I was talking about.

For my patient, I had made a fateful decision. Over the next six months, her blood pressure was poorly controlled, despite my best efforts, and she was plagued with all the disabling complications that were the well-known side effects of the Aldomet and Clonidine that I had selected as alternatives to Reserpine. With her blood pressure constantly fluctuating, I wondered if my patient was non-compliant with her medication; she wondered if controlling her blood pressure was worth all this trouble. Although I did not wish to acknowledge it myself, I thought she may also have lost confidence in me. We were both struggling with this unhappy situation when, astonishingly, my fragile medical confidence evaporated on the very day that the *New England Journal of Medicine* published two new papers in a single issue contradicting the results of the papers previously published in *The Lancet*. Remarkably, using the same case-control methods that previously indicted Reserpine as a possible cause of breast cancer in women, these new papers now suggested that Reserpine was exonerated. My patient now had poorly controlled hypertension, a (false) positive anti-nuclear antibody, and severe postural hypotension. I had done that to her because I did not know how to interpret the claims from unfamiliar research designs that Reserpine was a cancer risk. And to make matters worse, I now had no idea whether the old studies or the new studies were the "truth." Had I stopped the Reserpine needlessly? I didn't know.

I was frustrated and embarrassed. Over the ensuing weeks I read voraciously about case-control designs in my determined effort to avoid similar circumstances in the future. More importantly, I realized that I wanted to learn more about how research could improve medical practice in general. As a result of this experience, I made the decision to pursue fellowship training in the field of study that seemed most closely related to case-control research. Thus, I boldly announced my plan to the faculty at McGill to pursue study in epidemiology and biostatistics, unaware of how foreign the discipline was from the practice of medicine that had captured me so thoroughly. Fortunately, I was surrounded by people wiser than I was.

At the same time that I figured out that I wanted to learn about how research could improve the practice of medicine, I also discovered that study design and biostatistics were the nearly exclusive domain of epidemiologists in schools of public health who worked in isolation from the patients who motivated my interests. The Chair of Medicine at McGill, John Beck, had helped to initiate a new program of research training intended for physicians. The Clinical Scholars program was sponsored initially by the Carnegie Commonwealth Foundation before it was adopted by the Robert Wood Johnson (RWJ) Foundation. One of the Clinical Scholars programs was located at Yale University under the leadership of Alvan Feinstein (Fig. 20.1). Beck knew that Feinstein was helping to create a new discipline of clinical epidemiology, which was rooted not in public health but in clinical medicine, and

Fig. 20.1 Alvan Feinstein

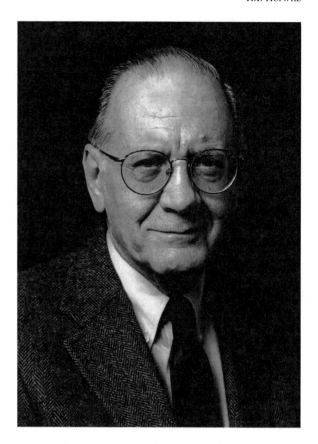

that his newly established training program was ideally suited to my own interests. Ironically, Feinstein was scheduled to visit McGill, and Beck arranged for Feinstein to interview me for the RWJ Clinical Scholars program when he was in Montreal.

Feinstein's visit took place as planned, but under remarkably adverse circumstances. Just two days before his visit to McGill, Feinstein's wife had given birth prematurely and the child was hospitalized in the Yale-New Haven Neonatal Intensive Care Unit with respiratory distress and what was then referred to as hyaline-membrane disease. The prognosis for the infant was dire, and Feinstein planned to return to New Haven immediately following his lecture in Montreal to be present with his wife at the expected death of their newborn. What kind of interview could I expect from a man dealing with such powerful emotions?

I quickly discovered the answer. In a remarkable display of intellectual and emotional discipline, Feinstein conducted a rigorous, probing, analytical interview lasting nearly two hours. Feinstein put a wall around his emotional life and maintained his focus on the intellectual challenge at hand. When he accepted me into his program, I knew I was in for a remarkable two years.

I was not disappointed. Feinstein was the type of person who central casting would send you if you requested a curmudgeon. Fortunately for me, he was also a brilliant teacher who held everyone to the same impossibly high standards he held himself. Shortly after beginning in the program, I started to read about case-control studies and to offer critiques concerning their design or analysis. Feinstein wouldn't tolerate such anecdotal criticisms. With his insistence, I embarked on a systematic review of studies using the design, developed a taxonomy of bias that threatened the validity and generalizability of the method, and offered strategies to improve the performance of case-control research. The paper I prepared with Feinstein went through more than a dozen different drafts until he was satisfied with the product. For the first time since I began my medical education, I was being forced to think creatively and rigorously. The experience was exhilarating. I wanted more.

Among the lessons I learned working with Feinstein in clinical epidemiology was to value outstanding research regardless of its type. I came to recognize that "basic" research is not only something that is done at the cellular or molecular level. Rather, basic research is that which is fundamental to a discipline, rigorous in its methods, reproducible in its results, and enduring. Population and clinical research that met these criteria was a new basic science for clinical care, and it did not need to seek endorsement of its value from misleading labels such as basic, applied, clinical, or translational. I was hooked. I was ready to pursue a career in clinical research and to use the results to improve the practice of medicine.

Feinstein and I differed in our affection and commitment to clinical medicine. I had been a member of the third class of medical students at Penn State where medicine was taught at the bedside by senior physicians who were both scientists and clinicians. When I graduated, I eagerly ventured north to McGill because it was a mature medical school and was notable for both excellence in research and the quality of its clinical instruction. Although my experience at Yale convinced me to pursue a career focused on population-based research, I was just as powerfully motivated by a love of clinical medicine. When I completed the fellowship in the Clinical Scholars Program with Feinstein at Yale, I accepted a position as a senior resident at the Massachusetts General Hospital (MGH), where I learned that clinical medicine and clinical epidemiology could also be reinforcing.

I am not sure we ever fully determine or shape our own career path. After completing clinical training at MGH, I returned to Yale as an Assistant Professor of Medicine and Co-Director with Feinstein of the Robert Wood Johnson Clinical Scholars Program. Unexpectedly, the ensuing 15 years were consumed by nearly an exclusive focus on clinical research and research education. I was having too much fun and success to notice how far I had drifted from clinical medicine. I also failed to notice how much more sterile my work had become: the epidemiologic methods I was using in my research had taken precedence in my mind over the clinical context that was so central to its relevance, until an accidental research finding set me on a new course.

In the early 1980s, the Coronary Drug Project was designed to test whether lipid-lowering drugs, compared to placebo, would reduce the risk of death in patients with coronary disease. Unhappily, analysis of the data showed no significant difference between patients who received active treatment and those who received placebo. When the investigators analyzed the actively treated patients further, they discovered that mortality was significantly reduced in patients who were highly adherent to treatment compared to those who were poorly adherent. Surprisingly, they found the same reduction in mortality among patients highly adherent to placebo compared to those who are poorly adherent.

An accompanying editorial pointed out that the use of post-randomization data, such as adherence, to test for treatment effectiveness was a test for bias, not effectiveness. The independent effects of adherence on clinical outcomes were dismissed and were largely ignored until my colleagues and I found a similar result among the placebo patients in the Beta Blocker Heart Attack Trial (BHAT). Indeed, good adherence to placebo in the BHAT was associated with a larger reduction in mortality than that observed with beta-blockers. This singular observation led me to develop an affiliation with a MacArthur Foundation network on Health and Human Behavior (at the invitation of Judith Rodin, then Chair of Psychology at Yale and now President of the Rockefeller Foundation) and later on social class and health. The experiences in the MacArthur network with social scientists enriched my understanding of the determinants of both health and disease. I became an advocate for a more inclusive medicine research program that integrated biology, behavior, and the social environment to understand better both the risk for developing disease and the response to treatment. In my roles as Chair of Medicine at Yale, Dean of the Medical School at Case Western Reserve, and Chair of Medicine again, this time in my current position at Stanford University, I have been able to nudge medicine in this direction.

These concepts are not new, of course. In the latter half of the nineteenth century, Europe was the center of excellence in both research and clinical care. At the pinnacle of celebrity was Rudolph Virchow, the eminent German physician and pathologist who is sometimes referred to as the Father of Social Medicine. Virchow was celebrated for his emphasis on the unitary theory of the cell (all cells come from cells) among many other notable contributions. He described the left-sided supra-clavicular node that heralded gastro-intestinal cancer (Virchow's node) and postulated the factors that contribute to thrombotic risk (Virchow's triad). When Virchow was asked to investigate an outbreak of typhus fever in a community of Poles in northern Germany, he reported that the epidemic was encouraged by poor nutrition and filthy living conditions. Virchow famously stated, "... Wealth, education, and freedom are the requirements for the health of a nation."

One of Virchow's devoted followers was Leon Eisenberg at Harvard, who wrote about Virchow and his view that medicine is both a biological and a social science. I was influenced strongly by Eisenberg's powerful advocacy for the appreciation that disease was rooted in social and behavioral determinants of health. However, the social medicine movement that Eisenberg so powerfully represented never integrated the critical importance of either clinical research or clinical experience in shaping both research and practice. Fortunately, early experiences in medical school and residency influenced me greatly and prepared my mind for the possibility that a new kind of basic science could inform the practice of medicine.

As noted earlier, I entered in the third class of students at Hershey. The curriculum was bold and the faculty members who taught us in the classroom and at the bedside were almost entirely senior professors. Anatomy (Bryce Munger), Biochemistry (Eugene Davidson), Pharmacology (Elliot Vessel), and Physiology (Howard Morgan) were all taught by senior professors. So too was Clinical Medicine. The Department Chair, Graham Jeffries, was classically trained in gastroenterology and hepatology, but only after he was deeply competent in general internal medicine. In General Medicine, John Burnside set an example for the bedside examination that inspired my interest in clinical medicine.

Training in Internal Medicine at McGill, then, was no accident of co-occurring match lists. Residents learned medicine from senior physicians at McGill whose clinical excellence was forged in rigorous clinical environments and honored in clinical experience. I went to Montreal to learn clinical medicine. I was not disappointed.

Everyone called him "Stubby," but I could not bring myself to join in the chorus. He was Dr. Stubbington to me, a British-trained cardiologist whose bedside rounds were clinically sophisticated and notable for their attention to the patient's story and his detailed and expert clinical examination. I was delighted to be rounding with him in the coronary care unit early in my internship along with a resident, a cardiology fellow, and Stubby's nurse in tow. Standing at the bedside of a patient admitted with a large anterior wall myocardial infarction, the team heard a large rush of air and the powerful odor of stool. The resident, fellow, and I all stepped back from the bed. Stubby and the nurse stepped forward, silently cleaning the patient and changing the sheets. I was humbled yet inspired by this simple act of kindness from a great physician who was unimpressed with his status. I attached myself to Stubby to learn the clinical exam of the heart and to emulate not just his clinical skills but also his humanistic approach to the patient.

It is not enough to claim that graduation from medical school earns you status as a physician. Medical school does not make you a doctor. Residency training does, but the knowledge and skills gained there require regular reinforcement. Clinical research in medicine is most vibrant when it emerges from authentic clinical experience. Without that legitimate context, many of my physician colleagues carry out research that could easily be done by their non-physician peers, and often is. The work may be superb, but the loss in opportunity is great.

Many of us were inspired to pursue academic careers by clinicians who were also researchers and whose work was closely linked to the problems we encountered on the wards. I can recall many times when a patient in the hospital with a disorder in acid–base balance would elicit an excited discussion from a nephrologist whose career was devoted to renal physiology, or when the illness of a patient with heart failure was understood best when a cardiologist explained the relationship of symptoms to pathophysiology. Physicians like Jerry Kassirer (Nephrology and Clinical Decision Analysis), Rick Lifton (Human Genetics), Gary Schoolnik (Infectious Diseases), Jerry Klatskin (Hepatology), and Helen Hobbs (Cardiology) encouraged young people to see the connection between profound scholarship and excellent clinical care. Many of the leading scientists in our contemporary departments of medicine today carry out their research at the cell or molecular level. Although their science is elegant, they often feel alienated from the patients who are cared for by our students and residents. I have always felt fortunate that I have been able to develop a career in clinical research in which I study the strategies of clinical care. By investigating patient-based problems in diagnosis, prognosis, and therapy, I have kept my research close to my patients.

I am also fortunate to have been mentored and inspired by some remarkable individuals throughout my career, including those discussed above. Not to be forgotten in the story of my career in medicine is the profound influence of two individuals who have not been professional colleagues of mine but who, in different ways, constantly remind me of the meaning of medicine.

Anna Deavere Smith (Fig. 20.2) is a playwright and actress whose one-woman shows have illuminated the American character. Whether in *Twilight Los Angeles* or *Fires in the Mirror*, Ms. Smith would portray the experience of people often caught in the most intense personal crises of their lives. I saw Ms. Smith in performance at the Long Wharf Theater in New Haven, CT while I was Chair of Medicine at Yale. Her work captured an essential part of the experience of every physician who

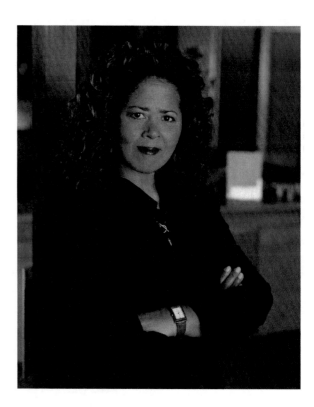

Fig. 20.2 Anna Deavere Smith

seeks to heal an ill patient, and that every patient has who needs to place their lives in trust of that physician. Patients who are seriously ill are often forced to deal with an intense personal crisis precipitated by illness. What were they feeling? I was so taken with her performance that I asked Anna to come to Yale to interview patients, their families and doctors, and to give a medical grand rounds performance based on those interviews. To my delight, she agreed.

The vignettes that Ms. Smith presented at our medical grand rounds that day were electrifying. Over the ensuing months and years, she deepened and expanded the work into a majestic play, *Let Me Down Easy*, that tells the story of life and loss and the extraordinary resilience and vulnerability of the human body. And at the very same time, Ms. Smith gave expression to the powerful emotion that so often sweeps across the relationship between doctor and patient and binds us tightly together in a common embrace.

At nearly the same time, I discovered Abraham Verghese (Fig. 20.3). Actually, Abraham did not need to be discovered. What I discovered was *My Own Country*, an anthem describing the early years of the AIDS epidemic in the USA written by this celebrated physician author who had experienced the epidemic first hand. I invited Dr. Verghese to Yale to give medical grand rounds. He was riveting, reading from the book and telling stories of patients dying from AIDS and seeking to reconcile with their families before their deaths. But he also managed to weave together a series of interconnected stories that plumbed the depth of his topic, the search for meaning in the life of a physician. For me and many of my physician colleagues who were present that day, Verghese succeeded in shining a light on the meaning of medicine. Its meaning was there for us in the experience of our dying patients and of the value of a physician who helped to heal patients with comfort when he could not offer them cure. Verghese went on to write other great works, including

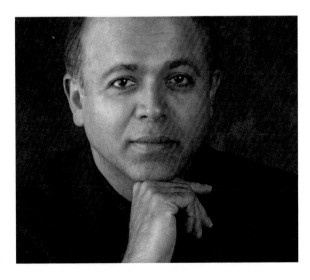

Fig. 20.3 Abraham Verghese

The Tennis Partner and most recently a novel, *Cutting for Stone*. Cumulatively, his work has created a medical narrative that gives expression to the value of doctoring and captures the rich and meaningful lives physicians are privileged to experience.

In this essay, I have chosen not to tell you the story of my journey to medicine but rather my journey through medicine. For me that journey continues. In my current role at Stanford as the Chair of Medicine, I once again have the opportunity to work with extraordinary students, residents, and faculty who make a difference daily in the lives of our patients. Along the way, I hope to shape medicine to reflect the values that have long endured in our profession and that I have long embraced. I can only hope that I have miles yet to go before I sleep.

Index

D.A. Schwartz (ed.), *Medicine Science and Dreams*,
DOI 10.1007/978-90-481-9538-1, © Springer Science+Business Media B.V. 2011

Watson, Jim, 193
Weber, Jim, 193
Weed, Lawrence L., 115
Weekly Reader, 109–110
Wegener's granulomatosis, 151
Weidenslaufer, 3–5, 12
Weiland, Stephan, 203–205
Weizmann Institute, 274, 275, 277
Weizmann Institute of Science, 275
Weltanscauung, 44
Westchester County Department of Health, 244
Westchester Science Fair, 19, 21, 23
Western culture, 93
Western red cedar asthma, 262, 265
Western Union, 35
West Germany, 203, 205–206
Westheimer, Frank, 25
Westinghouse Science Talent Search, 24
Westport, Connecticut, 219
White blood cells, 51
White, Gilbert, 156
White House, 169, 280–282, 284, 286–287
White, Paul Dudley, 275
Whitman, Walt, 286
Wichita Falls, Texas, 272
Wilchek, Meir, 278
Willcox, Mary, 121
Williams, Robert H., 269
Williams, Robert W., 293
Williams, R. Sanders, 91–106
Wilmington, Delaware, 270
Wilson, John, 130
Winsor School, 49
Wittgenstein, 8
Wittich, John, 290
"Wizard of Oz", 32
Wolff-Parkinson-White syndrome, 98
Wolff, Sheldon, 148–150, 157
Wolf, Sidney, 278
Wolters Air Force Base, 272
Woodrow Wilson School of Public and
    International Affairs, 283
Woodrow Wilson School (WWS), 93–94, 283

Woods Hole Oceanographic Institution, 273
Woolf, Sheldon, 175
Workers' Compensation Board, 265
WorkSafe BC, 266
World Health Organization, 236, 244, 255
World Series, 276
World War II, 48, 83, 111, 199, 230, 242, 244,
    289–290
Wyngaarden, James, 153
Wyngaarden, Jim, 97
Wyoming, 17, 239

X
X-box binding protein 1 (XBP1), 56–57
XBP1 signaling pathway, 57

Y
Yale, 28, 31, 33–34, 37, 44, 50, 60, 70–72,
    221, 227, 229, 238, 273–274, 305–308,
    310–311
Yale Bowl, 227
Yale, Jim, 238
Yale-New Haven Hospital, 31
Yale-New Haven Neonatal Intensive Care
    Unit, 306
Yale Old Farts Rowing Association, 238
Yale University, 305
Yalow, Roslyn, 17
Yalta Conference, 289
Yaoita, Hideo, 173–174
Yat-sen, Sun, 260
Yeast one-hybrid, 56
Yeast two-hybrid, 56
Yeshiva, 160–161
Yiddish, 160
Ykaterinberg, 231
Yorktown Heights, New York, 37
Young, Quentin, 278
Yurchak, Peter, 97

Z
Zedong, Mao, 219